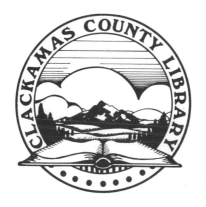

The Complete
Morgan Horse

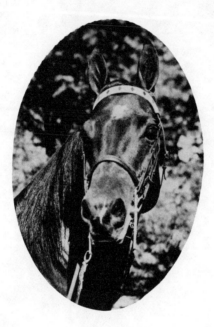

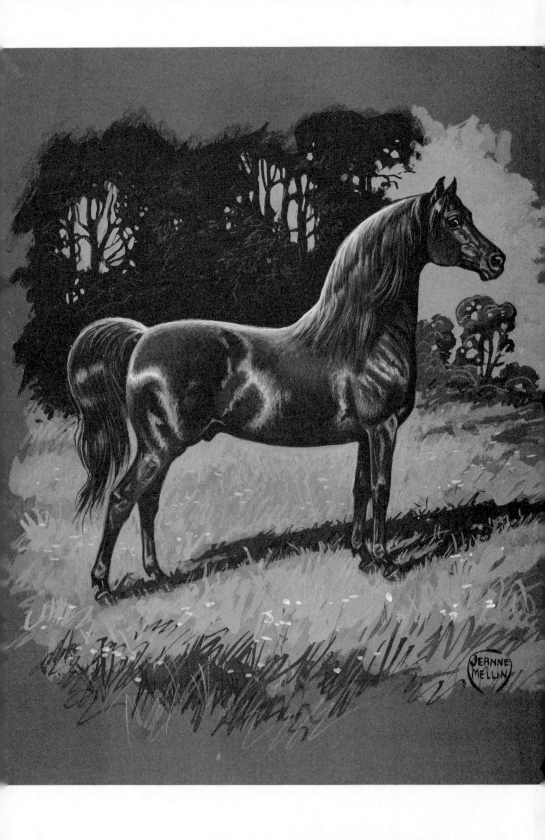

THE
COMPLETE

Morgan Horse

Jeanne Mellin

WITH ILLUSTRATIONS BY THE AUTHOR

The Stephen Greene Press

LEXINGTON, MASSACHUSETTS

First published in 1986 by The Stephen Greene Press, Inc.
Published simultaneously in Canada by Penguin Books Canada Limited
Reprinted 1988
Distributed by Viking Penguin Inc., 40 West 23rd Street, New York, NY 10010.

This work is derived from two earlier books by the author, *The Morgan Horse*
and *The Morgan Horse Handbook*.

All line drawings are by the author unless otherwise indicated.
Illustration credits appear on page 363.

LIBRARY OF CONGRESS CATALOGING IN PUBLICATION DATA
Mellin, Jeanne, 1927–
The complete Morgan horse.
Includes index.
1. Morgan horse.   I. Title.
SF293.M8M38   1986   636.1′7   86-7582
ISBN 0-8289-0590-8

Printed in the United States of America by
R. R. Donnelley & Sons, Harrisonburg, Virginia
Set in Baskerville

Foreword

"THE MORGAN horse is one thing: every other kind of horse is something else." This is an old statement—originating who knows where—with which, after you have owned a Morgan, you will undoubtedly agree.

Although this may sound pretentious, actually it isn't. We interpret it to mean that a Morgan horse is an entity unto himself . . . like no other breed . . . individual both in type and temperament.

Why are Morgan people such a fiercely loyal lot? Why do they all declare, "Once you have owned a Morgan, no other horse will do"? There are many reasons, and owners happily will expound upon them in detail at the slightest provocation and with sparkling-eyed enthusiasm. As you will discover, for many people not the least of these reasons is the tremendously interesting history of the Morgan breed.

And what a story it is! As one delves ever deeper into it, the more fascinating it becomes. It is heartily recommended reading on a cold night by the fire, or any other time, if you wish to lose yourself in another less frantic era. For it is not only the stories, bordering on legend, of Justin Morgan himself that enthrall every lover of fine horseflesh, but also the entire account of the breed that sprang from a single progenitor to become America's first native breed. The unlikely chance that one stallion could have gotten stock which to this day has retained his distinct characteristics is a miracle in its own right, and is apparent to all who see the Morgans of today and study the descriptions of their forebears. But in addition the Morgan horse emerged as a breed despite human frailty, arduous physical conditions, and often extremely indiscriminate breeding.

It is said that when one becomes thoroughly acquainted with the background and history of Justin Morgan and his progeny and ferrets out each fascinating circumstance for oneself, the fact that the breed has managed to survive the endless whims of Man and capricious Nature will be truly appreciated.

But how, in fact, did *you* discover the Morgan? And why have you become convinced that he is your kind of horse? Were you smitten by his beauty and sparkle? Or his tremendous versatility? Or his apparent easy-keeping qualities? Or his wonderfully tractable disposition?

Whatever the reason might be for your growing interest in the Morgan horse, time out to study his history and the things that "make him tick" is time well spent. And an amazing history it is! How the Morgan has retained his special characteristics for almost two hundred years of human vagaries is nothing short of phenomenal.

It cannot be stressed enough that the Morgan is a *type* breed. His type is his hallmark and his heritage. Without it we have just a group of horses that, with training, are versatile, but are Morgan in name only. The "Morgan look" is a distinctive and individual thing. As you familiarize yourself with this look, you will come to understand why it is so important for breeders and judges to have a thorough comprehension of Morgan type and character. Our judges set the standard for breeders, in a way. So often what is pinned in the show ring is what is desired in a breeding program, especially for the newcomer to the breed. Therefore, our Morgan judges should always be well aware of their responsibility when they place their classes.

All the photographs and drawings here of the Morgan in his various endeavors show horses of excellent or at least above-average Morgan type. I have, with these illustrations, tried to give the tyro a clear idea of the importance of retaining type, as well as of training the horse to excel in the many facets of the Morgan world.

The Complete Morgan Horse incorporates the history pertinent to today's Morgan from my book *The Morgan Horse* and the instructional and practical information from my *Morgan Horse Handbook* into one comprehensive volume. I have updated and revised both text and pictures where necessary to reflect the changing trends in horse-show standards regarding the Morgan. At least half of the illustrations that follow are new; the rest are the best from the two previous books.

As with my earlier works on the Morgan, I offer this book as a tribute to the breed that becomes greater with each turn of the seasons. My hope is that *The Complete Morgan Horse* will serve as history book, handbook, guidebook and reference book to all those who either already know and love the Morgan or who are about to discover the beauty and uniqueness of a breed that knows no equal among light horses.

JEANNE MELLIN
Hamilton, New York
January 1986

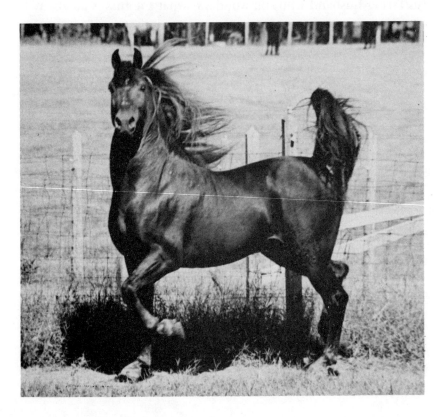

Acknowledgments

The author is grateful to her many dear friends on both sides of the Atlantic who have contributed so much to this book: with photos, ideas and, most of all, moral support for this project. And to a long-suffering husband who still wonders "what the fuss is all about"!

Contents

	Foreword	v
	Acknowledgments	viii
1	Justin Morgan: The Beginning of a Breed	1
2	Justin Morgan's Progeny	19
3	The Influence of the Morgan Horse on Other American Breeds	88
4	The Morgan Horse Club, *Register* and Farm	110
5	Growing Pains and Breeders' Guidelines	138
6	The Morgan Stallion, Mare and Gelding	176
7	Versatility and the Show Ring	209
8	The Morgan Park Horse and Pleasure Horse	233
9	The Morgan Roadster, Road Hack and Hunter/Jumper	288
10	Fitting and Showmanship in Hand	303
11	Pleasure Horse—Fun Horse	322
12	Further Points on Dress and Equipment	336
	Horsemen's Terms: A Glossary	356
	How the Author "Judged" Them	361
	Illustration and Photo Credits	363
	Index	365

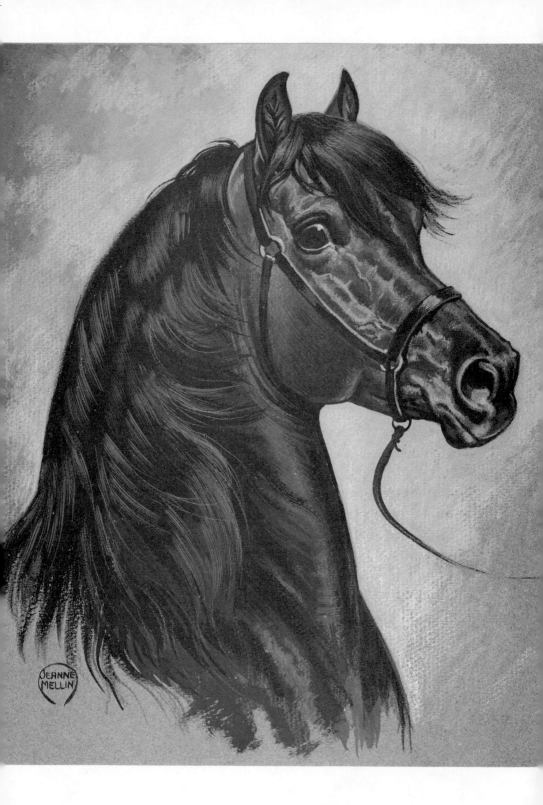

1

Justin Morgan:
The Beginning of a Breed

L OOKING AT him, not by the wildest flight of fancy could anyone have imagined that the small two-year-old colt that accompanied an impoverished music teacher back to Randolph, Vermont, one late summer day in 1795 was destined to become, as Justin Morgan, a horse unique in all equine history.

One wonders about the thoughts of the frail singing master as he trudged the long, lonely miles back to Vermont. The big three-year-old gelding that he led and the diminutive two-year-old bay colt that frisked along behind undoubtedly seemed scarcely worth this trip from Randolph to West Springfield, Massachusetts. A debt owed the poor fellow had been paid, not in the money that he so badly needed but in these two horses instead. Surely he was far from optimistic as he journeyed homeward.

Yet in the context of these commonplace happenings, Fate touched Justin Morgan, the man, in an unimagined way. Not for the few hymns and other music he composed for his church, nor for his short simple life as a singing master, will he be remembered. Instead, he will be known forever because he once owned a small bay stallion who acquired his name. The fame of Justin Morgan's little horse has spread from the green hills of Vermont to all of America and the world!

The few references to the trip taken by old Justin Morgan almost two hundred years ago and the reason for it could quite possibly be a part of the many legends that sprang up around the undersized colt that, by himself, founded the first American breed of horse— the Morgan. No accurate records have ever been found to substan-

1

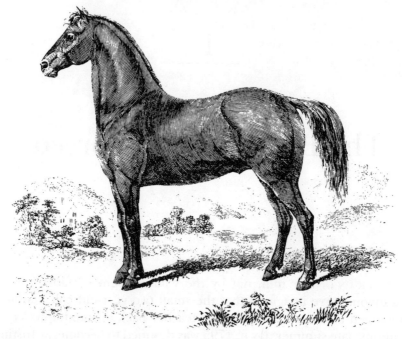

An unknown artist's conception of Justin Morgan—the only authenticated likeness—as it appeared in D. C. Linsley's Morgan Horses, *published in 1857.*

tiate absolutely the date of birth or the exact ancestry of the bright-eyed colt that Justin Morgan brought home to Vermont.

People intrigued by the breed have tried without success to trace the background of this amazing horse. They have attempted to tag him Thoroughbred, Arabian, Dutch, even French (Canadian), but despite all research and endless heated arguments, no positive record has ever been found that can conclusively prove his lineage. In breeding terms, he was a sport, or mutant, different from his parent stock and a type unto himself. No other stallion in history has stamped his own superlative characteristics and type on his descendants so thoroughly, and he holds the exclusive distinction of having a whole new breed named in his honor—an honor he fully deserves.

It is generally felt, and the breed *Register* goes along with this supposition, that Figure (as Justin Morgan called the colt that was later to bear his own name) was the son of a horse called True Briton, who was known to have traveled around under a number of assumed names—the best remembered of which was the flattering Beautiful Bay. But since the many stories and legends have made proof quite impossible, Figure's paternity will always remain a mystery.

True Briton was said to have been predominately Arabian or Thoroughbred (which in those days were similar in many respects, since the early Thoroughbred was not very far removed from the Arabian and Barb in the latter part of the eighteenth century). But, most assuredly, whatever his actual bloodlines, he was a fine horse of aristocratic breeding. He was owned by Colonel James Delancy of New York. The colonel, an ardent horseman and a rather adventurous soul, took great pride in his fine stallion and availed himself of every opportunity to parade him before admiring eyes. In those early days, when Americans sought good horseflesh in the same manner as we look over a showroom of shiny new automobiles, a horse of True Briton's caliber hardly went unnoticed. Delancy, unquestionably a Tory because of his decidedly Tory sympathies, naturally had many enemies among his neighbors in New York City. On several occasions his men raided local farms, running off the livestock and engaging in other mischief. This sort of behavior didn't set too well with the local inhabitants, and in retaliation a Continental soldier, finding an opportune moment, relieved the colonel of his pride and joy and skedaddled into Connecticut with True Briton. You can just bet that a horse thief's fate was probably considered much too easy and humane for this fellow; but neither he nor the horse was retrieved, so the colonel was cheated out of a fine spectacle of retribution, much to his enemies' glee.

From here it is difficult to follow the adventures of the horse True Briton, for his name was changed on several occasions (for obvious reasons!), and he was traveled about the countryside, and he acquired different aliases in just about every hamlet. Traveller was one—and quite appropriate under the circumstances—and Hero was another; finally he was given the elegant name of Beautiful Bay. He was sold on one occasion to Joseph Ward of East Hartford, Connecticut, for $300, a sizable sum in those lean years, and finally fell into the hands of one Sealy Norton, also of East Hartford. It was the imaginative Mr. Norton who pinned the name of Beautiful Bay on the horse and proudly stood him at stud at the stable of a John Morgan in West Springfield, Massachusetts, a mere hoot-and-a-holler from Hartford. Apparently, this John Morgan was the cousin of Justin Morgan, who had been late of West Springfield and had retired to Vermont in 1788. When Justin returned to West Springfield to collect on a debt owed him by John, the latter, it seems, unloaded the gelding and the bay colt on his country cousin and, undoubtedly in the manner of most horse traders, assured Justin that they would certainly double in value with "a bit of good feed and a year's growth." We wonder whether Justin was convinced of this as he trod homeward or whether he felt that he had been duped—and by a blood relation, too!

Another theory advanced by many researchers concerning the ancestry of the colt Justin reluctantly led home was that he was a Dutch horse and, using the vernacular of the day, "of the best blood." Justin Morgan was alleged to have always referred to the colt, which he always called Figure, as being a Dutch horse. To substantiate this is the fact that there was a Dutch stallion standing in Springfield in 1792. It is quite possible that Figure's dam was brought to the court of this horse, whose name was Young Bulrock, and who was large and a bright bay in color.

Now, the date of Figure's birth—which everyone argues about but no one can prove—at first glance would seemingly determine his breeding. If, as some would have us believe, he was by True Briton, it is quite likely that he was foaled in 1789, because that worthy animal was known to have been standing at stud for the season of 1788–1789. On the other hand, if he was indeed by Young Bulrock, the Dutch horse, his foaling date would more than likely be about 1793. This date seems to tie in better if we are to believe that Justin Morgan made his historic trip to Springfield in 1795, when the colt was supposedly two years old.

About Figure's dam there seems to be much agreement. She was described as a "native of the Connecticut Valley," which if you are a student of geography, you know takes in quite a stretch of territory, but which we assume in this case means in and around Hartford, Springfield and vicinity. She was called the Wildair mare and was supposedly of the same blood as True Briton—Arabian or Barb. Her sire, called Diamond, definitely had an "imported from England" background. We raise an eyebrow at his description, however, as it doesn't put one in mind of either Thoroughbred or Arabian breeding. He was of middle size—which isn't much help, since we're not certain what was then considered large and small—and heavy-bodied, with a thick, bushy mane and tail. He was called a smooth traveler, a trait that he is said to have bestowed upon his daughter, the Wildair mare, Figure's dam. She was a light bay in color and of medium size, having long hair on her legs and fetlocks and a bushy mane and tail like her father's. She was undoubtedly a good-looking mare and a good mover as well.

In regard to the possibility of Dutch breeding in Figure, it is in-

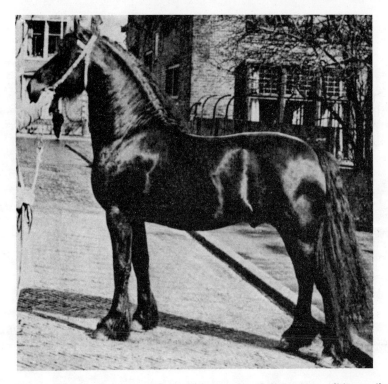

This Frisian stallion seems to personify a striking number of distinctive qualities ascribed to Justin Morgan.

teresting to note that the Dutch breeding was highly regarded at the time. Further evidence of what was apparently considered to be known fact can be found in part in the Introduction to Volume II of the *American Morgan Horse Register* (1900), where sons of Figure are referred to as having been sired by "the old Dutch horse." A stud poster of 1827 extolling the attributes of Bulrush (one of Figure's three best-known sons) said: "Morgan Bull Rush—The Famous Dutch horse . . . Morgan Bull Rush was actually sired by old Morgan, or the old Dutch horse, or Goss horse, [who] was perhaps more noted for fine stock than any horse in New England. The blood and stock [of] old Morgan [Figure] is generally so well known throughout the country, that we need say but little about them, they show for themselves."

Further, the *American Morgan Horse Register* also refers to the Fenton and Hawkins horses, Bulrush's half-brothers, as having been sired by "the old Dutch horse."

For "Dutch" it would seem logical to substitute "Frisian." From the Middle Ages to about 1770, the Frisian, a breed native to the northern

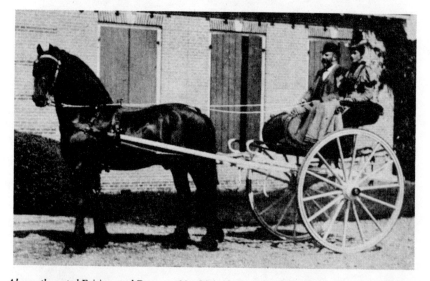

Above, the noted Frisian stud Regent—No. 32 in the Stamboek—*at ten years, in 1893. Below, a modern "Dutch" horse shows the natural high action and style for which his breed is famous.*

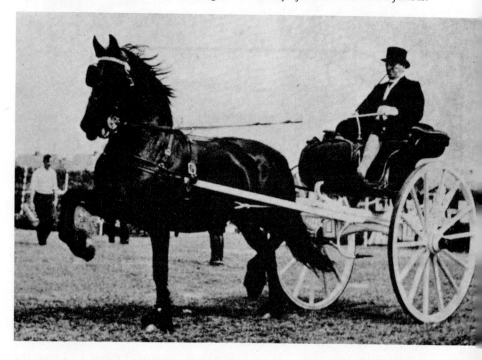

Dutch provinces, was crossed with Arabian and Andalusian blood (the latter being considered by some authorities to have been responsible for the Frisian luxurious fetlocks, manes and tails, which by tradition are never cut). It was in the eighteenth century that this breed—until then used primarily for military or agricultural purposes—became famous throughout western Europe for the height and speed of its trot: it was sought both as a carriage horse and for trotting races. And indeed, trotting competitions became established as a typical sport in Friesland at this time.

Because I think they will be of interest to Morgan fanciers, I quote several passages from material kindly provided by L. E. Huijing, Secretary of The Royal Frisian Society, who published *The Frisian Horse Studbook*.

First, from the Society's description of the modern Frisian, which now is only black: "It has a gracefully arched neck, a small head with small ears, and a slightly concave nasal bone. . . . The Frisian horse has a cheerful disposition, is extremely manageable and trustworthy, and yet full of spirit. It has a very high trotting gait and is very intelligent."

Immediately after the Napoleonic Wars, Mr. Huijing writes, "The Frisian regulations set the height of stallions at 5 feet 2 inches for five-year-olds [15.2 hands]. . . . The colour had to be black over the whole body, or bay with black legs, mane and tail. If the owner of the stallions kept three, it was permissible for one of their number to be a red or blue roan."

Quoting an authority on the Frisian in 1854, Mr. Huijing continues: "This breeding is healthy, compact, with . . . neck held high, well-built forequarters, broad-chested and excelling all other horses in his erect stance on four finely shaped legs. . . . The back is handsomely hollowed, forming a graceful curve from the withers to the broad, round and sharply split crupper. Mane and tail are thick and heavy, the latter set in high."

And finally, quoting Mr. Huijing on the Frisian's influence on other breeds: "Less well known [than its influence on the Russian Orlov breed] is the influence the Frisian had in the forming of the American trotting breed (American Trotter). Leon de Meldert, a very well-known American authority on horses, living in Galveston, Texas, wrote in the 1920s that this American horse's aptitude for fast trotting emanated from the *Equus fricius,* the horse from Friesland, or the Dutch fast-trotting horse. The fact is, that *Equus fricius* is the forefather of the American Morgan breed, and also of the

Norfolk trotting horse, the fast English road-horse that was once so famous."

In addition to the Thoroughbred and Frisian theories, there also has been one—advanced in the 1880s—that the founder of the Morgan breed was of French blood (Canadian).

But whatever the time-shrouded facts, Figure was to become one of the most important horses ever foaled in America. And as he won greater renown in his home territory, people began to refer to him as the "Justin Morgan horse."

Figure's arrival in the little settlement of Randolph, Vermont, was presumably taken quite lightly at first. Indeed, one needs little imagination to conjure up the reactions of the townsfolk when Justin arrived home with his unexpected horse companions. A mere pony in size, his bay colt was just a mite too small for the work expected of a horse in that rugged countryside—or so quoth the local experts. "The gelding might be good for something," they allowed, "but that little runt ain't worth a hill o' beans. Sure as sap flows in the spring, skiddin' logs ain't for ponies." And Justin Morgan's new colt fell neatly into the pony category. So you see Figure scarcely took Randolph by storm. But it wouldn't be long before he put the big horses to shame all around the town, in a variety of ways, too.

The most accurate description of Figure made him about 14 hands high and weighing about 950 pounds. He was a rich, dark bay, with the customary black legs, mane and tail. There wasn't a white hair on him, and his mane and tail were coarse and heavy with no tendency to curl (this last could be an Arabian characteristic). His head was good but, contrary to some notions, it was not extremely small. However it was lean, bony and very clean-cut. His profile was straight, with a broad forehead, and his ears were very small and fine and set wide apart. His best feature was his very dark and prominent eyes. The expression in them was spirited but pleasant, and no white showed around the edge of the lids.

In conformation Figure was as distinctive as a race horse is from a Percheron, yet he resembled neither. His body was rather long, due to the extreme depth of shoulders and the powerfully muscled and long quarters. He was close-ribbed; his back was short from wither to loin, and his barrel was very round and deep with no tendency to lightness in the flanks. His chest was wide and deep, projecting a good deal in front. The crest of his neck was high-arched

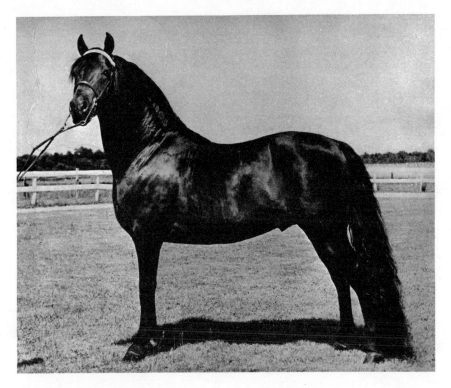

Modern Morgan stallion shows how the stamp of Justin endures.

and deeply muscled, an outstanding characteristic which has been a true Morgan feature through the years. The symmetry that this cresty neck, deep, well-rounded body and high-carried head gives the Morgan, is an appearance that is identifiable as Morgan in any group of horses.

Figure's legs were short and close-joined, with flat bone that was completely free from coarseness, although his fetlocks were a bit hairy. At all seasons of the year, however, his coat was soft and glossy, without the exceeding heaviness often seen on horses where the climate is cold at some season.

The remarkable point to remember as you read the description of Figure is that it tallies so closely with many modern Morgans today except for the matter of size—which even in his sons was varied. It is remarkable, considering that the average Morgan nowadays carries only about 10 percent of Figure's blood, that the stamp of his fabulous progenitor is present still, and is as recognizable as it was in the earliest days of the breed.

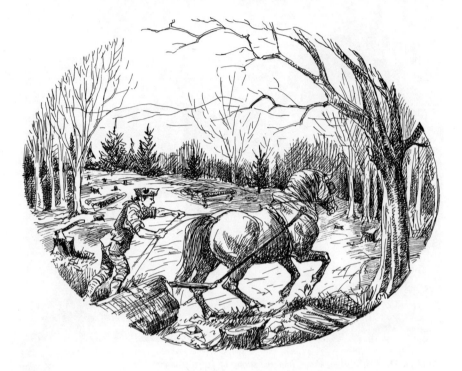

HIS PROWESS

From the very moment that he was fitted into a work harness, Figure's life was one work-a-day task after another. And work in that time and place was from dawn till dusk. Even so, Figure's day's work didn't always end when the sun had slipped down behind the Green Mountains.

By the time he was about four years old Figure really knew what the pinch of a collar and the tug of trace chains meant. For Justin, always in dire straits moneywise, leased him out to a local farmer named Robert Evans for $15 a year, a sum for which the little horse was put to work clearing a hillside woodlot. And the hillside woodlots in Vermont are rock gardens in the most literal sense of the word: they are so steep and rough that it almost seems that the unrelenting soil is staging a bitter tug of war with the men who come to till it. Into the woods, then, went Figure with a farmer at the lines who, I'm sure, was very dubious about the ability of his "team"—the team being Figure alone. But imagine his astonishment when he discovered that his pint-sized companion was a veritable dynamo of energy and strength!

No secret is ever a secret very long in a small village, and it was only a matter of the time it takes to fill a skidway that Figure's prowess in the woodlot made a topic of conversation around the general store of an evening. "He's right handy—might just amount to somethin' after all." It wasn't long at all before it was common knowledge that Morgan's horse, Figure, made up in ability and spirit for what he lacked in size.

One story that sprang from who knows where, but one which an actual eyewitness, Nathan Nye, claims is true, every bit of it, was the account of a test of strength among the village horses. It concerns an occasion when a particularly large pine log was defying all comers to pull it from its resting place near the sawmill in Randolph. All the local horses had found it just too heavy for their liking, and failed at all attempts to skid the log even one foot. Finally, down the street at dusk came Evans with the little bay stallion. He was just returning from a full day's labor on his piece of property over the ridge; but when he heard that there was a little logging still left undone in the village, he chirruped to Figure and strode down to see what was what. His confidence in the horse knew no bounds, so, sizing up the situation, he challenged the whole company gathered to see the sport, betting a gallon of spirits (in this case rum) that Figure could draw the log onto the way in three pulls. Now, Vermonters are always game for a little harmless diversion. Laughing and scoffing, they accepted the challenge. "Not even the Runt can budge that piece of timber," they said, for even though Figure was known by all as a resolute puller, this was asking just too much of the little fellow. Good-naturedly they heckled Evans as he fastened the tug chains to the log. But now Evans, a bit miffed at their jokes at his expense, stated that he was ashamed to hitch his horse to such a small log, and if three stout men would sit astride it, he would forfeit the rum if Figure didn't draw it at least ten rods. Agreeable to anything at this point, three of the brawniest men present clambered onto the log while Nathan Nye held the lantern in the gathering darkness. Warning the men to look out for their legs, Evans snapped up the lines and roared to Figure, "Git up!" The stallion instantly bent his mighty neck, straining into the collar. The laughing crowd grew silent as the swelling, powerful muscles flexed and rippled under the satin coat. With a mighty lunge, Figure, all his weight leaning into the harness, started the log. A cheer arose as, drawing it and the men, he didn't stop until he had gone halfway the distance to the sawmill. In the next pull he landed the load at the spot agreed upon.

Morgan's horse Figure had many an admirer after that night. Having worked hard in the fields and woods all day, he had outdrawn all the horses in the village that same evening!

But not only at pulling did Figure excel. Evans knew a good thing when he had it, and he had it in the bay stallion. He would ride the stallion into the village in the evenings with the work of the day behind him, looking for some form of relaxation. It might have been relaxation for him, but it certainly wasn't for the little horse. There was always some challenge floating around unanswered, or some record to beat. It mattered little whether the proposal was for a race at the trot or the gallop, or even at the walk: he would always accept on Figure's behalf. And he won with regularity. Up and down the countryside the horse gained fame. "Morgan's horse," people said, "can toil all day and win races at dusk!"

D. C. Linsley in his *Morgan Horses,* published in 1857, gives a stirring description of Figure (called by his later and well-known name throughout the book), and the type of races he won. Because the facts are interesting and the book is rare, a portion of the text is quoted here:

He [Figure, or Justin Morgan] was a fleet runner at short distances. Running horses short distances for small stakes was very common in Vermont fifty years ago. Eighty rods was very generally the length of the course, which usually commenced at a tavern or grocery and extended the distance agreed upon, up or down the public road. In these races, the horses were started from a 'scratch,' that is, a mark was drawn across the road in the dirt, and the horses, ranged in a row upon it, went off at 'the drop of a hat' or some other signal. It will be observed that the form of Justin Morgan was not such as in our days is thought best calculated to give the greatest speed for a short distance. Those

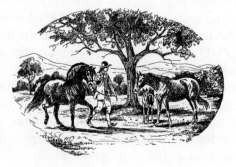

who believe in long-legged racers will think his legs, body and stride were too short, and to them it may perhaps seem surprising that he should be successful, as he invariably was, in such contests. But we think his great muscular development and nervous energy, combined with his small size, gave him a decided advantage in the first start over taller and heavier horses; just as any ordinary horse can distance the finest locomotive in a ten rod race. At all events, the history of racing in this country and in England, proves conclusively that small horses may have great speed. In such a race, a horse of great spirit and nervous energy derives a decided advantage from these qualities, especially after being a little accustomed to such struggles. When brought up to the line, his [Justin Morgan's, or Figure's] eyes flash and his ears quiver with intense excitement, he grinds the bit with his teeth, his hind legs are drawn under him, every muscle of his frame trembles and swells almost to bursting and at the given signal he goes off like the spring of a steel trap. His unvarying success in these short races may perhaps be partly accounted for in this way, though he was undoubtedly possessed of more than ordinary speed, and was a sharp runner.

So far afield did Figure's fame spread that on at least one occasion two Thoroughbreds were imported to race against him. In Brookfield, Vermont, so the records show, on June 26, 1796, Figure accepted the challenge from a horse called Sweepstakes, brought to the small Vermont town all the way from Long Island. Also, another horse, a gray mare called Silvertail from St. Lawrence County, New York, was to try her luck against his.

Everyone gathered at the little country track feared that this time Morgan's horse had met his match. Nevertheless, the cheers were with him, even if the money might have rested elsewhere. The distance of the race, or, as it turned out races, was eighty rods; not a long race but probably all the primitive little track would allow. The most interesting thing was, however, that Figure was to take on each of his challengers separately! Now, both challengers were used and trained solely for racing, having no other use in life; yet here was the small Vermont logging horse going to take them both on—one at a time.

Imagine the great surprise and chagrin of the racing men when the diminutive work horse from the back country of Vermont soundly beat both their champions handily! Morgan is said even to have given the defeated parties a chance to win back some of their losses by matching their horses against Figure in a walking race and/or a trot-

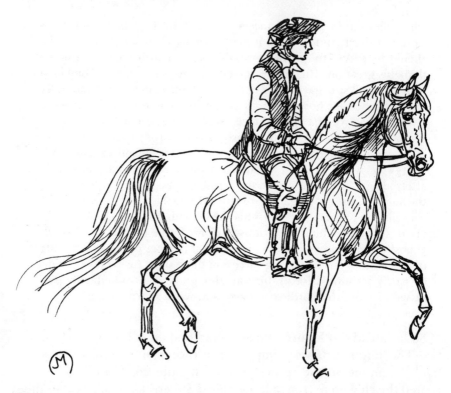

ting race if they preferred, but undoubtedly they'd seen about enough of Figure's heels and declined any further sport. Without a doubt there was much celebrating by the Vermonters that evening.

When Robert Evans's lease on Figure was up, the stallion was returned reluctantly to the stable of the singing master, Justin Morgan. It was on the back of this dashing young horse that the sickly Morgan, racked with consumption, made his rounds to teach music and singing in the little villages around Randolph. In those days people considered it of prime importance that their children learn singing as well as the three R's, and they allotted funds to pay the singing master to come to their community. Thus, on many a blustery day Justin Morgan, old in health if not in years, rode out into the countryside, earning his small, much-needed fees. The sprightly Figure carried him easily over the miles, and many travelers on the road could recall seeing the wasted man and his robust little stallion moving away down the empty roads as he went about his lonely rounds during the winters of 1796, '97 and '98.

But Justin's health had been growing steadily worse, and on March

22, 1798, he fought back no longer. Since his wife had died and his family had been split up into foster homes, Morgan, during his last illness before his death, lived with Sheriff Rice, a friend in Woodstock. It was to this man that he gave his well-loved young stallion as payment for expenses incurred while he was ill in the sheriff's house.

The town records of Randolph show that Justin Morgan left no valuable papers or documents to reveal answers to the tantalizing questions about the original Morgan horse. Indeed, all his worldly goods at the time of his death amounted to the pitiful sum of $160.13. Thus passed the simple Vermonter who will be remembered not for great deeds, but because he once owned a little bay stallion he called Figure. He had written many hymns, some of which were published and can be found in old collections of sacred music, but these have long since passed out of use. Yet the breed of horse established under his name yearly increases in numbers and popularity.

It was after the death of the singing master that Figure became known as the "Justin Morgan horse" and, finally, as simply Justin Morgan. His days were to be filled with endless hard work and a succession of owners both good and bad.

Sheriff Rice of Woodstock found a number of chores for the Morgan horse to do when he owned him, and the young stallion found no slackening of pace with his change of ownership. The sheriff, however, gave him good care during the years that he was in his barn. But old Bob Evans had his eye on the horse, biding his time until the stallion might come up for sale. He'd never had another horse like him before—or since!—and needless to say he was itching to get his hands on the Morgan again if the opportunity ever presented itself. His chance came sooner than he thought: the sheriff decided to sell, and back to the Randolph woods went the bay stallion, to labor from dawn to dusk without respite.

Not only were his hours in harness as long and tiring as they had been before, but the old racing and pulling bees were as frequent as ever. His reputation firmly established, he was attracting much attention now as a sire, and folks began to bring their mares to him. And what a varied lot they were! Draft mares of Canadian blood, big mares, small mares, sound mares and lame mares; mares of all colors and types were brought to the Morgan, who was expected to perform miracles. And he did not disappoint the owners of this varied group, for the foals that arrived each spring resembled their dams not at all, but their sire. The farmers and the horsemen—even the young folks who had been allowed to borrow the family mare to raise a colt from—were delighted. Regardless of the conformation of the mare they had hopefully sent to Justin Morgan, the foals always resembled their dad! They had the same round, close-coupled bodies, the same bold expression, the same sprightly gait and, best of all, the same gentle disposition.

For a number of years this situation remained unchanged, and the little stallion enjoyed the admiration and respect of the countryside. Then everything changed. Robert Evans, not making quite as much of a success of his business as the horse was making of *his,* fell into bankruptcy, was sued for debt in 1804, and was put in the pokey. Colonel John Goss, a good man and a keen judge of horses, took the Morgan horse as security against Evans's bail; by paying the farmer's debts he became the legal owner of the stallion.

Under his new owner, Justin Morgan's horse continued his previous occupations and, although worked as long and as hard, was given good care and wasn't abused. As well as the usual farm work which was his daily lot, he was ridden and evidently driven occasionally for pleasure as well. Linsley gives a brief description, which I think is worth quoting here:

> His proud, bold and fearless style of movement and his vigorous, untiring action, have, perhaps, never been surpassed. When a rider was on him, he was obedient to the slightest motion of the rein, would walk backward rapidly under a gentle pressure of the bit and moved side-ways almost as willingly as he moved forward; in short, was perfectly trained to all the paces and evolutions of a parade horse; and when ridden at military reviews (as was frequently the case) his bold, imposing style, and spirited, nervous action attracted universal attention and admiration. He was perfectly gentle and kind to handle and loved to be groomed and caressed, but he disliked to have children about him and had an inveterate hatred for dogs, if loose always chasing them out of sight the instant he saw them. When taken out with a halter or bridle he was in constant motion and very playful.

In 1811 little Justin Morgan's luck began running out, and he came onto the proverbial hard times. How often we wonder how a horse of his obvious greatness could have been so unappreciated as to have been served as he was! It has always seemed cruel and heartless that he was made constantly to suffer in the closing years of his life, with no compassionate person to rescue him from the rigors and hardships of the life he was forced to lead. There was Jacob Sanderson, who bought him in 1811 and then sold him. There was William Langmaid,

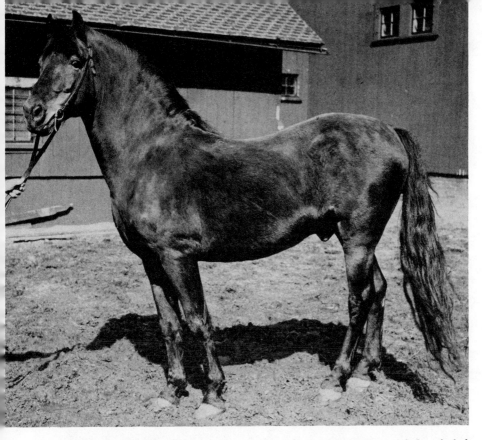

The old stallion Sonny Bob, foaled 1928, reminds us of how Justin Morgan might have looked in the twilight of his life.

a cruel taskmaster who used the aging little stallion in a six-horse hitch hauling freight between Windsor and Chelsea. How unfeeling and dull these men must have been to subject not only a well-known horse but an old one as well, to the afflictions of the road! Treated roughly, with no regard for past performances or fame, the Morgan horse became poor and worn; when he could be of no further use he was again sold down the road, this time for a pitifully small sum, to a man in Chelsea. A succession of owners followed, each seemingly anxious to pass him along for fear he would die on their hands. He returned to Randolph around 1816 under the ownership of a Samuel Stone, but after two or three years he left his old home for good and was kept at the farm of Clifford Bean, about three miles south of the village of Chelsea. It was here that he was to end his days.

Turned out in a small pasture with other horses to shift for himself without benefit of shelter or care, he was kicked in the flank by one of his companions. Since no one apparently saw or cared what happened to him, his injury was left unattended and inflammation set

in. Alone and completely unmourned, in 1821 old Justin Morgan
breathed his last. He was about thirty years old when death ended
his suffering.

It is a sad note indeed that the sole founder of America's first great
breed of horse should come to his end in this manner, but the legacy
he left behind him in the many sons and daughters cast in his image
has spread his fame from ocean to ocean and to other lands. As
Linsley writes:

> Before receiving the injury which caused his death, the Morgan
> horse was completely sound and free from any description of blemish
> despite his amazingly arduous life. His limbs were perfectly smooth
> and free from any swelling and very limber and supple.
>
> Those who saw him in 1819 and 1820, describe his appearance as
> remarkably fresh and youthful. Age had not quenched his spirit, nor
> dampened the ardor of his temper; years of severest labor had not
> sapped his vigor, nor broken his constitution; his eye was still bright
> and his step firm and elastic.

2

Justin Morgan's Progeny

ALTHOUGH THERE were undoubtedly many direct sons of old Justin Morgan (as we shall refer to the stallion henceforth), no authentic account of more than six which were *kept at stud* in New England has ever been found, despite endless research into the subject undertaken by students of the breed.

D. C. Linsley was the most noted authority on the subject of the origins of the Morgans, and the facts he unearthed during his lifetime have been invaluable to anyone and everyone interested in the breed. He states, concerning the sons of Justin Morgan: "Between all the stallions left by him there was a very close and striking resemblance, in size, form, and general character, and they also bore equal resemblance to their sire; indeed, the power of transmitting to his progeny his own form, constitution and temperament, was a very distinguishing trait of Justin Morgan, and we believe no horse ever lived that possessed in a higher degree the power of stamping upon his offspring his own great leading characteristics."

Justin Morgan's important characteristics, which he passed on to his sons were: his compactness of form, his high and generous spirit, combined with perfect gentleness and tractability, and his sinewy limbs, his lofty style and his easy but vigorous action.

The fact that not only did his valuable qualities descend unimpaired to the next generation, but apparently with little diminution to the second and third, thus establishing a new breed of horse, makes Justin Morgan undeniably just about the most important horse ever foaled in America. His legacy was the fine and enduring breed which helped to develop New England, and subsequently all America.

SONS OF JUSTIN MORGAN

Although many other stallions sired by Justin were kept for breeding, the four which became most celebrated were Sherman, Woodbury, Bulrush and Revenge. These four, with the Hawkins horse and the Fenton horse, were the sons of old Justin whom Linsley was able to trace with accuracy. Possibly other sons of Justin were just as valuable or well known in their own time and place, but often fate deals with a horse unfavorably, so that he is lost in obscurity though he may possess all the qualities for fame. Such seems to have been the fate of the unknown sons of old Justin Morgan and they have remained anonymous through the years.

Without any doubt the three most important sons of Justin Morgan were Sherman, Woodbury and Bulrush, and since each was responsible for a family in his own right much more detail is known about the lives of these three. Each became the progenitor of an immediate family, with his descendants being bred back to produce *third and fourth generation* horses more like the original Justin Morgan than any of his sons. Perhaps because the mares which produced them were so dissimilar, each of the three was known for his distinction from the others.

That the important features that characterize Justin Morgan were strongly and strikingly impressed upon his offspring can be seen in the following descriptions of his known sons. Yet not only did his unique qualities go almost full strength to the next generation, but apparently they did so practically undiluted to the second and third. Where pains were taken to select both sires and dams possessing most of his blood and characteristics, the resulting foals closely resembled Justin in all important respects—except, perhaps, in size, in which there was a decided increase.

SHERMAN

The first of the three most outstanding sons of Justin Morgan was Sherman. It was felt by many that Sherman was the greatest of them all, for he sired a prominent line down through Black Hawk 20 and his son Ethan Allen 50. His daughters, when bred to his half-brothers Bulrush and Woodbury, contributed greatly to the success of the Morgan breed.

Because he was a highly esteemed horse in his own day, it is a

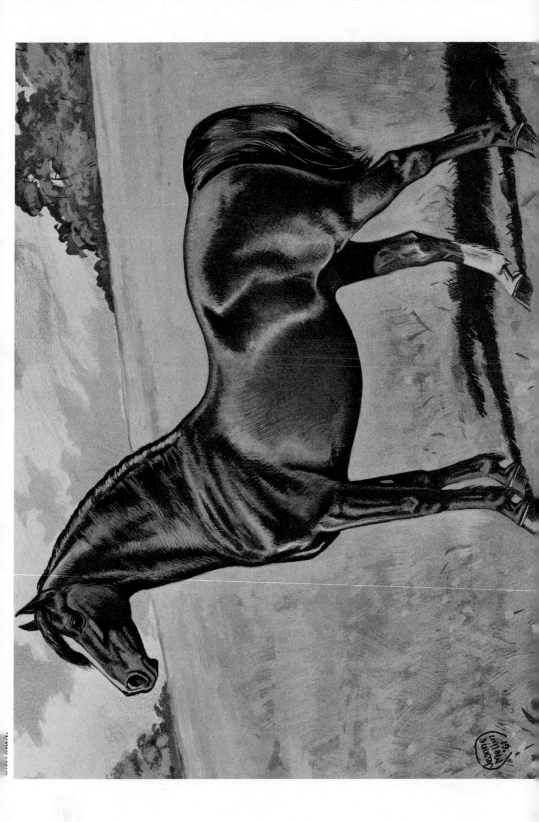
Jeanne Mellin '61

matter of some interest that the actual birth date of Sherman is not known. Consensus seems to put it either about 1808 or 1809.

Appearance and Early Years

By way of description, Sherman was a bright red chestnut, standing slightly under 14 hands and weighing about 925 pounds. His off hind leg was white from the foot halfway to the hock, and he had a small white stripe in his face. His head was lean and well shaped, with small, fine ears; and his eyes, although inclined to be small, were prominent and lively. He had the legs of his sire, including the same long hair at the fetlocks and the back of his cannons. He had an excellent deep chest with the prominent breastbone similar to his sire's, while his shoulders were large and well laid back into good withers. His neck was well crested and embellished with a full mane, but one not so heavy as Justin's. He had quarters which were long and deep, with broad and muscular loins. He was, however, a bit hollow-backed, a trait which occasionally he passed on to his get. But this tendency never seemed to indicate a weak back, for the horse worked hard all his life and never suffered from any weakness or breaking down.

Sherman's dam was a mare of high quality, some records stating that she was a full-blooded Spanish Barb. She was a light chestnut with a star, strip and snip, and three white legs. She stood over 15 hands. Her head was good; ears small, neck rather thin and long. She always carried her head high, exhibiting a marked degree of high-spiritedness, although her nature seemed pleasant enough. She was a good mare in harness, but seemingly at her best under saddle, and was used at the latter by most of her owners.

When brought from Rhode Island to Vermont by John Sherman, the mare unfortunately slipped her hip and was never quite sound again. She was subsequently given to his brother, James, of Lyndon, Vermont. James's son, George Sherman, was given the colt resulting from the crossing of this mare with Justin Morgan. This was in 1811, when the colt was three years old.

George Sherman was a hard-working man, and the horses in his keeping were compelled to keep their noses to the proverbial grindstone as he did. Like his sire, Sherman, only a pony in size, was required to labor long and hard at work meant for horses twice his size. Beginning at the age of four he was worked singly, and occasionally in a team with a large brown draft mare, on the stoneboat and at pulling stumps. But also like his sire, he never shirked any work asked of him, and was always willing and agreeable.

In the winter Sherman usually ran a team steadily between Lyndon and Portland, Maine. For several years this team consisted of Sherman and a half-brother by Justin Morgan who was a year older and a bit larger. This horse never gained the fame of his brother, never being named and probably never used at stud. Little is known of him except that he was a son of old Justin and was a heavier and slightly coarser horse than Sherman. Along the route between Lyndon and Portland, George Sherman was known as a man who would never be outdone in any kind of sport or wager, especially anything involving horses. He was always ready to match his team against any he met, either to draw or run, for a small wager. And his little team soon became famous at every inn on the route.

The races were always at catch weights, and usually for the distance of about eighty rods or about a quarter of a mile. As in Justin's time, the starting line was a scratch drawn across the road, and at the given signal the horses were off. Sherman soon became as adept at this sport as his sire had been, being alert and eager and able to reach his full stride in a matter of a few feet. It wasn't very long before other teamsters became reluctant to match their horses against the Morgans, and only strangers who hadn't heard of George Sherman and his team offered any competition.

Record at Stud

Such was the life of Sherman Morgan from his fourth year until he was about ten. At this time he was sold to Stephen C. Gibbs of Littleton, New Hampshire, to be used at the stud. He remained there for three seasons; afterwards he was traveled extensively by various owners around the Granite State, and many a stud poster tacked on a livery stable wall advertised the qualifications of Sherman Morgan. After several prolific seasons in New Hampshire, Sherman was returned to Vermont in the ownership of John Buckminster of Danville, who also stood the horse at stud in St. Johnsbury and Danville in 1828.

In 1829 he returned to Littleton with John Bellows as his owner and Gibbs providing the stable and care. He became a well-liked and highly regarded stallion—never unappreciated, as Justin had been during his lifetime.

For five more years under the ownership of Bellows, Sherman Morgan sired fine foundation stock of the breed that was to sweep New England and the growing America. Bellows stood the horse

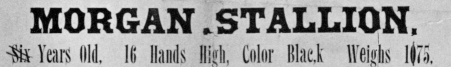

A stud poster extols the virtues of Sherman's line.

each season in a different location and was known to have leased Sherman every season to a qualified person who could handle the stud and take the responsibility of him. In 1830 he stood in Dover, New Hampshire, and vicinity; in 1831 he was at Colonel Jacques's Ten Hills Farm in Charlestown, Massachusetts. The colonel, liking the horse and the colts sired by him very much, tried to persuade Bellows to let him keep the stallion another season. However, he failed to do so, and this fact and Sherman's making the season of 1832 in Dover, Durham and South Berwick, New Hampshire, instead, resulted in the stud's being bred to the mare that produced his best son, Black Hawk 20.

In 1833 and 1834, he remained in the vicinity of Dover. Records state that he sired twenty-seven foals in 1833. In 1834, his last year, he was bred to fifty-seven mares, but no record can be found of the number of live foals resulting.

Sherman Morgan was probably the most popular of old Justin's sons, and the family he founded was very much like the old horse himself. His offspring were very tractable and easily broken to any use. They had their sire's short, nervous step and were also tough and courageous. That some of them also inherited their sire's hollow back could never be considered too much of a fault, as no weakness was ever apparent from this cause. Of his twenty sons left stallions, most were chestnut, although there were several grays, bays and blacks, and one brown. His other offspring were generally chestnut, with white markings on face and legs quite common. They ranged in height from 13.2 to 15.2, the average being 14.3.

Sherman Morgan died January 9, 1835, in the stable of John Bellows in Lancaster, New Hampshire. The actual cause of his death is unknown, although a heart attack was suspected. After appearing as usual in the morning, he was found dead in his stall shortly after one o'clock in the afternoon. With the exception of some slight indications of age, he was apparently as free from every species of blemish or infirmity on the morning of his death as on the day when he was foaled.

In stature Sherman was small, but like his sire he had a heart as big as the Green Mountain country in which he was foaled.

WOODBURY

If little Sherman Morgan was the hard-working, even-tempered individual of the known sons of Justin, then Woodbury could be called the show horse of the group, for he really enjoyed an opportunity to strut his stuff. He especially relished the noise and confusion attendant to the old Vermont muster days. The martial music and the flag-waving were meant for him, one would think, to see the horse on one of these occasions. He had absolutely no fear of the flashing uniforms or the pounding drums, but would prance and parade to the delight of all, and never was there a muster or a ceremony which he attended where he would go unnoticed.

Woodbury, at 14.3, was the largest of the three, and with his bold, fearless and showy ways seemed more like his sire than any of the others.

Qualities and Background

In color he was a rich, dark chestnut, with a white stocking on his off hind leg and an oddly shaped blaze on his face which ran from his upper lip to a little more than halfway to his eyes with no white between his eyes at all. He was a very compact horse with a broad chest, deep quarters and an excellent back and loin. His croup was nearly level with a high-set tail, which, after the fashion of the day, had been docked and was only ten inches long. His head was small and lean, bespeaking quality, and his large, dark, hazel eyes were set far apart and were very prominent and bright. His face was straight, his nostrils were very large and full, and he had the tiny ears that were to become such a positive characteristic of the Morgan breed.

In action Woodbury was very bold and fiery, with a nervous temperament that never allowed him to stand still. When led out in a bridle, he was restive and playful, tossing his head and dancing about and never seeming to be without motion. Surprisingly, he was good in harness despite his nervousness, but it was said that he always appeared at his best under saddle. Militia colonels and generals were always eager to ride him at the musters or reviews, for his showiness was also coupled with a pleasant disposition.

Woodbury was foaled the latter part of May 1816 in Tunbridge, Vermont, and was the property of Lyman Wight. Woodbury, too, had a couple of aliases, being sometimes called the "Burbank horse," and in Windsor County he was known as the "Walker horse."

Nothing has ever been learned about the blood of his dam. At the time the colt was foaled, Wight was a young man, about eighteen years old, and the mare belonged to his father, William Wight, who lent her to his son for the purpose of raising a colt. Woodbury's dam

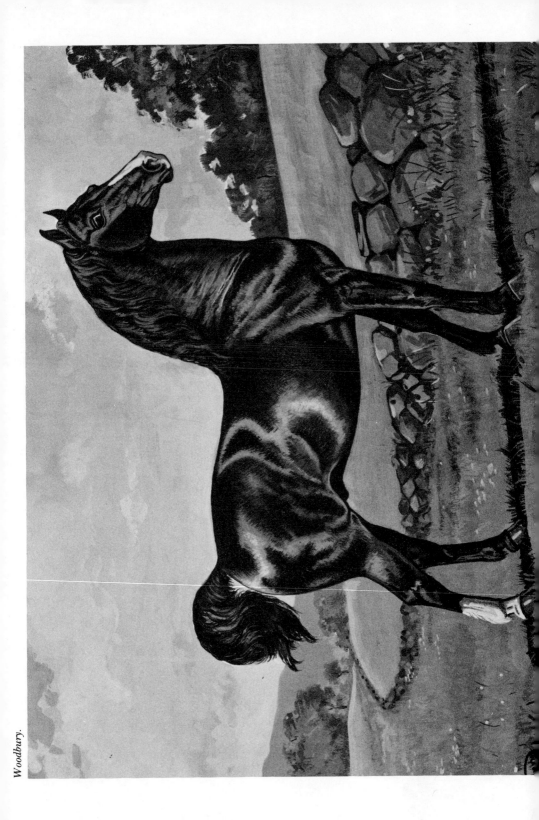

Woodbury.

was five years old when he was foaled. She was a large mare for those days, standing over 15 hands and weighing about 1,100 pounds. In color she was a deep bay with black points, and had a small star in her forehead but no other white markings. Although not very compactly built and with a tendency to be flat-ribbed, she nevertheless had an excellent chest, fine shoulders and good quarters. Her head, which was very fine, she carried high. She was known to be "good on the road and with a turn of speed." She nevertheless had a tendency to pace as well as trot (oh, how it's frowned upon in this day and age!), but she did not seem to pass this trait on to her son, nor did Woodbury's get show any inclination to pace. It was said that she made a fine appearance when trotting and attracted much attention for her speed.

At weaning time, the colt was sold by Wight to David Woodbury of Bethel, Vermont, for the sum of $50. Woodbury kept the young

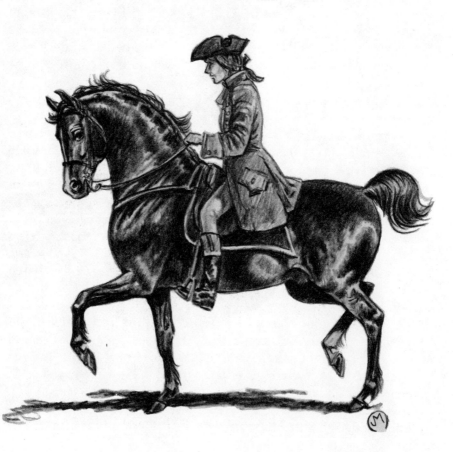

stallion until he was mature and trained him for both saddle and harness before selling him to his brother, John.

Reputation and Travels

John Woodbury was known as a keen judge of horses, and his new horse caused quite a stir in the community. For several seasons John kept the stallion at stud in Bethel and surrounding towns, where his get became quite favorably known.

When John Woodbury sold his horse to Ebenezer Parkhurst, the price received was high for those days. Parkhurst kept the stud until he was ten years old before selling him to Simon Smith and William Walker in March 1826. The price tag this time was $500. Shortly afterwards, Smith and Walker dissolved partnership and Walker became the sole owner of Woodbury.

Because Walker had a passion for horses and recognized the fact that Woodbury's fine qualities were inherited from his sire, Justin Morgan, he went to great pains to have the Morgan stock brought into the limelight. Unfortunately, after owning Woodbury only four years, the man's assets were too meager to make the venture pay, and he was forced to sacrifice the stallion for, in his own words, "the insignificant sum of four hundred dollars."

Woodbury's new owner was Peter Burbank, a lawyer of Newbury, Vermont. Burbank was not a breeder but was very fond of horses, and having seen Woodbury on one occasion at Keene, New Hampshire, became very taken with the horse and wished to buy him. He had a discriminating eye and knew a horse's good points. Still, he did not trust his own judgment, and consulted Jesse Johnson of Bradford, Vermont, about the advisability of buying the horse. Now, Johnson was an astute horseman with a close, critical eye that could take in at a glance all the minute defects of form that a more careless observer might fail to discover. However, upon seeing Woodbury, he was quite aware of the stallion's merit, and wholeheartedly advised Burbank to purchase the horse, which he did on the 20th of May 1830.

For six years the Johnson brothers of Bradford had charge of old Woodbury and he was kept at their stables during the winter and the latter part of the summer and autumn of each year, and, for one or two years, kept there all year round. He also stood at stud in Keene, New Hampshire, and Burlington, Vermont.

When Burbank died in September 1836, the administrators of his estate decided that the horse must be sold. It can be easily imagined

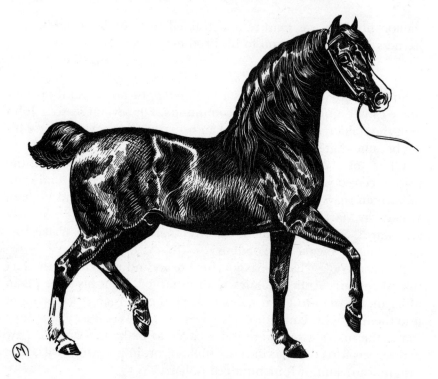

that there were many regrets when the well-known and well-liked Woodbury was sold at auction in Wells River, Vermont, only to be shipped away from his native state to Gainesville, Alabama.

He was purchased by Norman Baglee of that town and sent to sea aboard a small sailing packet from Boston. The trip was very rough and exceedingly unpleasant and Woodbury fared badly, arriving in Alabama in extremely poor condition. It is related that he unloaded with much difficulty from the boat, and some accounts state that he slipped and broke a leg at the time. This has never been verified, however, and seems rather unlikely as the horse lived two years more in Alabama. But he never regained his health and one wonders if the spirit he had always possessed had departed, too. There is no evidence of his leaving any stock at all in Alabama before his death at the age of twenty-two in 1838.

BULRUSH

All three of the outstanding sons of Justin Morgan were used in about the same capacity all their lives and were similar to their sire

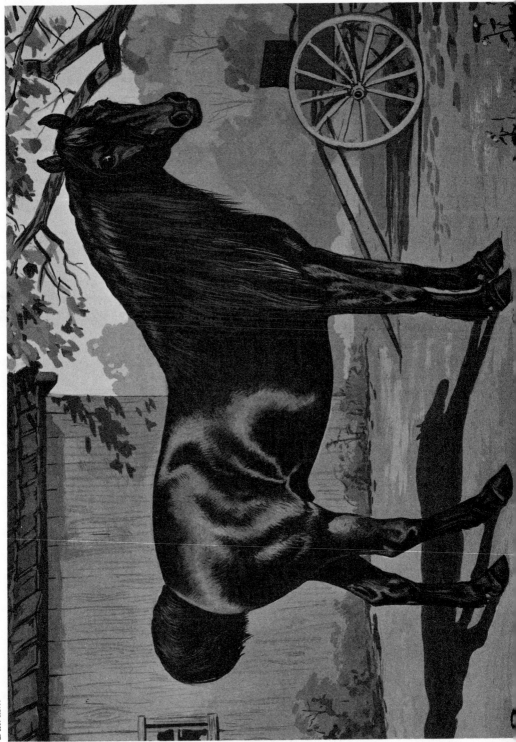

Bulrush.

in many ways, yet each left his own mark on the breed known as Morgan, and Bulrush was no exception.

Bulrush was foaled in 1812 and, again like the others, little is known about his dam. She was a dark bay with a heavy black mane and tail; she was built low to the ground, compact, and had heavy limbs with large joints. Her neck was rather long and, though her head was good, she did not carry it high. She was a fast trotter but inclined to be lacking in spirit. Her appearance indicated that she was of French (Canadian) blood and she was said to be probably of this breeding.

At the time Bulrush was sired, his dam was owned by Moses Belknap of Randolph, Vermont. Belknap was known to have obtained her from a teamster from Montpelier by the name of Boutwell, who had worked her in a six-horse hitch hauling merchandise and produce between Montpelier and Boston. Even though the mare was rugged and hardy, with great endurance, Boutwell thought her too small for his business, and he exchanged her for a larger horse from Belknap.

Late in the winter, when the mare was heavy in foal to Justin Morgan, Belknap sold her to Ziba Gifford of Tunbridge. The deal that went with her was that Gifford was to keep the foal until it was four months old, and then return it to Belknap; or, if he wished, he could keep the colt and pay $13 for it. Thirteen dollars for a Morgan foal—and by Justin, too! But evidently Gifford was short of cash, for he chose to return the colt.

Belknap kept Bulrush in Tunbridge and vicinity until 1819. At an early age the young stallion was broken to harness and saddle and he became a popular stud in the countryside around Tunbridge, leaving many sons and daughters there. The uniformity of type and tremendous endurance of his offspring gained him much patronage.

Like Sherman, Bulrush was a small horse, standing only 14 hands and weighing about 1,000 pounds. He was a dark bay in color with a few white hairs on the forehead, but no other white at all. His black mane and tail were exceedingly heavy and coarse: he must have made quite a picture, as it was said that his mane came down nearly to his knees, while his forelock fell to the tip of his nose! His tail had been docked when he was a colt, yet the hair was bushy and full even though short in length. His legs, like Justin's, were large, powerfully muscled and had the feathering of hair at the back of the cannon. His back, while not so short as either Sherman's or Woodbury's, was broad and straight, with no inclination to be hollow as the others' were. He was very deep in the chest, with shoulders which were powerful though possibly not so well placed.

Speed and Endurance

Although Bulrush lacked Woodbury's boldness and proud manner, and the short, nervous step of his brother, he was a sharp and speedy horse in harness, and indeed a faster horse at the trot than either Sherman or Woodbury. He was said to be a bit cross at times, but in harness this tendency rarely showed itself. His most outstanding trait, however, was his remarkable endurance. In this he had no equal, and all the local folk were well aware of the fact when sending their mares to be bred to him.

Of all Justin's sons, Bulrush probably got a more uniform group of colts, for they resembled their sire in color, type and weight. They were almost all dark bay or brown without white markings, and never a chestnut or sorrel. Almost all of them, too, had the same thick, luxurious mane and tail, and were extraordinarily good-legged and hardy.

Standing in New England

In his lifetime Bulrush had many owners and traveled around his native state and neighboring New Hampshire much the same way as old Justin had, always leaving behind him the finest of stock to aid in the development of a new and growing land.

His owners included the same partnership of Smith and Walker which had owned his brother Woodbury. When this partnership dissolved and Walker became the sole owner of Woodbury, Smith kept Bulrush. After a season in Maidstone, Vermont, and two years in the state of Maine, Bulrush was sold in 1833 to Jesse Johnson of Bradford, Vermont, where he was stabled with his brother Woodbury, then owned by Burbank. In 1833 Bulrush made a circuit season between Bradford and Bath, New Hampshire; 1834 found him in Keene, a hundred miles away. In 1835 he stood in Lyme, also in New Hampshire, and then back to Bradford. The next season found him far in the western part of Vermont in Burlington. Considering that there were no means of horse transportation as we know it today, and a horse went everywhere on its own power, it is an undisputed fact that little Bulrush scarcely suffered from lack of exercise. Records state that he was either ridden or driven on all his rounds.

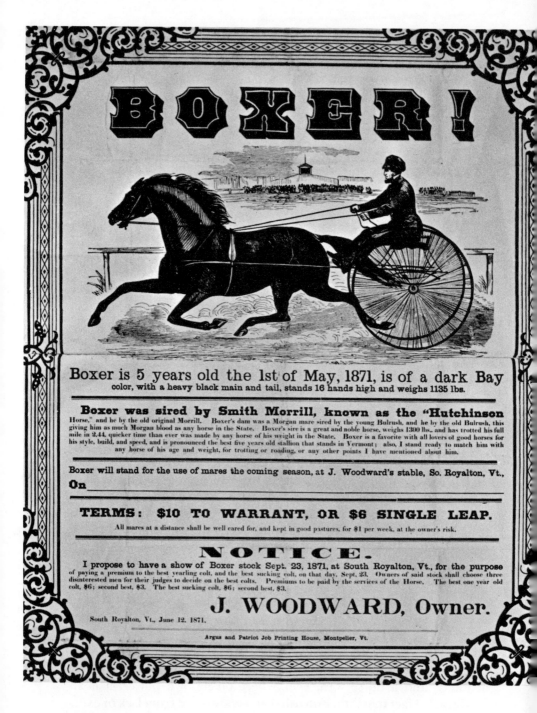

Bulrush blood promises stamina for Boxer's get.

The Johnson brothers kept Bulrush until 1837 when they sold him to the partnership of Blake and Foss in Chelsea, Vermont. He remained in their possession until 1842 and then at the ripe age of thirty he was sold to Lewis Jenkins of Fairlee, Vermont, and finally to F. A. Weir of Walpole, New Hampshire.

When he died at the remarkable age of thirty-six in 1848, Bulrush was as sound and clean-legged as any colt, and he had never been known to have a lame day in his very long life. All his family were just like him: tough and dependable, and with a dash of speed to satisfy the sport-minded.

THE THREE STUDS COMPARED

Linsley in a discourse on the similarities and differences between the Sherman, Woodbury and Bulrush families, wrote in 1857:

> Sherman had not so bold and resolute a style of action, and was not so nervous and high tempered as Woodbury; nor was he, in the language of the stable, so well 'finished up'; but he was more tractable, was exceedingly spirited, and a keen, rapid driver, possessed of great powers of endurance, a free and noble spirit, that needed neither whip nor spur, and courage that never flagged. . . . We think the Shermans are generally smaller than the Woodburys. They are more inclined to be hollow-backed, but their backs are very short, with wide, full and exceedingly muscular loins . . . none were known to have weak backs. . . . They have a shorter gait than the Bulrushes, and do not raise their feet as high. . . . They have not so bold, eager and commanding a style as the Woodburys, but we think they have a better temper for driving. They have a more rapid walk than either of the other families. . . . They are easily broken to harness. . . . The Shermans, like the Woodburys, are generally chestnut, being more common in this than the other families. A white stripe or star in the face and white hind feet are common. We think the Shermans have the best action in harness, and the Woodburys the best action under saddle.
>
> The founders of this the Woodbury family and of the Bulrush family were bred close together and remained near each other most of their lives; hence their descendants are found in the same vicinity [along the Connecticut River between Brattleboro and Newbury]. The average size of the Woodburys, we believe to be greater than either of the other families. They are deeper in the flanks with heavier quarters but not so heavy in the chest. Some are inclined to be hollow-backed and in this respect differ from the Bulrushes. They have an exceedingly bold, lofty and resolute style of action and are overflowing with spirit and

nervous energy. They are generally very tractable but eager and restless; are full of ambition and cat-like activity and they make excellent parade horses. Their prevailing color is chestnut or bay with a white star or stripe in the face and white on one or both of the hind feet. Only a few of this family have long hair on the legs above the fetlocks and they do not generally have as heavy mane and tails as the other families. They have a shorter gait than the Bulrushes and are spirited and pleasant drivers. The limbs, with the exception that they are freer from long hairs, closely resemble the limbs of the Shermans, being not so large as the limbs of the Bulrushes. They have generally a softer coat than either of the other families. The Woodburys have the largest, most prominent and brightest eyes of any of the Morgans. The forehead is also very broad and the muzzle good, but in some of them the jowls are not so well shaped as the others. . . .

[The Bulrush family] are almost invariably deep bays and browns with black legs, manes and tails; in this respect they differ from the other families and also in their general freedom from any marks: such as white feet or white spots in the face. They have large limbs, wide, flat and muscular, sometimes inclined to be a little coarse, but joints are good and the whole limbs very large in proportion to the size of the animal. We do not recollect ever seeing a spavin or a ringbone on a Bulrush horse. They exhibit great development of muscle and in point of size are fully equal to the average of Morgans. They have not so bright, lively and intelligent eyes as the other families, though the eyes are by no means dull or stupid. They do not carry their heads as high, nor do they have as bold and eager an expression as the Woodburys or as graceful and easy motion as the Shermans, but for lastingness and power of endurance, we believe they have no rivals in this or any other country among Morgans or any other breed. There is really some ground for the assertion once made that "a smart, active boy would wear out a wrought-iron rocking pony sooner than a grown man could break down the constitution of a Bulrush horse." In addition to this power of endurance, they are generally sharp, keen drivers and many of them are fast. They are not excitable, never fret upon the road but are busy industrious workers. Some of the family have considerable long hair upon the legs and others are entirely free from it. Most of them have very heavy manes and tails.

The above was written when men were numerous who had known the horses spoken of and could give eyewitness accounts of the Morgans of those early days. While Linsley tends to repeat himself on a few occasions and comes a bit close even to contradicting himself, still his account of the Morgans at the time of their birth as a breed

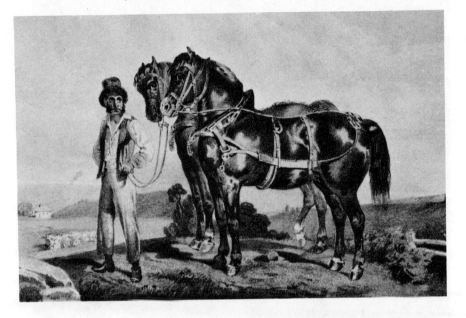

is the most thorough and detailed of anything that has ever been written about them.

REVENGE

The fourth of Justin Morgan's sons known to have been kept at stud was Revenge, whose history is far less complete than that of his famous brothers. He was a dark bay or light brown, foaled in Claremont, New Hampshire, in 1815, and was the property of Cyrus Moore of that town. His dam was a brown mare, marked with a white stripe and white hind socks. She was smart enough in harness, despite an inclination to be low-headed and an unattractive tendency to pace. No one seems to know anything about her sire, but her dam was thought to have a bit of Narragansett pacer blood in her veins, which would account for her daughter's gait.

Moore sold Revenge the autumn after he was two years old to Nehemiah Rice. Rice kept him two or three years, and then sold him to a Mr. Tyler who kept him in the vicinity of Claremont until the horse was nine years old. He had a number of owners after that. In April 1837 he had been driven to Chester, Vermont, by his current owner, who had intended to drive on to the western part of

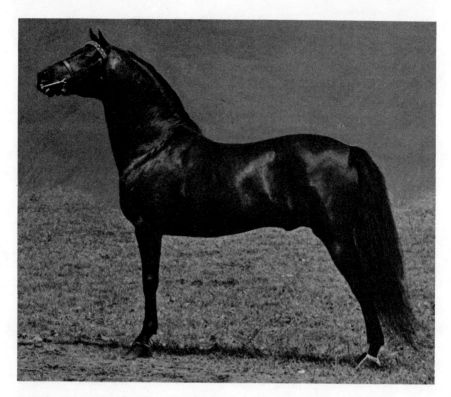

A modern Morgan fits the old descriptions.

the state; but in Chester the horse became sick and died suddenly.

Revenge was about 14.2 hands high and weighed a substantial 1,000 pounds. He did not have an overabundance of action or a very smooth gait, yet despite his mother's breeding he never paced or hitched. It was reported that he had plenty of get up and go and great endurance to boot, and was "hard to get away from on the road." He is reported, however, to have had one fault in harness. He had been frightened as a colt when a portion of his harness parted company with the buggy and he was known to have taken off. He never really recovered from the effects of this frightening experience, and would "take an awful hold" when driven singly and something spooked him.

His stock were dark bay or brown and sometimes chestnut. They had good size, were strong, hardy and enduring. They were generally free going in harness, although some of them would both pace and trot. None of his get approached the fame of his three notable brothers' offspring.

THE HAWKINS AND FENTON HORSES

The two other sons of Justin which Linsley was able to trace with accuracy were the Hawkins horse and the Fenton horse.

The Hawkins horse was foaled in 1806 or 1807, the property of a Mr. Melvin of St. Johnsbury, Vermont. His dam was a bay, standing about 15 hands, and with good conformation and excellent action. She was sired by a black horse brought from Connecticut and said to have been an imported Thoroughbred racer. When the colt was three years old, Melvin sold him to Olney Hawkins, a near neighbor. Hawkins was the captain of a troop, and bought the colt to use as a parade horse. He kept the horse five or six years and then sold him to his brother Stephen. Stephen stabled the stallion at St. Johnsbury for a period of two years and then took him to Stanstead, Quebec, not far over the border from St. Johnsbury. While in Stanstead, the horse was bred to some of the local mares, and left some stock in the surrounding countryside. From that locality he was taken to northern Canada and all trace of him seems lost thereafter, for no record has been found of where he was kept or when he died.

The Hawkins horse was a jet black, about 15 hands, and not quite so compact as his sire, being a little taller and a bit heavier. His shoulders, back and loins were excellent. He carried his head high, had a bold, smart way of going, and was said to be the fastest of Justin's six known sons. He was a good trotter and extremely speedy at the gallop. His eye was a little fierce in its expression, and he was inclined to be cross and not so tractable as the rest; however, he was one of the best-moving and finest-looking horses under saddle ever seen in Vermont.

Richard Fenton of St. Johnsbury was the owner of Justin's sixth known son at stud, foaled in 1808. His dam was bay and of unknown blood. The only particulars known about her were that she was a familiar horse in the neighborhood and was supposedly an excellent individual.

The Fenton horse was a bright blood-bay with black points, and stood about 14.2 hands high. He was the image of old Justin: very compact and muscular. Linsley refers to him as being one of Justin's best sons, but fate had other plans for him than to sire a line of Morgans. He bit his owner (as some studs have a habit of doing at regular intervals) quite severely; the owner decided he would be happier with a gelding, thus ending the horse's potential as a sire.

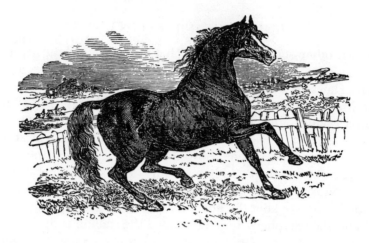

DESCENDANTS OF SHERMAN

Sherman's line comes down to us today in greater abundance than that of Justin's other sons not so much because he himself was superior to his brothers Woodbury and Bulrush, but because his siring of the famous racer Black Hawk put him into the public eye. Horsemen throughout New England, recognizing Black Hawk's greatness, sought out individuals which traced to Sherman's blood. Hoping for speedy, stylish colts, breeders looked to this line, and thus in retrospect the scales were tipped numerically in Sherman's favor.

BLACK HAWK

Probably the best-known son of old Sherman Morgan was the famous stallion Black Hawk. For many years he was the *beau idéal* of horsemen everywhere, and he founded a family which almost became a breed unto itself. His name was almost a household word, obscuring all others for nearly all his lifetime; meanwhile he established himself in his day as the head of the largest and most popular branch of old Justin Morgan's family.

That old Black Hawk was "bred in the purple" has been proved almost conclusively by students of the Morgan breed. Despite references which tend to disagree as to the origin of his dam, the majority state that she was of English or Thoroughbred blood, and that she first saw the light of day in Nova Scotia. All who knew her were quick to admit she was a fine animal and were always ready with their praise of her. We must go along with their statements and conjure up our own picture of the dam of Black Hawk, however, for there has never been discovered any likeness of her in the old engravings although her son was the subject of many. At the time Black Hawk was foaled in the early spring of 1833, the black mare was the property of Ezekiel Twombly of Durham, New Hampshire. Previously she had been owned by Benjamin Kelly of Durham, who is said to have gotten her from a peddler; and goodness knows where the peddler had acquired her. Actually, except for the Nova Scotia story, nothing else really has much basis in fact.

In every way the dam of Black Hawk was supposedly a fine animal. She is described as being a large mare, standing about 16 hands; jet black in color, with a white stripe in her face being her only marking. She had a good head and she carried her ears alertly although they were a bit long. Her neck was a good length, her throat clean and cut up under the jowl. She had a strong back, good croup and quarters. Her legs were clean and "breedy looking" and free from long hairs at the cannons.

In 1832 she came into the possession of Twombly in a horse-trading deal with Benjamin Kelly of Durham. The mare had been bred to Sherman Morgan early in the spring with the agreement that, should she prove safely in foal, Twombly owed Kelly a load of hay to seal the bargain!

The mare foaled right on schedule the following April, despite the fact that Kelly had used her extensively in harness and had even driven her a measured mile on the turnpike at a three-minute clip while she was in foal; Twombly had also driven her, after becoming her new owner, up until the time she foaled. All who knew her attested to the fact that she was a mare with unusual endurance and excellent wind. She was safe for anyone to drive and was comparatively alert and high-headed in harness. It is suggested by some authorities that she had a tendency to pace, but most sources indicate this to be unlikely. More mention is made of the fact that she was a fast trotter than that she would pace when urged. In short, throughout the vicinity of Durham she had the reputation of being an outstanding roadster.

The black mare remained in the possession of Twombly's family after his death, but in 1841 when the old lady became lame, Shadrack Seavey, a nephew of Twombly's who had acquired Black Hawk in the meantime, took over the selling of her for the family. She had had two colts by her son Black Hawk, but both of these died. As all

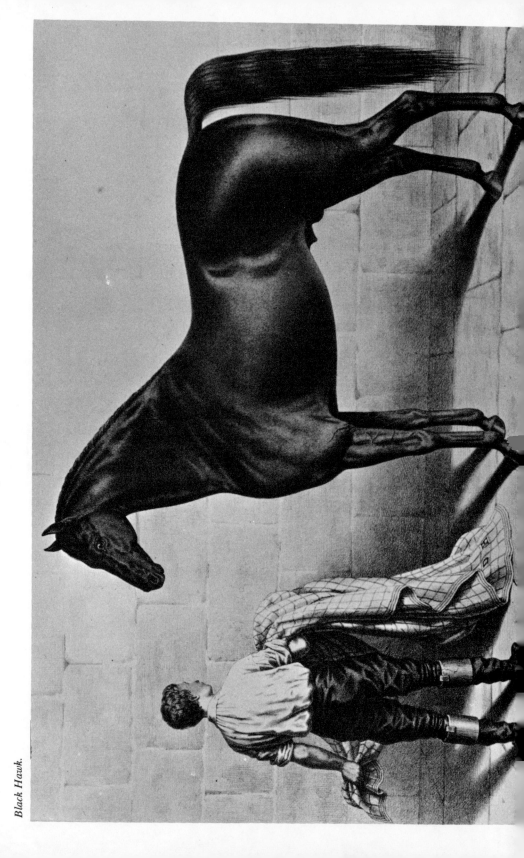

Black Hawk.

record of her was lost after she was sent down the road, it is anybody's guess whether she ever had any others.

When he was foaled, Black Hawk was as unpromising a colt as one could imagine. He was downright homely, and the neighbors assured Twombly that he'd be lucky if he got a hundred dollars out of him, grown!

The care, and soon the training, of Black Hawk became the task of Twombly's aforementioned nephew, Shadrack Seavey. Later the colt was given to Seavey; he was the first one to bridle him and train him to harness and saddle. When Twombly died in 1837 his property was appraised to include the value of the colt Black Hawk as $60. This sum Seavey paid to become the legal owner.

Black Hawk was always a square trotter from the very beginning, never showing any inclination to pace. He was amazingly intelligent and good-natured. Not once is it recorded that he offered to kick or run off even though the old harness would break repeatedly during his training. All the while Seavey owned him, Black Hawk was never passed on the road, and so strong was his trotting gait that he was never known to break no matter how tightly pressed. As well as being fast, Black Hawk had belied his early appearance by developing into an exceedingly handsome horse. In many ways he resembled his dam, especially through the head.

When he was two years old, the young rascal escaped his pasture on several occasions—and his first foals arrived the following year! Such a nuisance was this, and so annoyed were the neighbors by the clatter of hoofs in the night, that Seavey decided to have the young stallion gelded. But when the deed was arranged for and about to be carried out, the man who was to perform the operation strongly urged Seavey to change his mind, stating that the horse was far too good an animal to geld. The loss to the Morgan breed had this operation been performed would have been of such magnitude as almost to have doomed the breed. Luckily, Seavey saw the light, as it were, and agreed that perhaps the stud was worth considering again.

Seavey kept Black Hawk until the horse was a five-year-old and then he traded him for a mare and $50 to A. R. Mathes, who reportedly lived in Connecticut. We wonder why he should have been so foolish as to let the good horse go, but can only surmise that perhaps he preferred a mare to the unpredictable ways of a young stallion. At any rate, who's ever to try to explain just exactly what motivates any horse-trading deal? Seavey made his trade and Mathes gained one of the best Morgan stallions ever to look through a bridle.

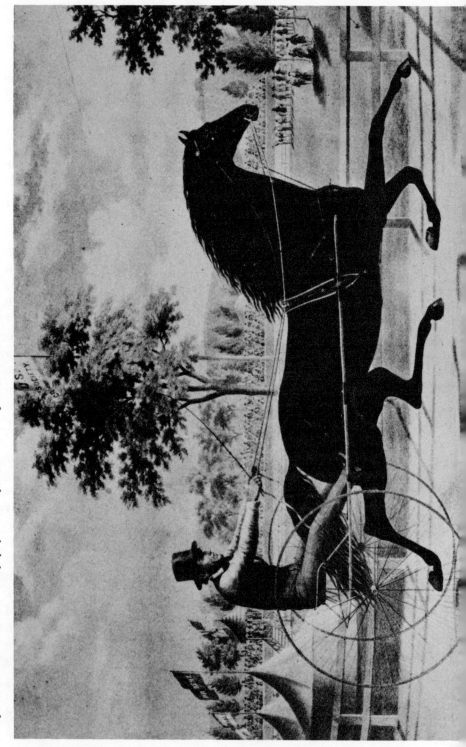

The fine Sherman Black Hawk always played second fiddle to his more famous brother Ethan Allen.

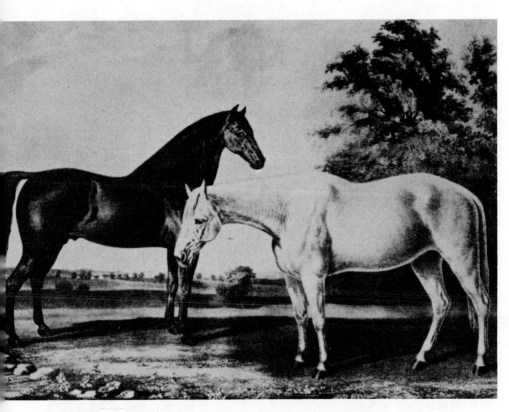

Black Hawk and Lady Suffolk, another well-known race horse of the day.

However, it seems that Mathes was, although an astute horseman, perhaps slightly more interested in the almighty dollar than in the ownership of a promising stallion; for after only a short time—approximately five weeks—he sold Black Hawk for $200, a sizable return on his original investment.

Black Hawk's new owners, Messrs. Brown and Thurston of Haverhill, Massachusetts, were interested primarily in the trotting speed of their new horse (which had increased noticeably even in the short time Mathes had owned him). Brown sold out his interest in Black Hawk to Thurston, however, after a short time. It was Thurston who gave the stud the name Black Hawk (he is known today as Black Hawk 20, in accordance with his registration number later assigned to him in Volume II of the *Register*).

At maturity this black son of Sherman was as handsome a horse as could be found anywhere. He stood 15 hands and weighed around

1,000 pounds. His finely chiseled head bespoke quality in every line. His eyes were large and very bright; his nostrils would flare to a size to hold a man's fist when distended. He had a short, strong back, being close-ribbed and compact. His shoulders were deep and well sloped, and his muscling was superb throughout. He was a symmetrical horse from all angles, each part blending into the other in the smoothest possible way. That such a horse as Black Hawk should have founded a fine line of Morgan horses is perfectly within the realm of understanding, for it is not from cold-blooded stock that equine stars find their beginnings.

Thurston, who was the first to bring Black Hawk out on the trotting courses, used the horse for six years as a family horse. He stated that Black Hawk was the finest horse he had ever owned in the considerable number which had come his way. He praised him as an excellent Roadster, saying that no matter how far or fast he traveled the stallion never showed any signs of fatigue. He praised his disposition as second to none, either for himself or any other member of his family, and he stated that the stock of Black Hawk were like their sire in all respects.

Thurston was known to have driven the horse in many trotting contests of the day, and so far as records show he was never beaten. The records may be few, but they show that in Boston in 1842 he won a race of five miles in sixteen minutes for a purse of $1,000; a year later, at the age of ten, he won in straight heats a best-three-in-five race of two-mile heats for $400. His best time for the two miles was 5:43. His record for the mile was 2:42, a time he made on numerous occasions.

Black Hawk was not used at stud to any great degree until he came into the ownership of David Hill of Bridport, Vermont, in 1844. After the arrival of his first foals, however, his service became very much in demand. Mares from all over New England and New York, as well as some Canadian provinces, were brought to him. The fee he commanded was $100, the highest figure paid for stud service at that time.

His greatest son, of course, was Ethan Allen 50, whose virtues we shall extol farther along. But other foals with lesser reputation sold for between $1,000 and $3,000, with some prices even higher. His stud earnings exceeded $34,000. No record indicates that any of his offspring were inferior or did not command good prices.

Where or when he died has never been recorded, so far as I've been able to discover. It is strange and sad that a horse so venerated should have no monument, even a verbal one. However, because he was so valued he certainly must have spent his last days in comfort.

In Black Hawk's day, road horses and race horses were much in demand, and the influence of this famous stallion easily can be seen by tracing back the pedigrees of many well-known Standardbred horses. His influence on other breeds is also quite clearly apparent. Billy Direct, the Standardbred who held the world's record for the mile (1:55) traces to Black Hawk. A Black Hawk–line mare produced George Wilkes, one of the greatest trotting sires of all time. And his influence on the American Saddlebred horse can be traced through such offspring as his son Blood's Black Hawk and his grandson Indian Chief. Bourbon King and the great Edna May's King come from Black Hawk blood.

Few Morgans of modern times do not trace back to old Black Hawk in countless lines. Indeed, as high a figure as 80 percent go back through his sons to this prolific black grandson of Justin.

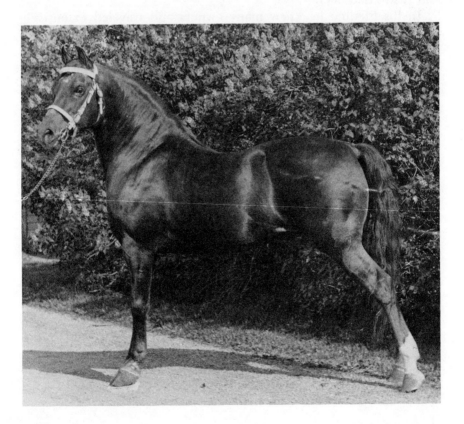

BILLY ROOT

A small, compact horse with a deep, cresty neck and a sprightly countenance was Billy Root. He would scarcely tip the scales by more than 950 pounds or stand more than 14 hands, but every atom of him was bubbling with personality and vigor. His back was round and short, with the smooth compactness of his sire and grandsire. In color he was a very dark chestnut, with a faint star and a bit of white on his off hind pastern. His legs and feet were exceptionally good, a trait noted in his offspring; no lameness was ever discovered.

Although he resembled his sire, Sherman, very closely, Billy Root had a personality all his own. He was quite mischievous in a playful way and delighted in making off with any blanket or strap left casually hanging over a fence or gate. Chasing hens or sheep were to Billy a sport to be indulged in whenever possible—undoubtedly to the complete chagrin of his owners. His antics, however, probably could be overlooked, because Billy Root was as willing a worker as his sire and old Justin had been.

In his lifetime he knew many owners and traveled extensively throughout New England, leaving behind progeny which were celebrated for their spirit, action, endurance and docility.

Billy's dam was said to be half French (Canadian) and sired by Justin Morgan. She was a fine road horse with undoubtedly amazing endurance, for she was said to have been driven the 120 miles between St. Johnsbury, Vermont, and Portland, Maine, in one day on at least three occasions! Little Billy was her only known foal; long before his

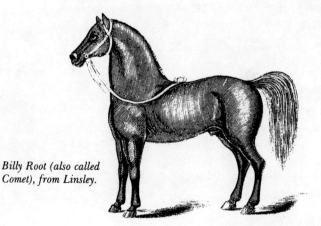

Billy Root (also called Comet), from Linsley.

value was realized, she had been sold down into southern Vermont, and all trace of her was lost.

Billy Root was foaled in St. Johnsbury in 1829, the property of a man by the name of Hezekiah Morton. Early in the horse's life he was known as Red Bird, but acquired the name Comet when purchased by Eldad Root in 1832 or '33. From St. Johnsbury he was taken by Root to the Genesee Valley in New York State. There he stood at stud for several seasons before returning to Vermont a few years later. His travels were quite extensive after that, and he made stud seasons in Lyndonville and Highgate in Vermont, where he remained four years. It was during this period that Root parted with the little stallion. His next owner's name was Stephens, and it was he who began calling the horse Billy Root.

But Billy didn't stay long with Stephens. Despite his being by then about twelve years old, he spent the next few years in the service of many owners in different parts of New England. He always was remembered in the different localities by the fine, strong colts with bright eyes and cheery dispositions; colts which, like their sire, would rather prance than walk and which, although small, were always ready and willing to tackle any load no matter how heavy.

In 1847 when the stallion was eighteen, the local farmers around the vicinity of Lyndon and Highgate requested that Billy be brought back to Vermont. And there he remained through the seasons of 1847 through 1851. Then, in April 1852, little Billy's unexpected death shocked the horsemen for miles around. It was said that his death was caused by the rupture of a blood vessel.

Billy Root was always noted for the quality of his daughters as well as of his sons. His name comes down to us in many modern pedigrees, while he himself will always be remembered as the personification of the old-time Morgan horse.

ETHAN ALLEN 50

Probably of all the now-legendary names within the Morgan breed during the nineteenth century, none can surpass the great Ethan Allen 50. This best-known son of the celebrated Black Hawk was perhaps the most famous horse of his day, and it certainly could be said safely that he even outranked his venerable sire in popularity, as well as overshadowing his second cousin, the widely shown Hale's Green Mountain. Ethan Allen's name also became almost a household word during his illustrious career—he was the epitome of America's ideal horse, a perfect horse in about every sense of the word: there was no finer example of beauty and symmetry coupled with lightning speed at the trot than could be seen in the form of this one Morgan stallion.

His fame extended from ocean to ocean, so publicized were his achievements. It is no overstatement to say that he was the darling of the racing public, and sports writers were hard put to keep from running out of superlatives to describe him. Win or lose, his style and speed were everywhere acclaimed. Cheers followed his every race; whether he was first under the wire or not, it made little difference. At four years of age, with a mark of 2:25½, he was named Champion of the World, and his phenomenal mark of 2:15, when matched against the mighty Dexter, topped a long list of honors in the trotting world. This famous race will be described shortly.

Just the appearance of Ethan Allen on any racecourse triggered the wildest applause, for even the most callous racegoer could not fail to be affected by his well-rounded Morgan conformation—which even in racing condition gave him the smoothness and symmetry for which Morgans were famous, then as well as now. His excellent disposition also made him a great favorite with his many owners and the men who worked with him.

S. W. Parlin, writing in the contemporary *American Cultivator*, describes Ethan Allen as follows:

No one ever raised a doubt as to his being the handsomest and most perfectly gaited trotter that has ever been produced. Horsemen will agree that no trotter has ever appeared upon the turf that excelled him in the style and beauty of his action, whether moving at a jog or flying at the rate of a mile in 2:15. His trotting instinct was wonderfully strong and his disposition the best imaginable, two qualities which enabled him when hitched with a running mate, to outstrip every competitor that could be brought against him in that rig. During the season of 1861, hitched with a runner, he won three races from the world-renowned Flora Temple, rigged in the same style, in one of which he placed his mark at 2:19¾. In May, 1867, at the Union Course, Long Island, he beat Brown George and running mate in straight heats, time: 2:29, 2:21, 2:19. The crowning event of his life, however, was the race in which, hitched with a running mate, he challenged the admiration of the world by defeating the great Dexter, which was then supposed to be invincible, at the Fashion Course, June 21, 1867, in

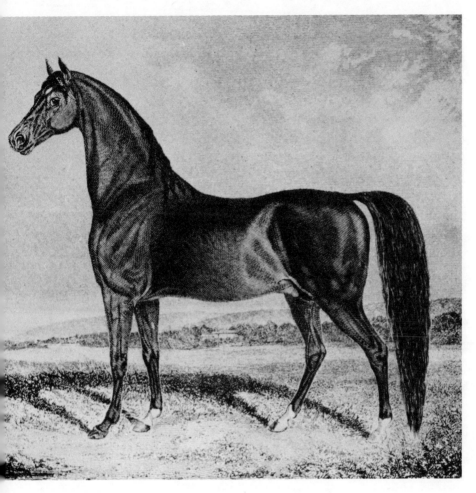

Ethan Allen 50.

short order, landing at the wire in 2:15, 2:16 and 2:19 respectively. Good judges estimated him capable of trotting the first heat in 2:12 had he been sent with that intention.

Ethan Allen 50 was foaled in Ticonderoga, New York, on June 18, 1849, and was raised, it is said, as a family pet. His owner was Joel W. Holcomb, who had acquired the colt's dam in the fall of 1844. She was a mouse-gray mare, foaled in 1830 and owned at the time by John Field of Springfield, Vermont. She was said to be by a small bay horse known as Red Robin, who was bred down on the Connecticut River at Weathersfield Bow at a time when Justin Morgan himself stood just across the bridge in Claremont, New Hampshire. Many authorities are quite convinced that Red Robin was by old Justin because of his marked degree of resemblance to the original Morgan.

Ethan Allen's second dam was a brown mare who also resembled the early Morgans, and according to local records was quite possibly out of a daughter of Justin. These opinions, if proved for a certainty, would give Ethan Allen a very strong percentage of the blood of Justin Morgan.

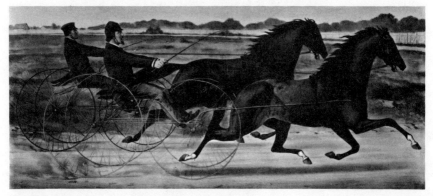

Detail from Ethan's race with George M. Patchen.

Volume I of the *American Morgan Horse Register* states, pertaining to Red Robin:

> We have given the substance of all evidence which we have been able to get relative to the history of Red Robin. It is probable that he was foaled in 1816 and that he came into the hands of Moses Bates before 1820. . . . At best, his breeder and breeding are purely a matter of conjecture, but the opinion of Mr. Bisbee, who knew him [Red Robin] well, that he was by the Justin Morgan, is very probably correct. It certainly is sustained by the character and appearance of the horse and by the fact that the original Morgan horse stood near where he was begotten and not improbably included in his circuit the town of Springfield itself in 1815, the year that Robin is supposed to have been bred.

The dam of Ethan Allen was used at regular farm labor until she was four years old. She was a willing worker despite a lack of size, and was a good mare on the road as well, being intelligent and docile in harness. At four, she was sold to F. A. Leland, who put her to a peddler's wagon. She was driven along a route in New York State in the vicinity of Hague, Schroon and Whitehall. Because she was likely to be nervous and frightened whenever goods were taken from the wagon, she was traded to Rufus Rising of Hague for a gray gelding. Subsequently, she was returned to heavy farm work, the result of which was a bad spavin, and was retired to the rank of broodmare in 1841. She produced three excellent colts from 1842 to 1844 and finally, in the fall of '44, became the property of Joel Holcomb. Previous to foaling the great Ethan Allen in 1849 (who proved to be her last offspring), this fine old mare produced a top mare of her day, Black Hawk Maid (2:37), by Black Hawk, as well as three other outstanding colts. She had foaled regularly for eight consecutive years and died in foal, again to Black Hawk, in 1851 at the age of twenty-one.

Ethan Allen 50 (his number, too, was assigned him in Volume III) was a remarkable colt even at an early age. That he truly was a family pet is proved by Mrs. Holcomb, who reportedly said, "You couldn't get him by the window but that he would put his head in to get a piece of cake." His beautiful conformation and kindly ways made him loved and admired by all who knew him even in those early days.

Ethan was a bright bay in color, with a small star and faint snip between his nostrils. He was liberally marked with white, having, besides the star and snip, three socks as well. At maturity he stood slightly under 15 hands and weighed 1,000 pounds in top condition. For a stallion, his head was remarkably fine, with large, bright and expressive eyes; sharply defined, small ears, and a full, flowing forelock to lend effect. His neck, with its clean-cut throttle, was of good length and not too heavily crested, blending smoothly into deep, oblique shoulders with well-defined withers. He had an excellent level back, with powerfully muscled croup and quarters. Despite his deep shoulders and long hipline—which gave him the look of being a bit long for his height—Ethan Allen was very symmetrical. With his lovely head carried high he was without a doubt one of the most beautiful of horses. His long flowing black mane and tail completed the picture.

Holcomb sold a half-interest in Ethan Allen to Orville S. Roe of Shoreham, Vermont, when the animal was still a colt, and during the earliest years of his life he was owned jointly by them both. The stallion was used for stud service both at Shoreham and also for a number of seasons at Cambridge, Massachusetts. Ethan Allen's greatest sons were sired during his seasons at Shoreham. Among them were Daniel Lambert, American Ethan, Holabird's Ethan Allen, DeLong's Ethan Allen and Honest Allen. Through Honest Allen his male line is carried down to us through Denning Allen, the sire of General Gates, who in turn became the foundation sire of The United States Morgan Horse Farm near Middlebury, Vermont.

During this same period Ethan was also put to racing nearly every season, and even in those early days he won most of his many contests.

As a Sire

From 1862, when he was sold to Frank Banker, Ethan Allen knew many owners and traveled many miles for both racing and stud service. His fame grew, and the demand for his services increased with his prestige. In 1869 at Medford, Massachusetts, his fee was $100. In 1870 at the same location it was raised to $200 the season.

Ethan Allen sired over seventy winners of the Trotting world, among them six sons which were listed as standard Trotters; of them, Billy Barr (2:23¾) and Hotspur (2:24) were the fastest. He also sired Fanny Allen, a bay mare with a mark of 2:28¼, and another bay mare, Pocahontas (2:26¾), for whom Robert Bonner paid the phenomenal price of $40,000. This mare was also a great Roadster and had an unofficial record of 2:17¾ when driven by her owner on the road. That she never produced a foal was a fact Bonner much regretted.

Probably the best known of Ethan Allen's sons was Daniel Lambert, a sire in his own right of speedy Trotters and snappy-going road horses. More about this stallion and his influence on Trottingbred and Saddlebred horses will follow.

Despite the fact that he was not unbeaten on the race track, Ethan Allen was the high-lighted personality of every race he entered. His well-balanced, brilliant action has been portrayed without exaggeration in many prints by Currier and Ives. He also reigns supreme over many a New England barn, as innumerable weather vanes carry his likeness. He was a point of comparison: if someone noted that a horse resembled old Ethan Allen, he was paying the animal the highest compliment. Even in later years when the lean, long-limbed (and homely!) Messengers and Hambletonians had taken over the racing scene and all Ethan Allen's records had fallen, old-timers still talked of the great Ethan Allen, and the Morgan beauty he brought to the race track.

The Race with Dexter

Ethan's greatest race, and the one which assured his permanent niche in the Racing Hall of Fame, was the famous match against the champion Trotter of the day, Dexter (2:19), a son of Rysdyk's Hambletonian.

This race is said to have been witnessed by an estimated forty thousand people. The following long passage by John H. Wallace, editor at the time of the *American Trotting Register* and an actual eyewitness, undoubtedly gives the most vivid description of Ethan Allen's greatest victory. Remembering that Ethan was at this time eighteen years of age and a veteran of many seasons at stud, as well as having been a participant in countless matches against the best Trotters of his day, gives added impact to his victory. Here is Wallace's account as published in *Wallace's Monthly* of April 1877 (note that it was accepted procedure to hitch a mate to the light racing vehicle to set the pace by galloping alongside; a strange practice to our modern notions, and possibly the origin of the political expression "running mate"):

On the 21st of June 1867, on the Fashion Course, it was my good fortune to witness the crowning event of his [Ethan's] life. Some three weeks before, Ethan, with a running mate, had beaten Brown George and running mate in very fast time, scoring one heat in 2:19. This made horsemen open their eyes and there at once arose a difference of opinion about the advantage to the trotter of having a runner hitched with him to pull the weight. This resulted in a match for twenty-five hundred dollars a side, to trot Ethan and running mate against Dexter, who was then considered invincible. As the day approached, the betting was about even; but the evening before the race, word came from the course that Ethan's running mate had fallen lame and could not go, but they would try to get Brown George's running mate, then in Connecticut, to take the place of the lame runner. As the horses were strangers to each other, it was justly concluded, the change gave Dexter a great advantage and the betting at once changed from even to two to one on Dexter. Long before noon the crowd began to assemble and sporting men everywhere were shaking rolls of green backs over their heads, shouting, "Two to one on Dexter." I met a friend from Chicago, who sometimes speculates a little and when he told me he was betting "two to one on Dexter," I took the liberty of advising him to be cautious, for I thought the team would win the race and that its backers knew what they were doing. Before the hour arrived, I secured a seat on the ladies' stand, from which every foot of the course and the countless multitude of people could be taken in at a glance. The vehicles were simply incalculable and the people were like a vast sea. The multitude was estimated at forty thousand!

Upon the arrival of the hour, the judges ascended the stand and rang up the horses, when the backers of the team came forward, explained the mishap that had befallen the runner, that they had Brown George's mate on the grounds, but, as he and Ethan had never been hitched together, they were unwilling to risk so large a sum and closed the race by paying one thousand, two hundred and fifty dollars forfeit. When this announcement was made, there was a general murmur that spread, step by step, through all the vast multitude. The betting fraternity were just where they started and every spectator realized a feeling of disgust at the whole management. As soon as this had had time to exert its intended effect upon the crowd, the backers of the team came forward again and, expressing their unwillingness to have the people go away dissatisfied, proposed a little match of two hundred and fifty dollars a side, which was promptly accepted by the Dexter party; and when it was known that there would be a race after all, the shout of the multitude was like the voice of many waters. This being a new race, the betting men had to commence again. The surroundings of the pool stands were packed with an eager and excited crowd, anxious to get on their money at two, and, rather than miss, at three to one on Dexter. The work of the auctioneers was "short, sharp and decisive," and the tickets were away up in the hundreds and oftentimes in the thousands. But the pool stands did not seem to accommodate more than a small fraction of those anxious to invest and in all directions, in the surging crowd, hands were in the air, filled with rolls of greenbacks and shouting, "Two to one on Dexter!" I was curious to note what became of these noisy offers and I soon observed that a quiet-looking man came along, took all one party had to invest and then quietly went to another of the shouters, and then another, and so on, till I think everyone who had money to invest at that rate was accommodated. The amount of money bet was enormous, no doubt aggregating a quarter of a million in a few minutes.

When the horses appeared upon the track to warm up for the race, Dexter, driven by the accomplished reinsman, Budd Doble, was greeted with a shout of applause. Soon the team appeared and behind it sat the great master of trotting tactics, Dan Mace. His face, which has so often been a puzzle to thousands, had no mask over it on this occasion. It spoke only that intense earnestness that indicates the near approach of a supreme moment. The team was hitched to a light skeleton wagon; Ethan wore breeching and beside him was a great, strong race-horse, fit to run for a man's life. His traces were long enough to fully extend himself, but they were so much shorter than Ethan's that he had to take the weight. Dexter drew the inside and on the first trial they got

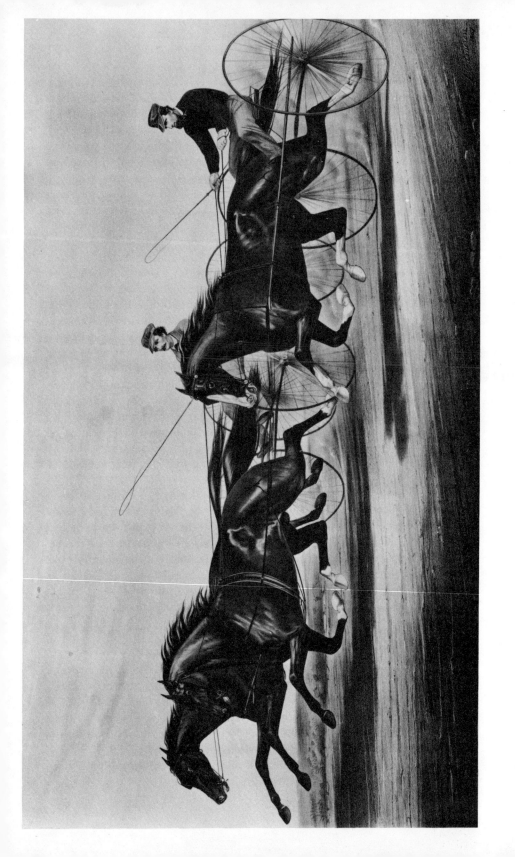

the "send-off" without either one having six inches the advantage. When they got the word, the flight of speed was absolutely terrific, so far beyond anything I had ever witnessed in a trotting horse that I felt the hair rising on my head. The running horse was next to me and, notwithstanding my elevation, Ethan was stretched out so near the ground that I could see nothing of him but his ears. I fully believe that for several rods at this point they were going at a two minute gait.

It was impossible that this terrible pace could be maintained long and just before reaching the first turn, Dexter's head began to swim and the team passed him and took the track, reaching the first quarter pole in thirty-two seconds, with Dexter three or four lengths behind. The same lightning speed was kept up through the second quarter, reaching the half-mile pole in 1:04, with Dexter still farther in the rear. Mace then took a pull on his team and came home a winner by six or eight lengths, in 2:15. When this time was put on the blackboard, the response of the multitude was like the roar of old ocean. Although some distance away, through the second quarter of this heat, I had a fair, unobstructed sideview of the stallion and of his action, when going at the lightning rate of 2:08 to the mile. I could not observe that he received the slightest degree of propulsion from the running horse; and my conviction was then, and is now that any such propulsion would have interfered with his own unapproachable action and would have retarded, rather than helped him. The most noticeable feature in his style of movement was the remarkable lowness to which he dropped his body and the straight gliding line it maintained at that elevation.

The team now had the inside and in the first attempt they were started for the second heat. Before they had gone many rods Ethan lost his stride and Dexter took the track at the very spot where he had lost it in the first heat. The team soon got to work and near the beginning of the second quarter, collared Dexter, but the stallion broke soon after and fell back, not yards nor lengths but rods, before he caught. Incredible as it may seem, when he again got his feet he put on such a burst of speed as to overhaul the flying Dexter in the third quarter, when he broke again and Mace had to pull him nearly to a standstill before he recovered. Dexter was now a full distance ahead and the heat appeared to be his beyond all peradventure. I was watching the team in its troubles very closely and my idea of the distance lost was the result of a deliberate and careful estimate at the moment; and the query in my mind then was, whether the team could save its distance. At last the old horse stuck his gait and it was like a dart from a catapult, or a ball from a rifle. The team not only saved its distance, but beat Dexter home, five or six lengths, in 2:16.

In the third heat Mace had it all his own way throughout, coming home the winner of the race in 2:19. The backers of Dexter, up to the very last, placed great reliance on his well-known staying qualities; but the last heat showed that the terrible struggle had told upon him more distressingly than on the team. It is said by those who timed Dexter privately that he trotted the three heats in 2:17, 2:18, 2:21.

If ever there was an honest race trotted, this was one, but there was such a specimen of sharp diplomacy, of "diamond cut diamond," in the preliminaries, as is seldom witnessed, even on a race course. It is not probable that Ethan's intended running mate fell amiss at all, the evening before, as represented; and if she did, it was not possible to send to Connecticut for another horse and have him there early the morning of the race, as was pretended. This was a mere ruse put out to get the advantage of the long odds. The backers of the team knew just how the horses would work and knew they had speed enough to beat any horse on earth. When the race was called and they came forward and paid forfeit, it was merely to give the "two-to-one-on Dexter" money encouragement to come out. It did come out most vociferously and was all quietly taken. It was said John Morrissey was the manager-in-chief and that his share of the winnings amounted to about forty thousand dollars.

After witnessing the second heat and studying it carefully, I am firmly of the opinion the team could have gone the first heat in 2:12 if it had been necessary.

Monument in Kansas

On October 17, 1870, old Ethan Allen was sold for the last time. His newest owner was Colonel Amasa Sprague of Providence, Rhode Island. The price reportedly paid for this famous stallion was $7,500. Ethan was kept in Providence for a time before being sent by his owner to the Sprague and Akers Stock Farm at Lawrence, Kansas. Here the venerable old campaigner and idol of millions spent his last years far from the noisy race tracks and their cheering throngs. At last, on the 10th of September 1876, in the twenty-eighth year of his life, old Ethan Allen died. He was buried at the entrance of the Trotting Park in Lawrence, where a monument was erected to his memory.

Thus passed one of the Morgan breed's brightest stars. But his greatness lives on down through the years in the breeding line of countless modern Morgans. Breeders today still point with pride to the crosses to Ethan Allen 50 in their horses' pedigrees, for even now his blood means a trace of beauty from the past.

DANIEL LAMBERT

During his lifetime, Daniel Lambert, the son of great-hearted Ethan Allen 50, was applauded and acclaimed for many things, but possibly his major contribution to the Morgan fame was the siring of so many superior Roadsters. The scores of sons and daughters of this prominent stallion, with their stylish mien and trotting speed on the road, gave their sire the vote of all New England horsemen as one of the greatest progenitors of Trotters that ever stood in the Northeast. Even though the majority of his offspring never saw a race track, it is said that "they could beat a 2:30 horse

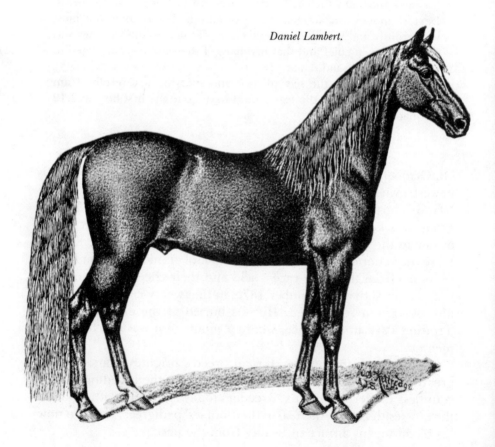

Daniel Lambert.

down the road with ease." And their elegance and spirit in harness were admired by anyone with a hankering for an outstanding horse.

The Lamberts were pure, open-gaited Trotters, needing neither boots nor weights; and, like all the Morgans, they were willing and cheerful in disposition. Many a chance brush on the road left the competition eating dust when a Lambert horse struck his gait.

The age of the fast road horse has passed now, with its throbbing of Trotters' hoofs gone from the open lanes, but there was a time when the ownership of a Lambert Morgan was equivalent to the possession of the snappiest, low-slung, roaring sports car made today. The folks by the general store in town were just as impressed when you drove down the dusty main street behind a sleek, smooth-gaited Morgan as the fellows by the drug store are nowadays when you pull up to the curb in your purring, chrome-trimmed, high-priced product of Detroit or Europe.

Time passes, progress changes our way of life, but I sometimes wonder which would give the greater thrill: holding the lines on a speedy Lambert colt when he overtakes a friend on the road and, to the music of flashing hoofs, leaves the other behind in a burst of speed born of heart and sinew—or sitting at the wheel of a roaring, ground-skimming sports car as its tires squeal out each turn in the road and the landscape blurs in the corners of your eyes. For me there could be but one choice. . . .

Foaled in 1858, the son of Ethan Allen and a fiery, bright red chestnut mare named Fanny Cook, Daniel Lambert was bred and owned by William H. Cook of Ticonderoga, New York. His dam was by Abdallah, a good son of Mambrino, who himself was by Messenger, the founding father of the Standardbred horse. His second dam was by Stockholm's American Star, by Duroc, the best son of Imported Diomed. Since Mambrino traces back to the Darley Arabian and the Byerly Turk, some of the same blood that is said to have produced Justin Morgan flowed in the veins of Fanny Cook.

The mettlesome Fanny Cook inherited her nervousness from her sire, who was so high-strung that he was never broken to harness, and was a decided departure from the usual farm mares that dot the distaff side of early Morgan pedigrees. Bred by Montfort Van Kleek of Dutchess County, New York, she was said to be an extremely fast mare at the trot and the gallop, although quite likely she was difficult to handle due to her peppery disposition.

His Qualities

Even as a foal Daniel Lambert had the fineness and quality which was later to dazzle horsemen everywhere, and he was sold at four months to John Porter of Ticonderoga for $300. Since weanlings of that day and age generally sold for about $50, the colt was considered high-priced; but when, at the age of five, this same young stallion was sold by Porter for $3,000 to R. S. Denny of Boston, the original outlay seems insignificant.

Denny took the horse—known up until that time as the "Porter colt"—to Watertown, Massachusetts. Denny renamed the stallion Hippomenes, and took him to Saratoga, New York, as his Roadster; and there the horse became the king of the road even in that famous mecca of fine horses.

When owned by Denny at Watertown, Daniel Lambert was not used at stud too frequently and so did not leave many offspring in Massachusetts. It would appear that he was used for the most part as Denny's own road horse, for the man would not permit him to be raced on the track, even though as a three-year-old colt Daniel Lambert had been driven to a mark of 2:42 by Dan Mace, the reinsman who had handled the lines on old Ethan Allen in the classic match against Dexter. At the time, Mace was so confident in the abilities of the untrained colt that he offered to trot him against any three-year-old in the world for $5,000 or $10,000 a side. But, undoubtedly, knowing Mace and his keen knowledge of horseflesh, no one quite dared match a horse against him.

In harness Daniel Lambert's manners were as flawless as his gait, for he had inherited none of his dam's nervousness. He was never put into competition on the race track, but was shown as a driving horse at the fairs. The classes, and the only ones for harness exhibition at that time, were judged on a basis of one-third for speed at the trot, one-third for appearance and presence, i.e., showiness, and one-third for manners. Needless to say, the golden beauty and matchless action of Daniel Lambert could not be bettered, and he was unbeaten in harness classes even when shown after his twentieth year.

As the horse was not having the opportunity of being used often at the stud in Watertown, Denny sold Daniel Lambert to Benjamin Bates when the stallion was eight years old. He made his first season at stud at the Cream Hill Stock Farm at Shoreham, Vermont, in 1866.

Each year for his next eleven years at Shoreham, Daniel Lambert was booked to an increasing number of mares. He remained at the Cream Hill Farm until 1877, when, upon Bates's death, he was re-

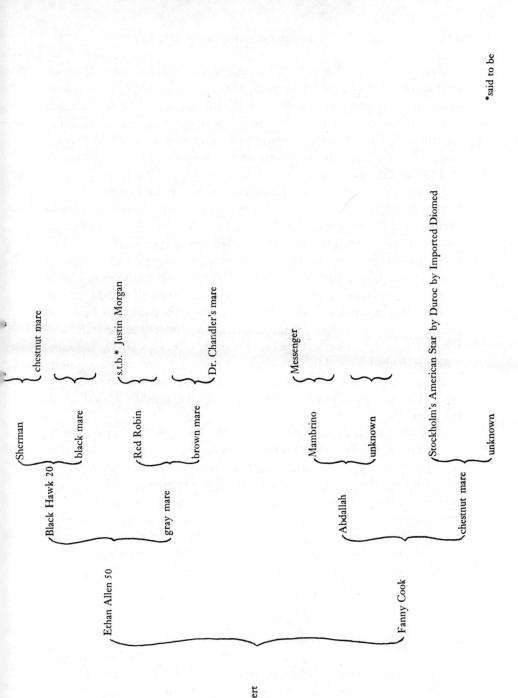

*said to be

moved to the Bates Farm back in Watertown, Massachusetts. He was sold to David Snow of Andover in 1880; later, in 1884, he was sold again to a company in Middlebury, Vermont, where he was stabled at the Bread Loaf Stock Farm, which was the property of Colonel Joseph A. Battell. There, enjoying a life of excellent health and vigor, and without a blemish or unsoundness, he remained until his death in 1889 at the age of thirty-one.

As with so many of the Morgans, age never seemed to fade the beauty of Daniel Lambert, and he remained a very handsome horse throughout his long life. He followed the Morgan pattern, too: he had a fine head, prominent eyes set wide apart, and short, alert ears; his clean-cut throttle, beautifully arched neck, deep shoulders, strong back, round barrel, broad, well-muscled loin and high-set tail were typical of his breeding. He had a lofty carriage, as do all true Morgans, and his bright chestnut coat, inherited from his dam, was fine and silky even in the winter months. His mane and tail were long and flaxen in color; he was marked with a narrow, even strip on his face, and a left hind sock. His forearms were long, broad and muscular; cannons short, with the bone being in good proportion to weight of body. He had excellent feet—a trait which he readily passed on to his offspring.

Colonel Battell in his Volume I of the Morgan *Register* quotes S. W. Parlin of Boston, who knew Daniel Lambert—and whose unreserved admiration for Ethan Allen has been noted—thus: "By common consent the Morgans have enjoyed the reputation of being the most beautiful horses, as a family, ever produced on this continent and Lambert, when in his prime, was one of the most beautiful of that family. Few horses have ever lived that possessed greater power of stamping their offspring with the above characteristics and imparting the ability to perpetuate them through succeeding generations."

Lambert's Offspring

It was to the Green Mountain State that Daniel Lambert left his greatest heritage, for during his two stays in Vermont he was bred to some 1,100 mares. Although few of his colts were developed or trained for the track, as mentioned earlier, 106 of them were winners of 465 races, 37 of these having marks within the 2:30 standard.

Without exception Daniel Lambert's get were pure Trotters. They ranged in size from 14.3 to 15.3, with a few measuring larger. All possessed the spirit, beauty and tremendous stride of their sire.

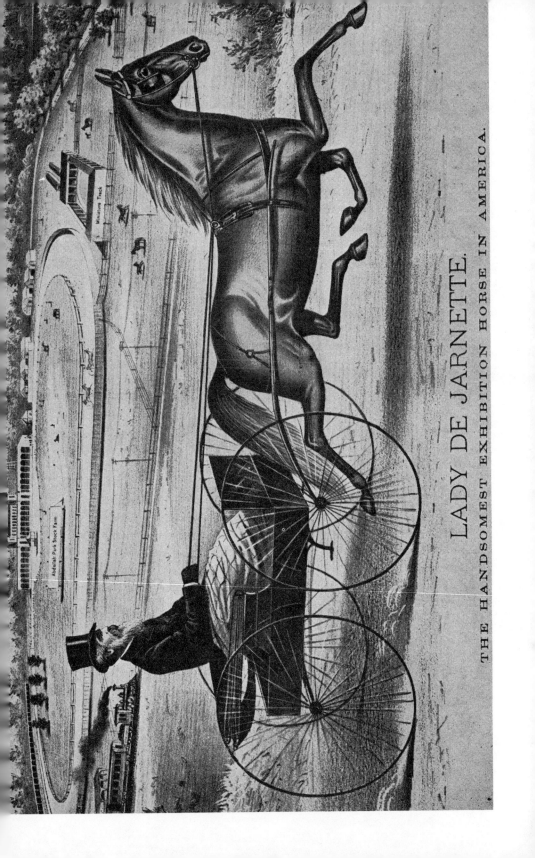

LADY DE JARNETTE.

THE HANDSOMEST EXHIBITION HORSE IN AMERICA.

One of his best sons was Jubilee Lambert, who was out of a grand-daughter of old Black Hawk. He was bred by John Porter, who had owned Lambert till the stallion was five years old. Jubilee Lambert was a 15.3-hand bay foaled in 1863, and most of his life was spent in the vicinity of Cynthiana, Kentucky, where he was known for siring colts with outstanding show ability and presence. Jubilee de Jarnette—out of the great show mare Lady de Jarnette by Indian Chief, a grandson of Black Hawk—was by Jubilee Lambert, and was considered his finest son.

Through the blood of Jubilee Lambert the early American Saddlebred gained much of its beauty and ability. Some of the greatest names in that breed trace back to Morgan through the sons and daughters of Jubilee Lambert.

DESCENDANTS OF WOODBURY

Of the three sons of Justin Morgan, undoubtedly Woodbury would enjoy the liveliest patronage were all three living today. With all the interest in the show ring now, breeders are striving to produce Morgans which exhibit an inborn showiness and an abundance of natural action. And Woodbury would be their ideal, for he certainly possessed all the symmetry, the bold eagerness and commanding style of action desired in today's show Morgans. Even in his own time Woodbury and his get were greatly admired for their style and beauty.

Although many of Woodbury's progeny were noted for the same beauty and performance of their sire, the fact should not be overlooked that speed, too, was inherent in Woodbury's line. He was the first horse foaled to leave three sons who each sired a 2:30 Trotter: Morgan Caesar sired Mac (2:28), a 15.2-hand brown gelding foaled in 1848; Morgan Eagle sired Lady Sutton (2:30), a fast brown mare who defeated the top mares of their day, Lady Suffolk and Lady Moscow; Gifford sired Beppo (2:28), a good chestnut gelding who also gained fame as a racing crack.

The *American Morgan Horse Register* in reference to Woodbury's siring of speed horses notes that "early were the grandchildren of Woodbury Morgan from three different sons engaging in brilliant and successful trotting contests with the fastest and gamest in the land. Two of these three famous sons were founders of trotting families. A son of Morgan Eagle, bearing the same name, got Magna Charta (2:33), that at one time held the four-year-old trotting record of the world, and became one of the foremost among the trotting sires in Michigan."

According to Linsley, Woodbury sired eighteen sons which became outstanding sires in their own right. Of these, chestnut seems to have been the prevailing color and the average height was 15 hands and weight 1,050. Besides the above-mentioned stallions, the Babbitt horse, the Putnam horse, General Hibbard and the Nichols horse were popular studs in their day.

GIFFORD MORGAN

As a model for old Justin, Gifford Morgan, too, could qualify almost without a change except for color. And all his stock were also very much like the get of the old horse.

Gifford was a small, dark chestnut replica of his grandsire, and the smallest of Woodbury's sons. He resembled little Billy Root in

One of Gifford Morgan's sons, Gifford Morgan, Jr. (Munson's), from Linsley.

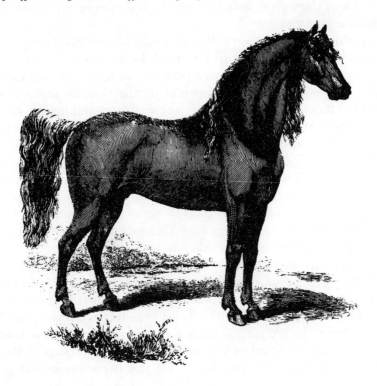

build, being pony-sized and short-legged. But despite his size Gifford's action and style and his spirited outlook were unexcelled by other horses of his time.

Gifford was foaled in Tunbridge, Vermont, on June 13, 1824, the property of Ziba Gifford of that town. His dam, a bright bay with a great deal of quality, was sired by Henry Dundas, who was by Woolsey, a large bay who was one of the first Thoroughbreds of proved ancestry in New England. There was no doubt as to the fact that Gifford's dam was a high-bred mare tracing to some of the best of the early imported Thoroughbreds; yet persons who knew the mare always stated that she resembled the Morgans of the time and was not typical of the Thoroughbred in appearance.

When mature, Gifford was a very much admired horse, for he possessed to marked degree the lofty head carriage and stylish action that made the Morgans so popular. He was a fine saddle horse who loved the parades and musters which gave him the opportunity to show off his fine action and appearance. Like his sire he was completely fearless in the vicinity of cannons or muskets; the din of them merely caused him to prance and toss his finely chiseled head with enthusiasm. However, he was a gentle and completely trustworthy stallion at all times.

Gifford measured an even 14.2 in height and weighed about 1,000 pounds in his best condition. His head distinctly showed the Thoroughbred-Arab blood which his pedigree indicated: it was exceedingly fine, with large lively eyes and flaring nostrils and a dished profile so typical of the Arab. His neck was short and heavily crested with a lovely arched line from poll to wither. He had a deeper chest than his sire and his quarters were heavily muscled and strong. His tail, in the style of the time, had been docked, leaving the bone only about seven inches long, but despite this, the hair was thick and wavy. He had the typical good bone and feet of the new breed and was never unsound or blemished even though, as with the other horses of his time, his life was far from easy. Gifford was not liberally marked with white, having only a small star and snip and white pasterns behind and a white coronet on his right forefoot.

At the age of four years Gifford was purchased by Ira Coolidge of Barnard, Vermont. He remained in Barnard for four years, and then was bought back by Gifford, his breeder. From then until he was sixteen years old he was ridden, driven and used at the stud by his owner. He returned to Barnard under the ownership of Russell Topliff, who kept him until the horse was twenty years old. Only

GEN. GIFFORD

106

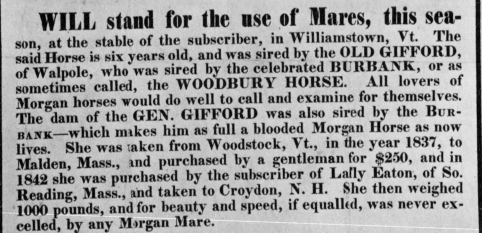

WILL stand for the use of Mares, this season, at the stable of the subscriber, in Williamstown, Vt. The said Horse is six years old, and was sired by the **OLD GIFFORD**, of Walpole, who was sired by the celebrated **BURBANK**, or as sometimes called, the **WOODBURY HORSE**. All lovers of Morgan horses would do well to call and examine for themselves. The dam of the **GEN. GIFFORD** was also sired by the BUR-BANK—which makes him as full a blooded Morgan Horse as now lives. She was taken from Woodstock, Vt., in the year 1837, to Malden, Mass., and purchased by a gentleman for $250, and in 1842 she was purchased by the subscriber of Lafly Eaton, of So. Reading, Mass., and taken to Croydon, N. H. She then weighed 1000 pounds, and for beauty and speed, if equalled, was never excelled, by any Morgan Mare.

It has been said by some French Canadian horse men who have sailed under the Morgan flag, that he was not as full a blooded Morgan horse as could be found. The subscriber would say that he will pay those men, or any gentleman, ONE HUNDRED DOLLARS if the blood of said Horse is not substantially correct. Now, Gentlemen, had you not better call and examine said Horse for yourselves, before putting your Mares other wheres, and losing the use of them and $25 with it.

ARIAL HALL.

Williamstown, May 18, 1855.

$100 was the price paid for the old horse when he was sold again, at twenty, and was taken into the state of New York. In his many years in the stud, old Gifford left much good stock all around the vicinity of his various homes. He commanded a very small fee and it is said that many a fine colt or filly cost its owner little more than fifty cents or a bushel or two of corn.

After the old stallion was sold into New York, F. A. Weir of Walpole, New Hampshire, became interested in the get of the horse and went to some lengths trying to locate him. He finally found Gifford in a little town near Lake George, New York. The old horse had come into hard times and was being used to draw slabs for a sawmill. He was weary, very poor and footsore, so Weir was able to buy him for the hundred dollars he'd sold for in the previous fall. Upon getting the old horse home to Walpole, he treated the animal for the lameness he suffered, the cause of which was a bad case of corns.

Weir is said to have secreted Gifford into the town late at night so no one would see the old fellow in such poor shape. Evidently he kept the old horse under wraps until such time as he was sound and feeling his old self again, for when Gifford had recovered from the corns and was back in condition, Weir had quite a lark parading the stallion through the streets of Walpole, astonishing the villagers with the horse's style and animation.

For the next four years Gifford was a very popular sire in the neighboring countryside. He was bred to more than twenty mares a year at a fee of $30 (some improvement over the previous bushel of corn!). All during the four years that Weir owned him Gifford was shown quite extensively despite his advanced age.

At the New York State Fair of 1847 in Saratoga, old Gifford, along with a cavalcade of other Morgans, was paraded by the grandstand for all to see. It is reported that he had even then all the sprightly action and gaiety of a horse of six instead of an old granddad of twenty-three. Behind him in the cavalcade was his most famous son, Hale's Green Mountain Morgan, as well as other fine sons and daughters.

Despite his spirit and animation, old Gifford was extremely gentle and easily handled. Weir took much pleasure in walking into a show ring with the old stallion moving along beside him without a strap or bit of any kind on him. Then he would put the horse through his paces by oral commands alone, while Gifford moved about the ring as full of fire and vigor as a colt. And after the show when Weir loaded his equipment, old Gifford would follow in the same way in the manner of a big friendly dog. Needless to say, the old horse had many fond admirers and was exceedingly popular.

As well as being popular, Gifford was also very prolific: his progeny have been estimated to number 1,300!

When he was twenty-four, old Gifford was sold by Weir to a stock company in Walpole for the considerable sum of $2,000. However, he got very few colts after he was sold and two years later, at the age of twenty-six, he died. His passing was a great loss to the Morgan breed.

HALE'S GREEN MOUNTAIN MORGAN

Perhaps the best known of the old-type Morgans was Hale's Green Mountain Morgan. A show horse in every sense of the word and a model for the so-called true type, his likeness appears on the top of today's Morgan registration certificate as the personification of the ideal. In the show rings of his time Green Mountain Morgan was known from Vermont to Kentucky to Michigan, for he was probably shown more extensively than any Morgan of his day. In the above-mentioned states, as well as in Ohio, he won championships at the state fairs, and his beauty and breeding were highly praised. Like his sire, he, too, created much interest when used for the frequent musters and military reviews in his home state.

Stockmen all over New England who knew the Green Mountain Morgan had nothing but the highest praise for the horse. He was said by many to be the best stock horse, i.e., breeding stallion, in all New England at that time, and his sons were in much demand with substantial price tags on them all.

Silas Hale, under whose ownership the horse gained his greatest fame, says in a circular about the Green Mountain Morgan printed in 1853:

> The proprietor several years since becoming familiar with the peculiar experience of the Morgan race of horses, their speed, bottom, fitness for general practical service, their high spirit combined with docility and tractableness . . . which makes [them] perfectly reliable in all situations, was induced to inquire for a high-blood Morgan stallion, for the purpose of sending mares to him and improving the breed of horses in his vicinity. The horse formerly known by the name, "Young Woodbury" and owned by John Woodbury of Bethel, Vermont, attracted his attention and he sent several mares to him, the colts from which gave early indications of valuable qualities. Afterwards, the pro-

prietor carefully examined the Young Woodbury and many of his colts in the vicinity of Bethel, which examination impressed him so favorably as to induce him to purchase the horse at a high price, which horse is now known by the name, "Green Mountain Morgan." Since said horse has been in the possession of the proprietor, he has had a liberal patronage and himself and his stock are become widely known and are highly valued. Several stallions begotten by the Green Mountain Morgan have been sold as high as fifteen hundred dollars each; many stallions of his get have brought prices ranging from eight to twelve hundred dollars each; numbers of geldings and mares of his get have been sold from three hundred to eight hundred dollars each; and many

Hale's Green Mountain Morgan.

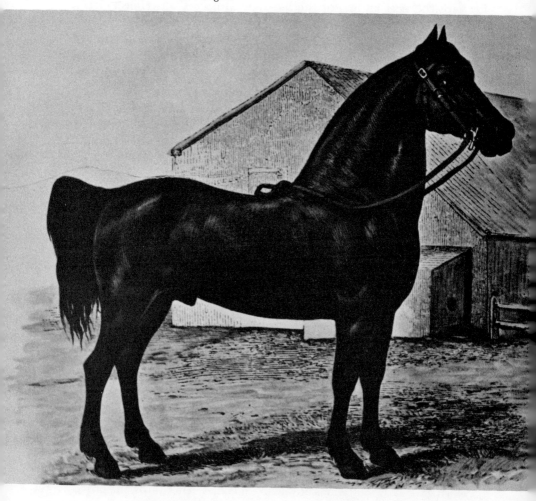

of them have proved very fast and but few of his colts, when matured, have been sold for less than two hundred dollars each.

With regard to the pedigree of the Green Mountain Morgan, the proprietor has to say that he has conversed with quite a number of elderly persons who were acquainted with the original or Justin Morgan horse, with the stock immediately descended from him and with the sire and dam of the Green Mountain Morgan and who say that the Green Mountain Morgan strikingly illustrates the peculiar qualities of the original stock.

Green Mountain Morgan was foaled around 1832. The exact date of his birth is not known. He was born the property of George Bundy of Bethel, Vermont, but was bred by Nathaniel Whitcomb of Stockbridge. He was seal-brown in color, and when mature was 14.2 hands high and probably weighed about 1,100 pounds. His dam was a dark bay and said to have been by Woodbury; but nothing definite is really known about her except that she was purchased at Nashua, New Hampshire, by Whitcomb. At the time Whitcomb took a fancy to her she was working on the canal there. She was a low, thick-set mare, exceedingly strong and well-muscled but not possessing much in the way of good looks. She was a bit long in the tooth when bred to old Gifford. After foaling Green Mountain Morgan she was sold and nothing more is known of her.

Green Mountain Morgan was only four months old when he was weaned and sold to David Gray of Stockbridge for $25. Gray kept the horse until the stallion was a four-year-old, when he made $50 on him by selling him to Hiram Twitchell of Bethel for $75. The horse became the property of John Woodbury shortly afterwards.

Someone had been remiss about the horse's training along the way, for Woodbury, on trying to drive the stallion, found him ugly and contrary. He made several attempts to straighten the horse out but to no avail. The following spring, however, Woodbury decided to have another go at educating his purchase. Again he tried to drive the stallion (what preparations were made we have no way of knowing). This time he hitched him to a harrow and began to work him in a field bordering a river. But the horse got away from him and plunged into the river, to be held fast by the harrow to which he was still attached. The cold water foundered him badly and he was very lame for several months. Meanwhile, Woodbury leased the stallion for stud purposes in Springfield, Vermont, where gradually he returned to a sound condition.

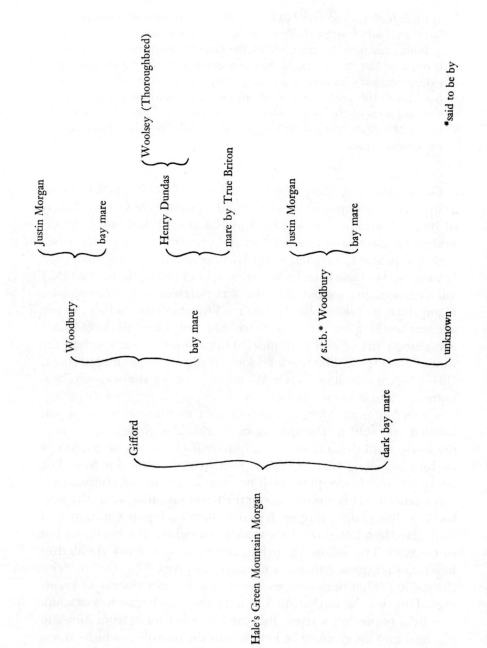

Hale's Green Mountain Morgan

Gifford
  - Woodbury
    - Justin Morgan
    - bay mare
  - bay mare
    - Henry Dundas
      - Woolsey (Thoroughbred)
    - mare by True Briton

dark bay mare
  - s.t.b.* Woodbury
    - Justin Morgan
    - bay mare
  - unknown

*said to be by

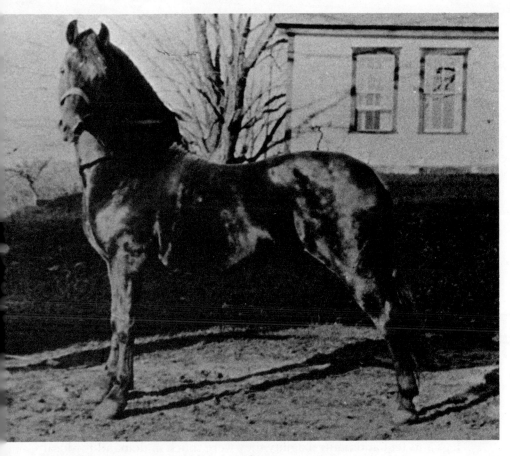

Descendant of Green Mountain Morgan, Sealect.

It was in 1842 when Silas Hale paid the $700 for him and brought the horse, now ten years old, home to South Royalston, Massachusetts. He kept the horse for eight years. The stallion must have improved much in appearance and way of going for it was during this time that he was shown so extensively.

Hale took Green Mountain Morgan west in 1853 and showed him at the state fairs of Kentucky, Ohio and Michigan where, as mentioned above, the horse won first premiums and much acclaim by all who saw him. In 1854 he won the first premium at the Vermont State Fair in Brattleboro. Only rarely was he ever beaten in competition, on one occasion by the famous Black Hawk at Rutland, Vermont.

When he was twenty-eight years old, Green Mountain made one

of his last appearances in the show ring in Woodstock, Vermont, in 1860. Heading a group of his best sons, the old stallion put on a great show for the spectators. He tossed his head like a colt and pranced about the ring, showing off all his fine qualities despite his advanced age. In his later years his disposition had mellowed and was such as to leave little to be desired. His manners also had improved to a point where he could stand or go through his paces on command without benefit of halter or bridle.

The best advertisement for the get of Green Mountain Morgan was the horse himself. Silas Hale evidently knew this full well, for everywhere the horse was shown, horsemen were putting in their orders for Green Mountain colts. Needless to say, the demand far exceeded the supply. Prices for the colts of this popular horse were far above the average of the day. A $1,500 horse would have the townsfolk goggle-eyed!

When you consider that the stud fee on Green Mountain Morgan was a mere $20 and that very few mature horses by him sold under $200 minimum (this being almost three times the general average sale price for the time), it is easy to realize the horse's great popularity as a stud.

Green Mountain Morgan's colts sold especially well on the farms and were considered the Vermonters' ideal. For the city markets they may have been regarded as a bit small in size, but with their good legs and feet and natural agility they were much in demand for local work. Of course, not to be underestimated were their bright good looks, which enhanced their value as well, for it was certainly no disgrace to drive to church behind a snappy Morgan even though all the week the same horse had been skidding logs or pulling a plow.

As far as beauty went, the Green Mountain colts had it aplenty. Their short, dished faces and big expressive eyes, their crested and smoothly arched necks and their close-ribbed, short, round bodies lent a symmetry which could not be overlooked. No wonder all who had seen the old Green Mountain were clamoring for his colts. And even with the beauty went the strong legs which were equal to any task: for they were known to be "all-day" driving horses who would come in at night with a spring in their step and light in their eyes. Small they were in stature, but with hearts as big as the new country they were helping to develop.

Years after his death Green Mountain was still considered the finest of the early Morgans. He lived to be thirty years old and left behind him some of the best examples of the Morgan breed to carry on for him in establishing a great line.

Even from its earliest beginnings in the rugged, windswept hills of New Hampshire and Vermont, the Morgan horse was never without its ardent admirers. The northcountry men of the soil, wise in the ways of the conditions in which they lived, knew instinctively that the qualities in evidence in the first Morgans were made-to-order for their way of life. As the Morgans increased in numbers through the efforts of these men, they found great favor with the folk of the surrounding countryside.

At this time, the Morgans were virtually confined in their useful-

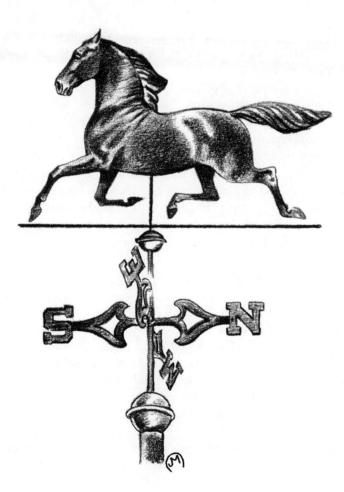

ness to the farm and the road. Endurance and strength mattered more than speed, and hardiness more than beauty, and these leading virtues the Morgans had in abundance. That the early horses of the breed also possessed beauty and a certain ability to burn up the road when necessary was another mark chalked up in their favor, for who could resist a bit of a contest on the highway when the occasion demanded? There was little enough recreation in a difficult life of trying to scrape a living from a rocky side-hill farm.

Farmers raised Morgans because the hardy little animals were their type of horse. They respected the Morgans' abilities, and cleared their land and plowed their tilting fields and yet never tried to conceal their pride in the fact that here were horses which could not only work so willingly and successfully but could, when hitched to the Sunday rig, hold up their heads and trot down the road with snap in their gait and a full measure of proud beauty in their every line. And knowing that a turn of speed was available when needed made many a farmer sit straighter in his seat when passing a neighbor on the road.

But speed, while appreciated, was nonetheless not paramount with the men of the northcountry. Farmers had little time for developing race horses; and as far as the roads were concerned, one has only to scan a topographical map of the area to see that the roads, such as they were, were hardly conducive to the racing of horses to any great extent. And as for race tracks, at that time Vermont had none worthy of the name. So the Morgan was bred for and became the all-purpose horse of New England. His great endurance became his greatest asset and he toiled with his equally rugged human companions in the development of a new and difficult land.

THE NEW DEPARTURE

This, then, was the condition of the Morgan horse during its beginnings as a breed, prior to the 1840s. Then gradually, with the improvement of roads and the demand for harness horses which could move at a faster clip, it became evident to breeders that in order to sell their horses profitably the animals would have to be able to show ever-increasing speed at the trot. The lanky Messengers were appearing on the scene to challenge the Morgans' position on the road, a position which had seemed so firmly established. The Messengers, offspring of an imported English horse of primarily Arabian (Thoroughbred) breeding, were becoming increasingly popular.

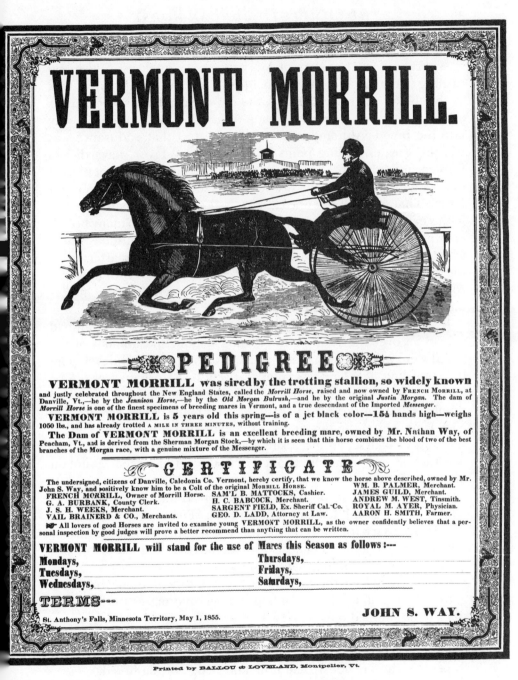

Outcrossing to Messenger blood is a selling point in this 1855 poster.

Now the trouble began.

Where, before, breeders of Morgans made attempts to keep returning to the blood of the original Justin Morgan by selecting mares of that blood wherever possible, the new demand for speed and its attendant cry for greater size caused outside blood to find its way into the breed. Although recognizing the fact that endurance was still the greatest selling point in the Morgans' favor, nevertheless farmers and others breeders were tempted to outcross to other blood in an attempt to satisfy the desire for horses which were larger and faster. That many of the fine characteristics of the Morgan were lost in this experiment was a source of great consternation to many breeders who considered tampering with the breed a grave mistake. Luckily, back in the hills there were enough farmers who, unaffected by the popular demand, continued to breed Morgans as Morgans and considered the original characteristics of the breed far more important than the craze for speed.

By this time—the late '40s and '50s—the fame of the Morgan had spread all over the young and growing nation, and animals of the breed were in great demand to assist in opening up and developing the sprawling new land. As comparatively few Morgans were to be had, due to the fact that they were being raised only in moderate numbers and for the most part in the back country of Vermont and New Hampshire, the demand greatly exceeded the supply. The result was, of course, an increasingly high price tag on good individuals such as has been noted concerning the get of Green Mountain Morgan.

Linsley, quoting from *The Maine Farmer* around 1850, says, pertaining to price and demand for Morgans: "For a seller of horses, it is only necessary for him to establish the fact that his horses are of the Morgan blood and he meets with a ready sale at good prices and the purchasers are more than satisfied."

Another result of the increasing country-wide demand for Morgans was the selling of outstanding stallions and mares for breeding stock to be shipped outside New England. The tour of Hale's Green Mountain through Ohio, Kentucky and Michigan was one example of how the excellence of the Morgan horse was successfully advertised to people who previously had little knowledge of the breed.

Buyers from the south and the west began trekking to Vermont to offer farmers and breeders very high prices for their best animals. Tempted by the jingle of silver, many a breeder parted with some of his best stock, an action which soon resulted in lessening the quality of his herd. It is an obvious fact that unless some of the best individuals raised by a stock farm are retained for use by that farm, superior animals can hardly be expected to appear in its future breeding program.

This fact soon became apparent to many wide-awake breeders of Morgans during this period and, by turning down all offers on their best animals, they began producing first-rate Morgans in large enough numbers to be able to spare some for market.

DESCENDANTS OF BULRUSH

THE MORRILL FAMILY

The Morgans of this period were used for the most part as road and business horses as well as for farm work. Some were occasionally raced. Their natural speed, which was a definite characteristic of the breed, was developed as had not been done in the early days and Morgans, more and more, became noted for this speed as well as for their endurance, spirit and beauty. The outcrossing of Morgans with the Messenger and later Hambletonian line also brought about a certain type of road horse that was different from the old-type Morgans and yet was still known as Morgan. These were used and trained as horses for the trotting tracks, and while some great individuals were produced they differed greatly from the original Vermont Morgans and were Morgans, really, in name only.

One family of Morgans which succumbed almost entirely to the influence of outside blood were the Morrills. Tracing in lineage to Bulrush, they possessed as a family the inherent substance and stamina which was so evident in Bulrush himself. They were bred from good road and work mares and were not high-strung and nervous as some lines tended to be. It is unfortunate, but all the good qualities of the Morrills are almost completely lost to the Morgan breed: after an all-too-brief day in the limelight they were bred to the lanky Hambletonians and, losing their identity, were absorbed by the new Standardbred breed. That they strengthened the Standardbred cannot be argued against, but they did so to their own eventual abdication as Morgans.

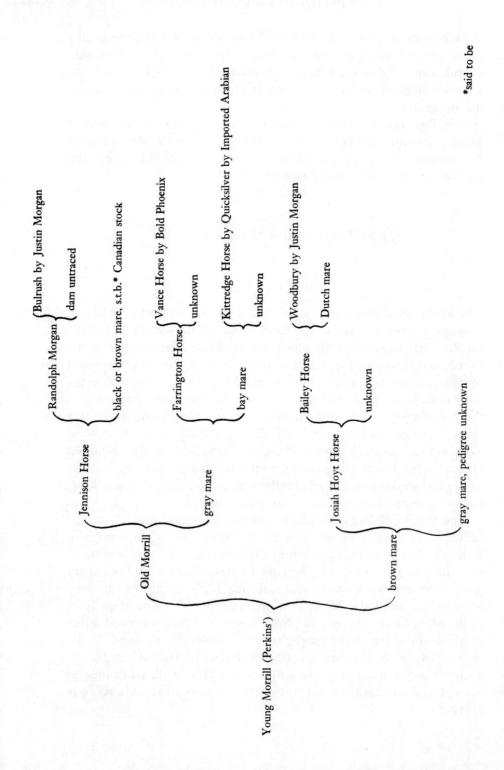

Young Morrill (Perkins')

Old Morrill

Jennison Horse

Randolph Morgan

Bulrush by Justin Morgan

dam untraced

black or brown mare, s.t.b.* Canadian stock

gray mare

Farrington Horse

Vance Horse by Bold Phoenix

unknown

bay mare

brown mare

Josiah Hoyt Horse

Bailey Horse

Kittredge Horse by Quicksilver by Imported Arabian

unknown

Woodbury by Justin Morgan

Dutch mare

unknown

gray mare, pedigree unknown

*said to be

Randolph Morgan

The beginning of the Morrill line was Bulrush's best son, the stallion Randolph Morgan. He had a string of aliases to rival any Post Office "wanted" poster, for he was also called Morgan Bulrush, Little Bulrush, the Weston horse, the Edson horse, etc., etc. He was very much like his sire, being a brown bay with a small star, and standing about 14.2. His mane and tail were thick and bushy, although in appearance he was possibly more finished and less drafty than Bulrush. But in endurance the Randolph Morgan could rival his sire, for no task, however tough, could wear him out. He was said to have drawn two men in a two-wheeled chaise eighty miles in one day without a sign of fatigue! A three-minute mile was considered lightning speed in the 1830s but the Randolph Morgan, boasting a great trot, could keep well within that time. All who knew him agreed that he was a very handsome horse of Morgan type and a great Trotter for his day.

Little is known about the dam of the Randolph Morgan. She might have been a daughter of old Justin, as she originated from the vicinity of Randolph, Vermont, where the old horse had left many foals. At any rate, her son, foaled about 1820, was the image of Justin—possibly even more so than Bulrush himself.

The Jennison Colt

When the Randolph Morgan was bred, in 1840, to a large Canadian-bred mare (of unknown ancestry but possessing a certain ability at drawing timber from the Randolph woods), the result was a cherry-bay foal called the Jennison colt. At maturity this colt, the spit and image of his sire but the size and weight of his dam, was considered a fine horse and the proverbial pride and joy of his owner, Abijah Jennison. To quote Jennison, speaking of his colt:

When he was foaled, well, the best description of him I can give is that he was perfect and he grew perfect. He weighed over 1,200 pounds and was a bright bay, no white on him but a little star, and he had the same little, short, sharp, quick ear of the little Morgan [presumably Randolph Morgan]. His mother had pretty long ears and they lapped some [an interesting note]; and he had a wide forehead and his eyes were large and stood out and he had just such a foretop, mane, and tail as the little Morgan. Oh, he was the little Randolph all over except his size; and he took that from his mother. I had the colt when he was two years old and that was the season he sired Old Morrill.

It is easy to see from the statement above that Abijah Jennison was very fond of the big bay colt. This fact must have made it quite difficult for him when, being a poor man, he was forced to sell his young stud as a three-year-old. Somehow he managed to buy him back two years later, only to have to part with him again due to a pathetic lack of funds. This is the last that is ever heard of the Jennison horse, although some say he was sold to a New Hampshire stock farm. At any rate, nothing is definite.

Old Morrill

Old Morrill, by the Jennison horse—whose stud fee it is reported was a pound of tea!—was foaled late in 1843. He was seal-brown in color, although some describe him as black with tan muzzle and flanks. He had a white right hind sock and at maturity stood 15.3 and weighed about 1,225 pounds. His dam was gray. She was a very well-bred mare, being seven-eighths Thoroughbred; she stood 15.2, had a long neck, moderately lengthy head and ears and a fine coat through which the veins showed prominently. She was purchased by James Heath of Walden, Vermont, as a two-year-old. Despite the fact that shortly afterwards she fractured one of her hind legs, which, though it healed, left her with a distinct hitch in her gait, she was very good in harness and was known to have cleared Heath's rough, side-hill farm. Some work for a crippled mare of Thoroughbred blood!

Morrill was a composite of the breeding behind him. He was fine-coated, and unlike his Morgan forebears had a scant mane and tail. His head was excellent, with fine ears and large eyes, although something of his granddam showed up in his hairy jaw and shaggy fetlocks. His feet were large and his pasterns a bit short, but he was a strong, energetic horse with a pure trotting gait that was as speedy as it was balanced. He was a rare combination of speed and strength and was considered at the time to have no equal in New England in this respect.

Morrill was sold as a weanling to Urban Perkins of South Walden, Vermont, and was later traded to French Morrill, in neighboring Danville, when four years old. Until he was seven Morrill was used as a buggy horse and worked in a team on the farm. He was used regularly at stud as well, before being sold for the rumored price of $1,000 to a man in Massachusetts. However, back he came to Vermont shortly afterwards, when the Massachusetts man proved unable to

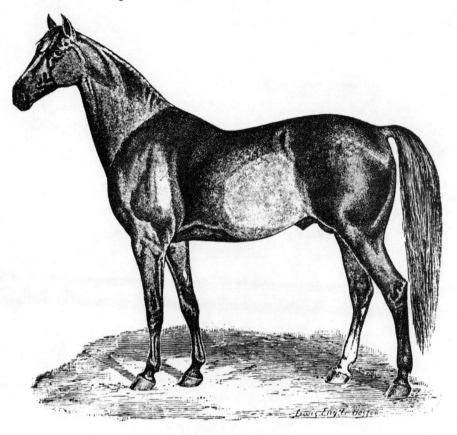

Winthrop Morrill by Perkins' Young Morrill.

pay for him. There he remained under the ownership of Morrill until he died at the age of nineteen in 1862.

Young Morrill, Winthrop and Fearnaught

Most of Old Morrill's Vermont sons and daughters lived out their lives on the farms of the region in the traditional Morgan manner: as driving horses and for farm work. But the old horse sired also a prolific line of race horses which subsequently were the ones to become absorbed into the Standardbred breed.

Old Morrill sired the bay Perkins' Young Morrill, his best son, who was foaled in 1850. Young Morrill in turn sired Fearnaught and Winthrop Morrill, two of the very best Trotters of the century. Winthrop Morrill, even though bred to ordinary farm mares, stood fifth

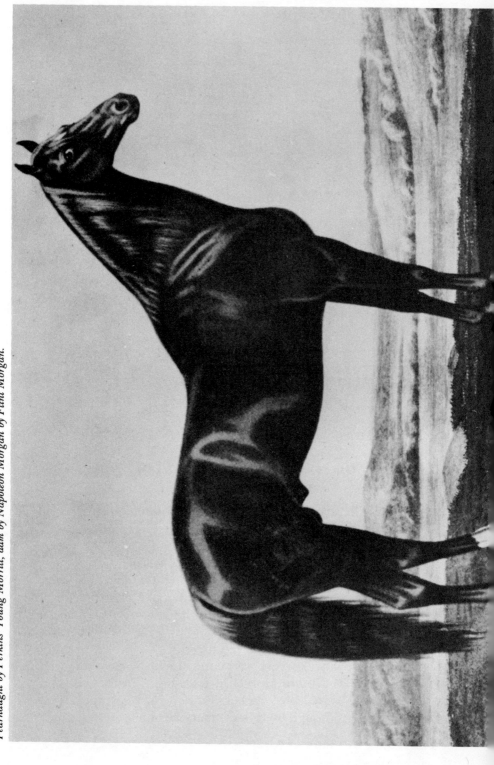

Fearnaught by Perkins' Young Morrill, dam by Napoleon Morgan by Flint Morgan.

on the list of sires of 2:30 performers (horses which could trot the mile in 2:30). Fearnaught at one time brought the fabulous sum of $25,000 and was Grand Champion Trotting Stallion of the World in 1868. He was a very successful sire and commanded a fee of $250, a substantial amount for any stud in those days.

Young Morrill also sired Draco (2:28½) and Danville Boy, two racing champions of the day.

As a family the Morrills were larger in all respects than the early Morgans. Their absorption into the Standardbred *Register* took place when breeders, finding the speedy, line-bred Messengers lacking in racing stamina, crossed them with the Morrills to make up the deficit. Gradually the Morgan blood, thinned by an ever-increasing amount of the Messenger-Hambletonian, was lost until it became unrecognizable. But the blood was there, though diluted, and the establishment of the Standardbred horse owes much to the Morgans of the Morrill line.

3

The Influence
of the Morgan Horse on
Other American Breeds

THE STANDARDBRED HORSE

Until the advent of Hambletonian 10 (Rysdyk's), foaled in 1849, the Morgan horse was the king of the road and the race track. Black Hawk and his descendants were *the* harness-race horses standing in undisputed favor throughout the racing world in the early nineteenth century. Gradually, however, the descendants of a gray English Thoroughbred named Messenger began appearing on the scene to steal some of the Morgans' thunder. Messenger, imported from England in 1788, traced to all three of the Eastern stallions which were the foundation sires of the Thoroughbred: the Darley Arabian, the Byerly Turk and the Godolphin Arabian. Like Denmark in the Saddlebred *Register,* Messenger became the foundation sire of a new breed, for he was recognized as the founding father of the American Trotter. Although he was a horse bred and trained for the running gait, Messenger sired horses with a peculiar proclivity for the trot. His offspring—sons and especially grandsons—were soon to whittle away at the stronghold of the Morgan, chalking up records that even the most pro-Morgan horsemen could not fail to recognize. Ethan Allen 50, the darling of New England and a racing crack who was admired wherever he appeared, was the last of the great Morgan stars; his retirement became the swan song of the full-blooded Morgan's supremacy on the track. Little by little the larger, faster Messengers, and subsequently the Hambletonians, drove the Morgans to the wall as far as racing was concerned—but not before the influence of the Morgan breed had left its indelible mark.

As mentioned earlier, a prominent Morgan family to influence the new breed—eventually to be known as the Standardbred—were the Morrills, a line descending from Bulrush, as we have noted in Chapter 2. The patriarch of the family was Old Morrill; his best son, Perkins' Young Morrill, carried the line on. Outstanding among the descendants of Old Morrill were Winthrop Morrill, sire of twenty-seven winners and founder of a great strain of Trotters, and Fearnaught (2:23¼), one-time Champion Trotting Stallion and head of a Trotting family second only to the Ethan Allens for speed. Winthrop Morrill, though bred to the plainest, run-of-the-mill mares, sired a great many speedy Trotters and despite the handicap of common mares stood fifth on the list of sires of 2:30 performers in 1877. Fearnaught, his half-brother, was a popular race horse and an equally popular sire and frequent prize-winner in the show ring. He had a number of owners, one of whom was reported to have paid $25,000 to possess him.

Draco, another grandson of Old Morrill, and his brother, Danville Boy, were two more Morgan stallions who, after successful careers on the track, forged still more Morgan links in the chain of the Standardbred family through sons and daughters bred for the track.

Walker Morrill, a son of Winthrop Morrill, was yet another prominent sire of Morgan blood. Foaled in 1861, he sired six known 2:30 trotters and was the winner of thirty-six races himself. And so it went: a list of the descendants of Old Morrill alone and the growing number of "2:30" horses would fill a volume.

But there were other lines and individuals that had their season of fame before being swallowed up by the Hambletonians.

One such individual was Golddust. From his description it would seem he had been rightly named, for he was said to have been "pure gold in color." Foaled in 1855, Golddust was the son of Vermont Morgan by Barnard Morgan, a son of Old Gifford. His dam was the Hoke mare, who was said to have been sired by Zilcaadi, a chestnut Arabian stallion which had been the gift of the Sultan of Morocco to the U.S. Consul, Mr. Rhind, who imported him.

Golddust was a stallion of extreme beauty; yet beauty alone did not win him the esteem and popularity accorded him all his life. He had a brilliant career although the short span of sixteen years marked his lifetime.

Foaled the property of Andrew Hoke near Louisville, Kentucky, Golddust was sold as a weanling to L. L. Dorsey. He remained at Dorsey's Eden Stock Farm all his life, so fond was that gentleman of

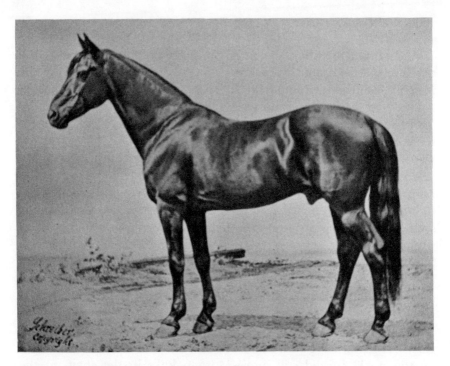

Draco, another example of an early Morgan stallion.

his golden stallion. Golddust was a large horse by Morgan standards, standing 16 hands and weighing 1,275 pounds. To quote Volume I of the Morgan *Register*: "Golddust was a most beautiful horse, and one of the very great sires of the country. In getting extreme speed he outranks Hambletonian, only three of whose more than 1,300 colts are found in the 2:20 list, the best of which is Dexter with a record of 2:17½ made against time."

In his brief lifetime Golddust sired 302 foals, yet two made the 2:20 list. His greatest offspring was Lucille Golddust, who had a record of 2:16½, which she made in a hotly contested race.

The Civil War years, and the ensuing turmoil caused by them, resulted in Golddust having fewer opportunities at stud than a less unstable situation might have offered. That, coupled with his all-too-early demise, put a limit to his successes. Nevertheless his place is assured and he stands strong on his accomplishments despite the adversities life meted out to him. He sired thirty-eight winners, and among his sons sixteen became outstanding in their own right.

Ethan Allen 50, whose story is found earlier in this book, was probably the most prolific of the Morgans in regard to production of outstanding harness horses. His line overshadows all others and, unlike some of the others, his contribution to the Morgan breed was as consequential as the legacy he left to the American Trotter. Ethan Allen sired seventy winners and was the winner, himself, of over thirty races against some of the top names of his day. His greatest sons were, in addition to Daniel Lambert, DeLong's Ethan Allen, Holabird's Ethan Allen, American Ethan, Superb, Woodward's Ethan Allen and Honest Allen.

Honest Allen, foaled in 1855, got Denning Allen, who was the sire of Lord Clinton, a black gelding who had a laudable race record and a mark of 2:10¼! Denning Allen was triumphant in the show ring, winning first premiums for Morgan Stallions Five and Over, and Sweepstakes for Morgan Stallions, All Ages, at the World's Columbian Exposition in Chicago in 1893. His full brother General Gates stood at the head of The United States Morgan Horse Farm breeding program in Weybridge, Vermont.

Daniel Lambert, Ethan Allen's best son, filled his sire's shoes to

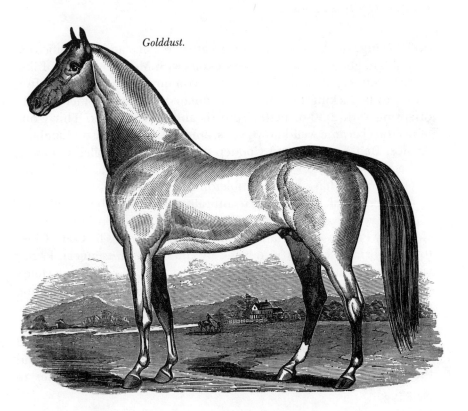

Golddust.

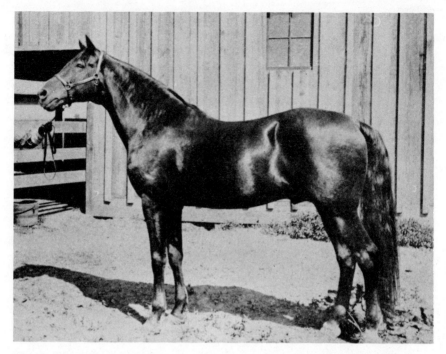

Ben Franklin by Daniel Lambert.

overflowing, for he was another great speed sire and a prolific one as well. He got a goodly number of colts with Morgan beauty of line and movement and speed to boot (a combination which was often found to be lacking in the Hambletonians). His family included 37 offspring with 2:30-or-better records and 106 winners. Thirty-one of his sons became well-known sires, among them: Addison Lambert, Aristos, Ben Franklin and Cobden in addition to Jubilee Lambert, and a host of others which wove the thread of Morgan blood intricately through that of the Hambletonian.

A stallion which probably technically could only be called half-Morgan, yet nevertheless traced to the blood of Justin Morgan, was Kentucky Prince. A bay stallion foaled in 1870, he was by Clark Chief (by Mambrino Chief by Mambrino by Imported Messenger). Prince was out of Kentucky Queen sired by Morgan Eagle, a son of Hale's Green Mountain. It might have been his breeding or his trotting ability or perhaps his sheer good looks: but at any rate, his name appears in more Trotting-horse pedigrees than that of any Morgan-bred stallion. Kentucky Prince sired winners of almost three hundred races, became the grandsire of about seventy-five more winners, and the great-grandsire of countless others. He was a half-brother to

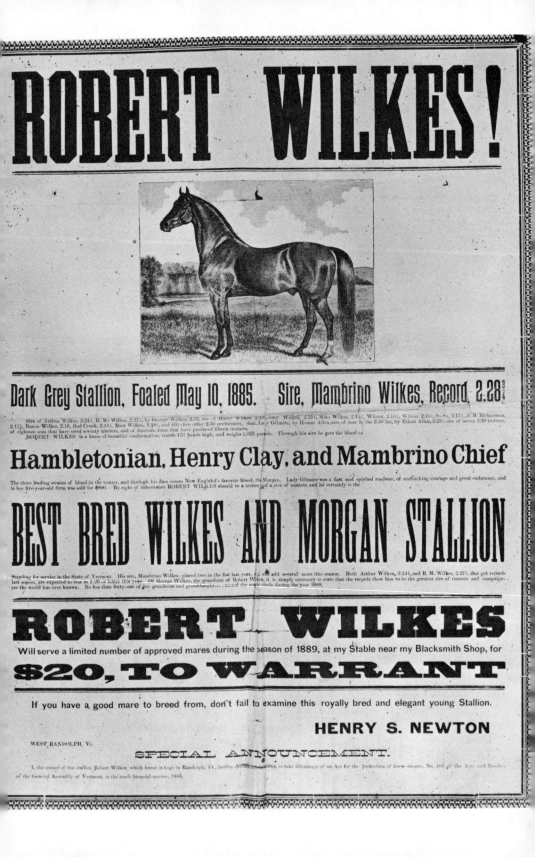

Harrison Chief, both being by Clark Chief. And while Harrison Chief went on to fame in the annals of the American Saddlebred, Kentucky Prince will be remembered as a prominent sire in Trotting-horse history.

Many Morgan fanciers, thinking of the lucrative race-horse market, began to breed for one characteristic: speed. Outcrosses were made to this end. In some cases, so diluted became the blood of Justin Morgan that it almost caused the demise of the Morgan horse as a breed in its original form. When animals with the blood of Messenger, the imported gray Thoroughbred, and others of this line were crossed with the Morgans, speedy horses may have resulted. But the Morgan type for which old Justin was famed, was lost. The Morrills were a Morgan family which gained fame as harness-race horses and were incorporated into the rising new breed then known as the American Trotter.

Still, the Morgans competed successfully on the track. Such undisputed stars as Black Hawk 20 (grandson of Justin Morgan) and his son Ethan Allen 50 (foaled 1849) kept the Morgan name bright. Although in the 1840s and '50s the Morgans commanded the roads and contributed so much speed and style to the racing scene, the tremendous development of the American Trotter as a breed began to see the Morgans outdistanced on the track by horses with often more size, and which were bred for speed primarily. Thus the Morgans—which had given so much of themselves in the formation of the Standardbred, as the Trotter came to be known—found themselves being overshadowed by the newer breed on the race track. On the road, however, they were still supreme, and remained in that position until the advent of the automobile again imperiled their future.

The names of Morgans woven in the tapestry of Standardbred greats is seemingly endless, and their numbers and their records if set down would surely make the reader's head swim. It is sufficient to say that although the Hambletonian blood has at last obscured all others today, still the heritage of those old Morgans will be there in the twentieth-century champions tracing to them. There are many Trottingbred all-time greats which carry crosses to Justin Morgan. Among them are Lee Axworthy, Uhlan and Hamburg Belle. The champion Trotter Greyhound (1:55¼) has five crosses to Justin Morgan, and Titan Hanover (2:00) has *no less than twenty-two* crosses to Justin. So be it.

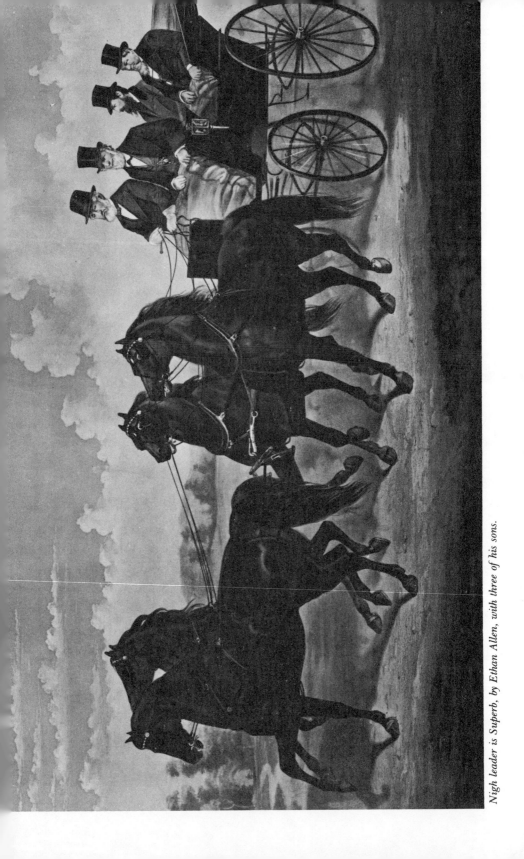

Nigh leader is Superb, by Ethan Allen, with three of his sons.

THE AMERICAN SADDLEBRED

For the admirers of the American Saddlebred horse, the credit for establishing their breed belongs at the feet of its recognized foundation sire, the immortal Denmark. The Standardbred enthusiast reveres Imported Messenger as the patriarch of the Trotting horse; and Allan F–1 has gone down in history as the foundation sire of the Tennessee Walking Horse.

Yet many are unaware of the fact that all three breeds share a common blood: that of the Morgan. Supporters of the Saddlebred and the Standardbred and the Walking Horse should pause and contemplate the contribution of the Morgan to each breed's success, for the thread of Morgan blood is woven inextricably through the pedigrees of their greatest stars.

The Saddlebred originated in Kentucky early in that state's history. A need for horses for light harness and saddle work resulted in breeders developing a type of easy-gaited animal, which, while it had the stamina and hardiness needed for a raw new land, also possessed the quality and refinement so sought after by the avid horseman. This utility saddle horse of early Kentucky soon emerged as the forerunner of what we now know as the American Saddlebred.

Thoroughbred blood was brought in and crossed on native saddle-type mares to give an increase in size and a generous measure of refinement and quality as well. Perhaps the most influential of the Thoroughbred importations to Kentucky was the seal-brown stallion Denmark, who had been foaled in 1839. Denmark was an extremely beautiful horse, although he had a racing record that was far from sensational, and it was soon discovered that his progeny were outstanding in the quality and beauty of their sire as well as in having the stamina so important to the times.

Denmark's best son was Gaines Denmark, whose dam was the Cockspur pacing mare known as the "Stevenson mare." A magnificent black stallion and a show horse of remarkable ability, Gaines Denmark became the founder of the Denmark strain of saddle horses. Through his four best-known sons—Washington's Denmark, Diamond Denmark, Star Denmark and Sumpter Denmark—the blood of Gaines Denmark had a profound effect on the advancement of the Saddlebred.

Then in 1863, there was foaled a Morgan-bred stallion, Cabell's Lexington, which was also destined to have a strong influence on the new breed being developed in Kentucky. Named on the original list

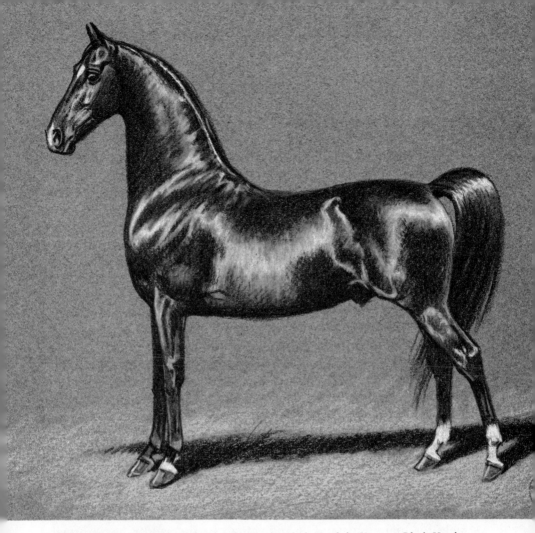

Cabell's Lexington by Gist's Black Hawk by Blood's Black Hawk by Vermont Black Hawk by Sherman by Justin Morgan.

of seventeen foundation sires of the *American Saddle Horse Register*, Cabell's Lexington remained on that list through two subsequent revisions and was dropped, as were all the others, only when in 1908 the National Saddle Horse Breeders Association voted to make Denmark the sole foundation sire of the breed. Another Morgan-bred stallion, Coleman's Eureka, was also retained on the list until it was decided to designate Denmark alone as the fountainhead of the breed.

Cabell's Lexington was sired by the little-known son of Blood's Black Hawk called Gist's Black Hawk. His dam was a good road mare by Tom Hal, a son of Green Mountain Black Hawk (also known as

Sorrell Tom), a show horse and Trotting stallion. Her dam was by Copperbottom (a Canadian pacer). The Canadian pacers were introduced into Kentucky around 1816 and the most famous of them were the original Tom Hal (according to Volume I of the Morgan *Register,* no relation to the Tom Hal above) and Copperbottom. Old Tom Hal was noted for his toughness and endurance; he is said quite possibly to have been of Morgan blood, as there were horses of this breeding in that area of Canada where he was foaled. The blood of both Tom Hal and Copperbottom was influential in the establishment of the pacing strains in the Standardbred breed as well as having its effect on the Tennessee Walking Horse. Both stallions were natural pacers and although a great many others found their way into Kentucky and Tennessee, these two were the most famous of those horses known in the 1800s as the Canadian pacers.

Cabell's Lexington, a dark bay with a star and three white socks, stood 15.2 and weighed 1,070 pounds. He had the beautiful head and the tiny ears of the Morgan, and was strong and compact of body with excellent legs and feet. During a long and very successful career in the show ring, Cabell's Lexington was beaten only once. And as a progenitor of outstanding saddle horses of the day, he had but one rival—Gaines Denmark. His get were noted for their fine dispositions and wonderful balanced action: traits which their sire had in abundance. They brought high prices and were in tremendous demand wherever there was an appreciation of fine horseflesh. The daughters of Cabell's Lexington, when crossed with such illustrious sires as Bourbon Chief and the great Harrison Chief, were responsible for many outstanding individuals of the saddle horse breed. Lexington's greatest son was Tom Boyd, a show horse of great brilliance and endurance (the latter being a trait often found lacking in today's show-ring performers—many a good horse is found to "run out of gas" nowadays when the workouts get too lengthy!). Cabell's Lexington himself had proved in his many successful onslaughts of the show ring that not only must a show horse have presence and action but, in the days when individual classes had fifty or more entries, it was necessary also that he have plenty of bottom and heart—plus a generous measure of the will to win. Some authorities state that old Lexington probably sired more fine saddle horses than any other sire of Morgan breeding. Certainly he was responsible for much of the greatness in several lines of American Saddlebred families.

Rivaling Cabell's Lexington in prominence as a Morgan-bred progenitor of saddle horses was another stallion whose name, as men-

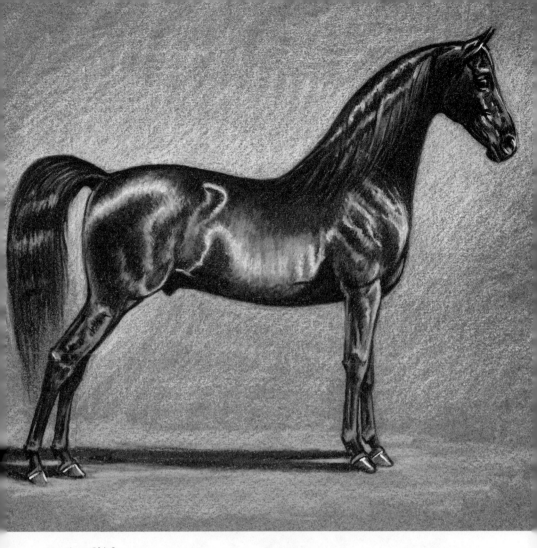

Harrison Chief.

tioned earlier, appeared on the original list of foundation sires of the Saddlebred. This was the dark chestnut, Coleman's Eureka. Although his dam, Mary Boston, was of Thoroughbred blood tracing to the great Sir Archy, and bred for the race track, she also was a great success in the show ring before she was retired to the breeding farm. None can deny, however, that notwithstanding her show-ring record, her most significant contribution to the horse world, particularly that of the saddle horse, was her son Coleman's Eureka. Foaled in 1868 in Trimble County, Kentucky, Eureka was by Young's Morgan, a grandson of Butler's Eureka. Butler's Eureka was by the cel-

ebrated Hale's Green Mountain Morgan and so was of the recognized
Morgan type. In the words of the Morgan *Register,* Volume I, he was
"as nice a chestnut horse as ever you saw, 15 hands, 1,000 pounds;
very stylish. . . ." His best sons were the sire of Young's Morgan and
Cox's Eureka—both sires of some of the finest horses in Frankfort
County, Kentucky.

Coleman's Eureka was 16 hands at maturity and a rich dark chestnut in color. He had a remarkable record in the show ring against
the stiffest competition that section of the country had to offer. In
1877 he won a first premium at St. Louis, Missouri, with forty-two
competitors. The *National Saddle Horse Register* says, "Coleman's Eureka was a horse of remarkable power to transmit his good qualities,
and Kentucky is full of good stallions and mares that trace to him.
Some of the finest saddle horses of the present time have much of

*Coleman's Eureka by Young's Morgan by Butler's Eureka by Hale's Green Mountain Morgan
by Gifford by Woodbury by Justin Morgan.*

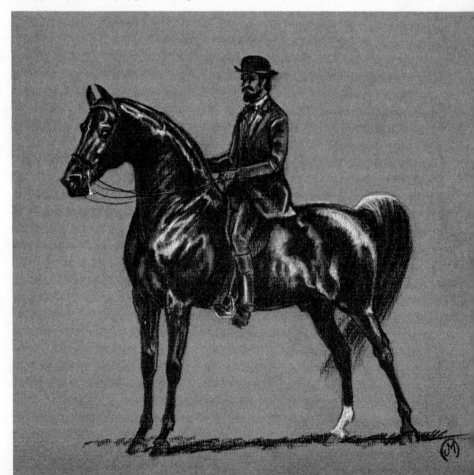

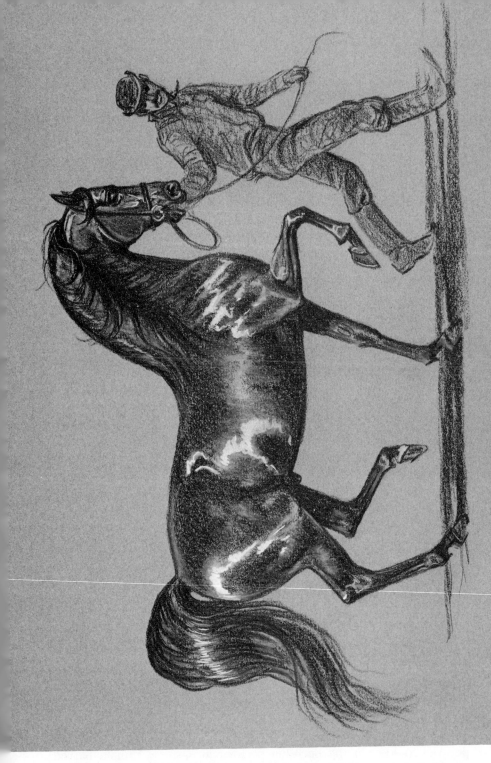

Indian Chief by Blood's Black Hawk by Vermont Black Hawk by Sherman by Justin Morgan.

his blood. . . ." Through his daughters, his blood flows in the veins of such great show horses as King Bourbon, Chester Chief and the stallion American Born. But the blood of Coleman's Eureka, while it is found in abundance in the Saddlebred, has been lost to the Morgan through absorption into the Saddlebred.

Indian Chief, by Blood's Black Hawk, a son of old Black Hawk 20, was another Morgan stallion who left his mark indelibly on the American Saddlebred. Foaled in 1858 in Cynthiana, Kentucky, he was kept most of his life in Harrison County, near Cynthiana. His sire, Blood's Black Hawk, was foaled in Wells River, Vermont, in 1847, and taken to Lexington, Kentucky, by a man named Blood, his breeder, in 1853. He won a first premium at the Kentucky State Fair in 1856 and was shown in harness singly and double, gaining himself a sizable record of wins. The dam of Indian Chief was Lou Berry, who was by Ned Forrest, he by Young Bashaw. She traced to Thoroughbred blood through both her sire and dam. Indian Chief was a bay horse with a stripe and a left hind stocking. He stood 16 hands and weighed 1,100 pounds. He had a lively patronage throughout his life, for he was not only a successful sire of "fine-styled roadsters and fancy drivers" but himself a show horse of distinction. B. J. Treacy, a prominent Kentucky breeder of the time, said of Indian Chief, "He was, in his day, one of the most beautiful horses that ever lived and almost invincible in the show ring." He won the Champion Sweepstakes at the St. Louis Fair in 1878; and there were sixty-three entries in the class! To quote from *Famous Saddle Horses:* "Indian Chief was built on stocky lines showing heavy muscles, with great substance and power. . . . There was a magnetism about his countenance, made up of a great big eye, neatly pointed, finely used ear, an expression—winsome and individualizing. His neck, beautifully crested, fitted rightly both onto his head and into his shoulder. Full barrel, ribbing out to his hips; quarters, such quarters! Full, round, well let down so that he filled his breeching when harnessed. . . . His tail was full, set on high and carried naturally waterspout fashion."

However, many feel that the siring of the incomparable Lady de Jarnette was Indian Chief's greatest claim to fame, for she was the undisputed champion of show rings the country over. One of the brightest stars of that or any era, the Lady remained undefeated throughout her career, and was called on numerous occasions the perfect harness show mare of all time. Since none of her contemporaries could even approach her performance, she was finally barred

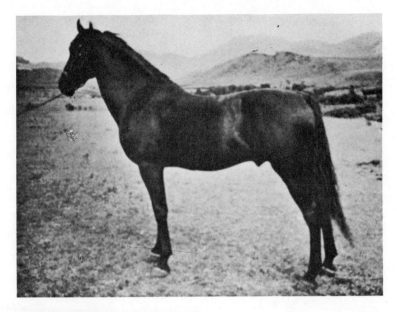

Jubilee de Jarnette.

from competition in the ring. Thereafter her life in the limelight consisted of exhibitions at horse shows and fairs where $500 a week was paid for her appearances. After her show-ring career was over, the Lady was sold for $5,000 to a gentleman in Boston who kept her until her death. Lady de Jarnette's only foal was the stallion Jubilee de Jarnette, a son of Jubilee Lambert, by Daniel Lambert. This stallion, sold to J. C. Brunk of Springfield, Illinois, was used on Morgan mares; thereby returning the blood of Indian Chief to this breed.

But except through his daughter, Lady de Jarnette, the blood of Indian Chief was responsible for greatness in the American Saddlebred instead of the Morgan, for like Cabell's Lexington and Coleman's Eureka, he was destined to become one of the outstanding foundation sires of the Saddlebred. Like the others, too, his daughters were important broodmares, for when bred to such great stallions as Bourbon Chief and Harrison Chief, they produced show horses of outstanding ability.

Indian Chief also got the brown stallion Richelieu, who was the sire of Kate, the dam of Annie C. Since Annie C. was the dam of three of the Saddle breed's greatest stallions—Bourbon King, Montgomery Chief and Marvel King—she was voted one of the most

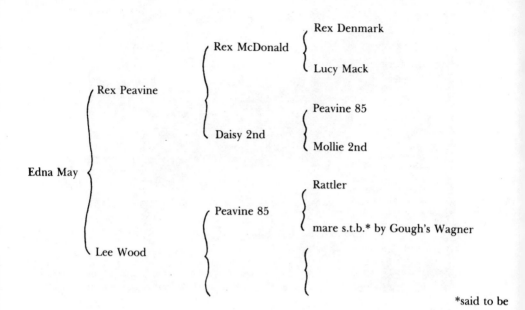

Edna May

- Rex Peavine
  - Rex McDonald
    - Rex Denmark
    - Lucy Mack
  - Daisy 2nd
    - Peavine 85
    - Mollie 2nd
- Lee Wood
  - Peavine 85
    - Rattler
    - mare s.t.b.* by Gough's Wagner

*said to be

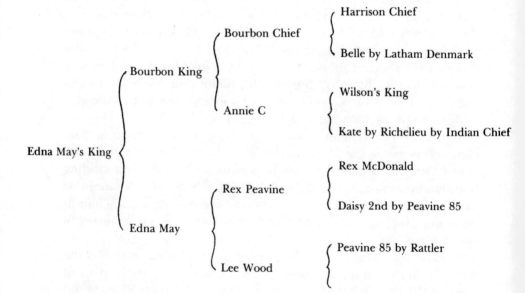

Edna May's King

- Bourbon King
  - Bourbon Chief
    - Harrison Chief
    - Belle by Latham Denmark
  - Annie C
    - Wilson's King
    - Kate by Richelieu by Indian Chief
- Edna May
  - Rex Peavine
    - Rex McDonald
    - Daisy 2nd by Peavine 85
  - Lee Wood
    - Peavine 85 by Rattler

eminent broodmares of all time. Bourbon King was considered among the horsemen of his day to be above reproach. In the show ring and as a sire he won the wildest acclaim. He was never defeated under saddle wherever he was shown even though his competition was the top show horses of his day. Bourbon King in turn sired yet another great show horse and family-builder with a nearly unequaled record in the breed, the remarkable Edna May's King. Out of Edna May, who traced to Morgan ancestry through both her sire *and* her dam, this famous stallion got Anacacho Shamrock (sire of Wing Commander), Anacacho Denmark and Cameo Kirby. Also by Bourbon King was the magnificent show stallion King's Genius, who undoubtedly has worn out just as many superlatives as his illustrious sire and grandsire! He was the finest example of the Rex Peavine–Bourbon King cross and became still another sire of a great line.

Now, of all the Morgan names in the Saddle breed, none is more familiar to those of us who admire Morgans than Peavine. The name had its origin in Peavine 85, a registered Morgan stallion foaled in Kentucky in 1863. Peavine was by Rattler, who was by Stockbridge Chief, a son of Black Hawk 20. A chestnut with a very heavy mane and tail, he stood 16 hands and weighed 1,150. A show horse in his own right, Peavine got a great many fine horses in his home country. He was also a harness-race horse and had a mark of 2:35½. Peavine sired Daisy 2nd, the dam of Rex Peavine, and this alone assured him a place in saddle horse annals. He also sired the dam of Edna May, whose pedigree and that of her son, Edna May's King, give a fair example of how Morgan blood has assisted in the production of outstanding Saddlebreds. Edna May's King sired Anacacho Shamrock, Cameo Kirby and Anacacho Denmark. Wing Commander, one of the greatest show horses of modern times, is by Anacacho Shamrock.

All the above-mentioned stallions of Morgan blood and innumerable others—as well as many, many unrecorded mares—have been of untold value in the development of the American Saddlebred. Both of the two most well-known families of the breed—the Chiefs and the Denmarks—have felt the Morgan influence. Especially through the Chiefs and Peavines has the blood of the Morgan had its greatest effect. These families are noted for their substance, style and brilliant action.

It is interesting to the Morgan enthusiast to note that of the 11,977 horses registered in the first four volumes of the *American Saddle Horse Register,* horses tracing in male line to Justin Morgan number

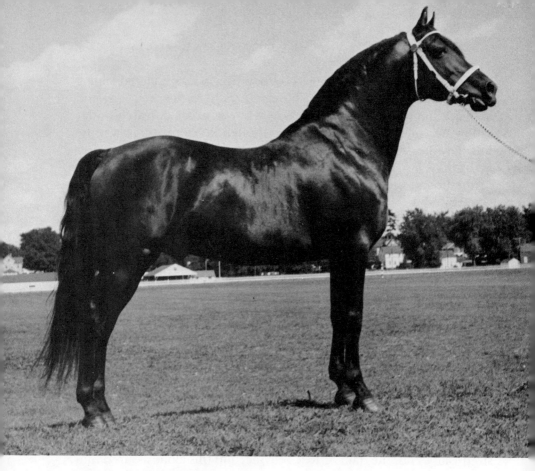

Upwey Ben Don.

714, or 6 percent of the total registered. And included in this number are some of the most venerated stars of the breed.

In the pedigree of one of our modern Morgans' most revered sires, Upwey Ben Don, you will find the blood of Peavine 85. And it is interesting to note that Ben Don, too, was a top broodmare sire, his most illustrious daughter being the incomparable Windcrest Dona Lee. Windcrest Nancy C, Harmony Brook, Windcrest Sentimental Lady, Miller's Adel, Green Meads Princess, Windcrest Rose Marie and Windcrest Madonna are but a few other top mares to perpetuate the blood of the great Ben Don.

Finally, to quote "Susanne" (the pen-name of Emily Ellen Scharf) in Volume I of her *Famous Saddle Horses:* "Very few pedigrees of Standardbred or American Saddle Horses are lacking the great name of Morgan. The Morgan imparted his strength and beauty to the Saddle Horse. The name Justin Morgan must be classed with those of Messenger and Denmark as founders of the two great American breeds of light horses. Without the prepotency of the Morgan horses, the present-day show ring would have lost some of its most attractive performers."

THE TENNESSEE WALKING HORSE

The Tennessee Walking Horse breed also owes some of its characteristics to the Morgan. Although Morgan influence was probably not felt as greatly as in the American Saddlebred or Standardbred lines, the Morgan does figure quite prominently in the development of the Walking Horse.

The little mare Maggie Marshall was the dam of the foundation sire of the breed, Allan F–1. She was sired by the Morgan horse called Bradford's Telegraph, a son of old Black Hawk 20.

A black horse himself, Telegraph was foaled in Vermont in 1849 (a banner year: both Hambletonian 10 and Ethan Allen 50 were also foaled in 1849!). Telegraph was said to have had a tremendous amount of style and speed as well as beauty and endurance. From Vermont he was taken to Ohio and subsequently to Augusta, Kentucky. There his daughter Maggie Marshall was foaled. In 1886 she produced the foal that would be known as Allan F–1.

Although plantation owners were always interested in horses with the natural running walk—the most suitable gait for their requirements—it wasn't until the appearance of Allan F–1 that any really significant advances were made to establish a breed based on this gait. When Allan was bred to the good Walking mare Gertrude, who through her dam traced to Gifford Morgan (a son of Woodbury), the resulting foal was the stallion Roan Allen F–38. A beautiful strawberry roan with a faultless gait and a proud, stylish bearing, Roan Allen was greatly admired, and with his sire became designated as a foundation sire of the Tennessee Walking Horse breed. Hence, this breed too, owes no small amount of its best qualities to the Morgans in its lines.

So prepotent was the blood of Justin Morgan that study and comparison of photographs of the four prominent American breeds show many striking similarities.

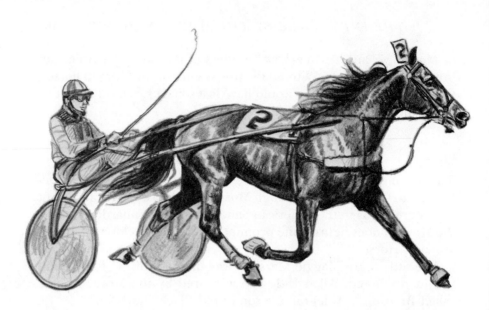

Standardbred.

Morgan.

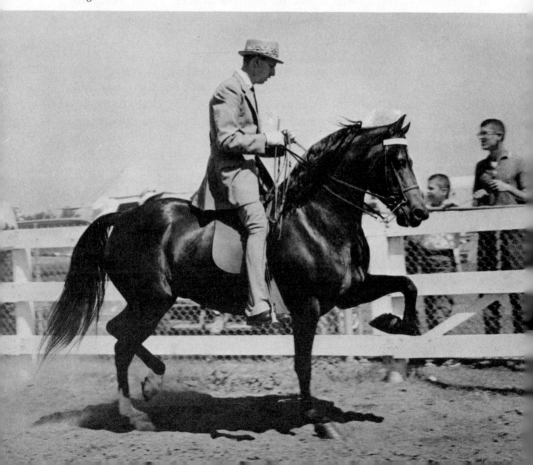

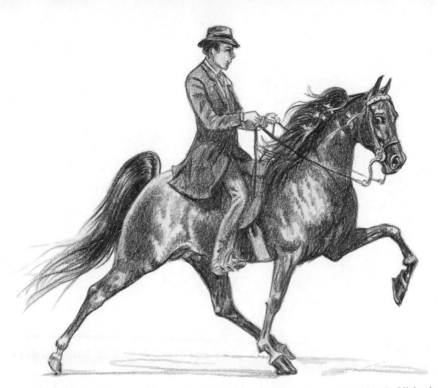

American Saddlebred.

Tennessee Walking Horse.

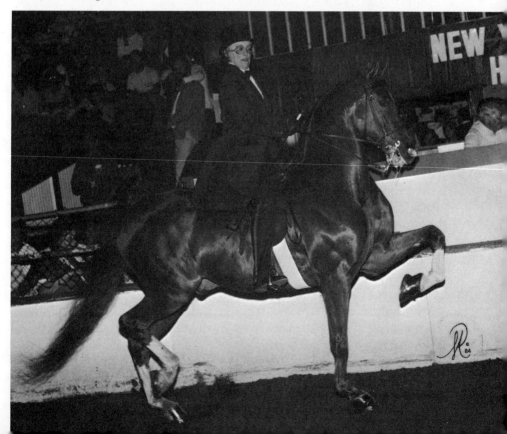

4

The Morgan Horse Club, *Register* and Farm

COLONEL JOSEPH Battell, a native of Middlebury, Vermont, had a tremendous admiration and affection for the Morgan horse all his life through. That this affinity for the breed was far from passive is evinced by the herculean amount of effort and seemingly endless research he put forth in compiling a Morgan history and *Register*. This was accomplished with the publication of *The Morgan Horse and Register,* Volume I, which he had privately printed in 1894.

Early in life Colonel Battell began to accumulate as much published information on the Morgan breed as could be found. His correspondence pertaining to the Morgan reached tremendous proportions; letters from hither and yon arrived at Middlebury to cast just a little more light on the subject. Anxiously he awaited the answers to his many queries, hoping as each one arrived that its contents would help untangle some of the early history of the Morgan. He wrote to men who had known some of the old horses and had actually witnessed their activities. He searched out musty records for any fragment of fact to further his cause. Remote pedigrees were ferreted out by him and his assistants, and no stone was left unturned that might shed some glimmer of light on his subject.

Probably his best source of information, and the foundation for the Morgan *Register*, was the excellent *Morgan Horses* by D. C. Linsley of Middlebury, Vermont. Written as an "essay" for a competition sponsored by the Vermont State Agricultural Society, Linsley's book

American Morgan Register
OFFICIAL CERTIFICATE

This is to certify that _Linda_ has been duly registered as entitled under Rule _Two_ in Volume _Three_ of The American Morgan Register, and the pedigree can there be found as follows:

Linda, black, solid color, 15 hands, 1000 pounds; foaled Oct. 1st, 1898; bred by Edgar Davenport, W. Chesterfield, N. H.; got by Madison Wilkes (dam Minna, by Red Jacket, 67, son of Billy Root, 4), son of Geo. Wilkes: dam Molly, black, bred in St. Lawrence Co. 1. Y., and said to be by Ben Franklin, 1508, son of Daniel Lambert, 62; and 3d dam by Henry Clay, son of Andrew Jackson. Sold to Louis D. Herrick, Brattleboro, Vt.; to Mrs. Louis D. Herrick, Brattleboro, Vt. by whom registered.

Given under my hand and seal, at Bread Loaf, Vt., this _12th_ day of _April_ A. D. 190_9_.

Joseph Battell
Registrar.

Typical early registration certificate signed by Colonel Battell.

received the award for the first premium in 1856. The work gave a graphic description of the Morgan family, its history to that time (1856) and pedigrees of about 240 stallions of the breed. The committee making the award to Linsley for his book declared at the time the award was made:

> In consequence of the peculiar merits of this treatise, the Committee feel authorized to commend it to the particular notice of the Society, as one eminently adapted to the wants of the people of this State and as supplying a desideratum long felt, both in regard to the true history of the Morgan horse and in respect to the best methods of its perpetuation. We believe Mr. Linsley has collected all the facts pertaining to his subject which intelligent research and thorough devotion can furnish; and that he has embodied them in an attractive form and with just discrimination. The information relating to the history of the Breed is important, and, we think, can be found in no work yet published; the style in which it is communicated is clear, spirited, and in perfect keeping with the subject discussed.
>
> When it is considered that the sources of information in regard to the origin and history of the Morgan horse, now obscure at best, are rapidly diminishing, and that Mr. Linsley has rescued so much, which in a short time would have been beyond the reach of the compiler, it must be admitted he has rendered a valuable service to the farmers of the State, and one which, in the judgment of the Committee, the Society ought not to leave unrecognized.

Considerable portions of Linsley's work are to be found in the first Volume of the Morgan *Register*, so valuable did Colonel Battell consider Linsley's researches. He reinvestigated Linsley's pedigrees and found them to be very accurate, and in his introduction to Volume I he stated that "neither trouble nor expense has been spared to learn all the pertinent facts concerning every pedigree. In the preparation of the present work and the inquiries and investigations connected therewith, extending over a period of eight years, we have used in correspondence nearly a hundred thousand letters and have personally visited most of the States in the Union, some of them several times, made repeated excursions into the Provinces of Quebec and Ontario and also visited Mexico."

Another source of Morgan pedigrees which Colonel Battell used extensively were the records of the American Trotting horse, of which the Morgan was then considered a family. He also consulted the

American Saddle Horse Register, where much of the foundation stock was Morgan or part Morgan.

OFFICIALLY A BREED

The publication of Volume I, which gave a history of the breed for the first one hundred years, stimulated much interest and enthusiasm among admirers and breeders of Morgans of the period. The Colonel encouraged all Morgan owners to trace and register the pedigrees of their horses. So contagious was his enthusiasm and so rewarding were his efforts that they resulted in Volume II being published in 1905. This volume was a supplement to Volume I and included many new pedigrees. The work of Joseph Battell had begun to bear fruit, and the Morgan was being preserved and perpetuated as a definite breed—not merely as an offshoot of another.

In 1909 several dedicated breeders and supporters of the Morgan horse called together as many owners as could come to a meeting, with the purpose of organizing a Morgan club. They met, sixty strong, on September 23, 1909, at the Vermont State Fair in White River Junction, Vermont. Here the purposes of The Morgan Horse Club were outlined and subscribed to by all. A president, Henry S. Wardner, and a secretary-treasurer, C. C. Stillman, were chosen at this time, with plans being made for a future meeting when a constitution and by-laws could be adopted.

Thirty-one attended the second meeting held at Hartford, Vermont, on November 27, 1909. The constitution and by-laws were subsequently voted in and the election of a board of fifteen governors and five vice-presidents took place.

Impact of the Club

For several years the newly organized club held an annual meeting at the Vermont State Fair. The meetings were paralleled by a great showing of Morgan horses at each fair. In 1909, 90 were entered for the show, but each year thereafter brought out added numbers of fine animals until reportedly there were 180 entries in 1914.

It seemed that the Morgan was on firm footing as a breed and on its way, at last. Membership in the club reached a high point of 289 in 1914, with the majority of members residing in New England. Many of those early members were men who had known Morgans all their lives, from the time when the Morgan held an enviable

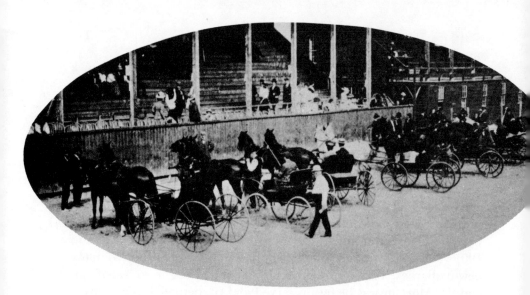

Judging matched teams at a Vermont State Fair.

position on the harness tracks and during the period when they were popular and outstanding Roadsters.

The 1917 meeting at the Vermont State Fair and its attendant fine showing of Morgans turned out to be the last one of its caliber for a number of years. However, after an absence of two years (during World War I) when the meetings and the shows were resumed, nothing seemed the same and a drastic decline was in evidence from previous years. The automobile had honked the Roadsters from the highways and the harness horse had followers only among the die-hards. Only *five* members attended the annual meeting in White River in 1925, a far cry from the prewar days of 1914. It seemed then as though the Morgan had really come to the end of the road this time. Colonel Battell's tireless efforts on behalf of the breed had been terminated by his death in 1915 just as his third volume of the Morgan *Register* was about ready for publication.

The Register *Revived*

Middlebury College in Vermont, receiving the *Register* as part of Colonel Battell's estate, completed the publication of Volume III. Then C. C. Stillman, the original secretary-treasurer of The Morgan Horse Club and a noted breeder of Morgans, purchased the *Register* from the college and incorporated it as The American Morgan Horse Register, Inc., with Colonel Battell's works as the first three volumes.

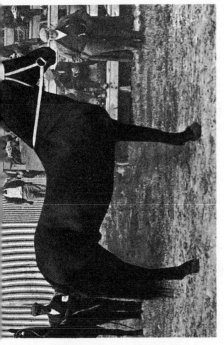
Bobby B.

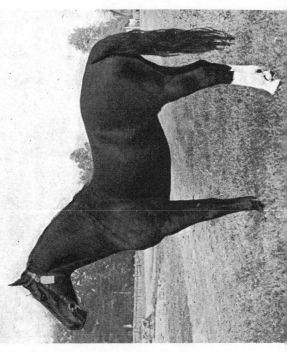
Scotland.

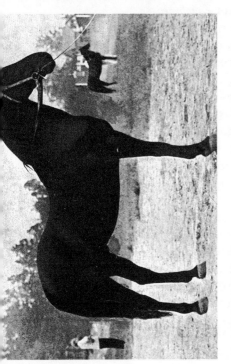
Bob Morgan.

Noted stallions circa 1910.

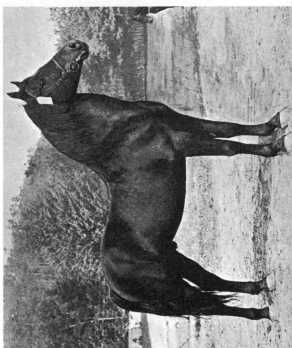
Prince Charlie.

In Volume III all the stallions of the first three volumes were assigned numbers. It was also Mr. Stillman who published Volume IV in 1921. This volume included registrations recorded from about 1912 to 1920.

In 1921, which marked the one-hundredth anniversary of Justin Morgan's death, Mr. Stillman, personally bearing the full cost, presented to the United States Department of Agriculture the beautiful statue of Justin Morgan, in behalf of The Morgan Horse Club. The fine statue by sculptor Frederick Roth stands now, as it stood then, on the grounds of the Morgan Horse Farm in Weybridge, near Middlebury, Vermont.

Mr. Stillman died in August 1926 after having devoted so much of himself toward the perpetuation of the Morgan, and the club lost yet another dedicated admirer. He had not only carried on the work of the *Register* but had maintained offices for the club at his own expense in New York City. His death left a great void, for the members had relied on Mr. Stillman to carry out much of the work of the club.

Club and Register *Combined*

His successor, Charles A. Stone, along with the other directors, felt that the club should properly own and carry on its register—which until that time it had not done. Since the *Register* had been set up as a corporation and the club had no corporate entity, being only an informal society, it was necessary to incorporate the club before it could receive the assets of the *Register* from the Stillman estate.

In August 1927 at the regular annual meeting, a plan, developed by Charles Stone, was presented to incorporate the Morgan club itself. Then, with acceptance of the assets of the *Register* corporation, that corporation would be dissolved as such and would become a part of The Morgan Horse Club, Inc. A committee was formed and on November 1, 1927, the club became incorporated and subsequently the *Register* became an integral part of The Morgan Horse Club, Inc., and subject to control by the membership.

It was a few years after this took place that the breeding of Morgans fell to its lowest point. In 1933 there were only seventy-eight registrations of horses and sixty-three transfers of ownership, and paid membership numbered only a scant fifty-two. However, a change for the better took place from the year 1934 on through World War II, when the general interest in pleasure riding gave many breeds of light horses the much-needed impetus.

In 1941, Charles Stone, who had been an active member and served as a director and officer since 1912, passed away, leaving yet another serious vacancy in the club roster. Like Mr. Stillman before him, Mr. Stone had also provided the club with office facilities in New York for the club work. Whitney Stone, club treasurer, followed the generous example of his father and continued to provide the offices for the club's business. Thereafter Frank B. Hills, secretary and registrar since 1931, continued to serve in this capacity until his passing in March 1961.

By the early 1940s the Morgan breed had made huge strides. In 1941, 402 horses were registered, as compared with only 78 eight years earlier, and membership in the club had tripled. Interest in the breed was in evidence from many different parts of the country. By 1947, registrations reached their highest point since the club was founded, with 697 horses registered and membership up to almost 300. Each year since then has brought ever-increasing registrations and club activities.

The Magazine

A breed magazine was introduced by Owen Moon of Woodstock, Vermont, in 1941. An officer of the club, Mr. Moon published the first number, called the *Morgan Horse Bulletin,* at his own expense. With the fourth issue the name was changed to *The Morgan Horse Magazine.*

Mr. Moon published the magazine with success until his death in 1947, when the publication was presented to The Morgan Horse Club by Mrs. Moon. With news and pictures of Morgan activities and articles of interest about the breed, the magazine was, and continues to be, very instrumental in introducing the Morgan horse and his virtues to a wide audience.

The Local Groups

Soon The Morgan Horse Club—with affiliated local clubs springing up all over America, and even in Canada—had attained the position envisioned by its founders. With membership climbing from the dismal low of less than forty in 1927 to thirty-five hundred in 1960, the club and the breed have advanced enormously over the years. Today, known as the American Morgan Horse Association, the parent body has a membership of more than ten thousand. And allied societies have been founded in Canada, Great Britain and Sweden to date.

The British Morgan Horse Society, with a growing membership, was founded in 1975 by Angela Conner of London and Hereford, England. With much dedicated effort, the membership has established the Morgan horse as a viable entity in the United Kingdom.

The success of the American Morgan Horse Association and the local groups—indeed the growing popularity of the Morgan horse—can be said to owe much to the dedicated men who have stood by it these many years. Since the inception of the club these men have, through faith and affection for the Morgan, given of themselves in both time and money to support the club in all its efforts. We are all very much indebted to: Colonel Battell, whose lifelong research made possible the founding of the *Register;* to C. C. Stillman, through whose help The Morgan Horse Club was organized and Volume IV was published; and certainly to Charles A. Stone and his son, Whitney Stone, who reorganized the club for the purpose of ownership and perpetuation of the *Register.*

To quote the late Frank Hills, who served the club so well as secretary and registrar for many years: "With this foundation, future generations must certainly carry on the good work, endeavor to improve the breed of Morgan horses and widen the circle of those who will have pleasure in their ownership and use."

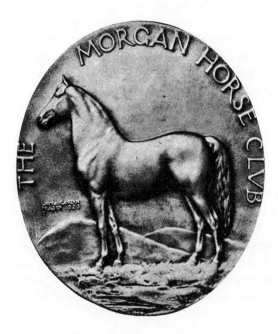

THE MORGAN HORSE FARM

After the turn of the century, despite the efforts of a few dedicated breeders, the Morgan horse was, as a breed, on extremely precarious footing. Indeed, the Morgan was almost on the brink of extinction, being sidelined by the advent of the automobile and the rise of the Standardbred horse. Therefore, the government of the United States, maintaining an experiment station at Burlington, Vermont, to test the breeding and feeding of livestock, was urged to step in to try to save the Morgan.

The first suggestion that the Department of Agriculture take over this work was made by Senator Redfield Proctor, chairman of the Senate Committee on Agriculture in 1904. In the fall of 1905, the breeding of Morgans was arranged at the experiment station farm, and the first purchases of Morgan stock took place in June 1906, when a board of competent men acquired seven mares and two fillies to be used in the government's work; the mares were in foal when purchased or were bred immediately thereafter.

AS A FEDERAL VENTURE

The aim of the project at the time was to produce true Morgan type, with stress also on an increase in size and quality over that sometimes in evidence in the old Morgans. However, type was to be adhered to and not sacrificed to size, as had happened previously. The department advertised for mares as follows: "They should be from 5 to 8 years old, and standing 15.1–15.3 hands and weighing 1000–1150 pounds. Colors preferred: Brown, bay, chestnut. Grays not to be submitted for inspection unless exceptional individuals. Mares submitted for inspection should be sound, with good conformation, style and action and a pure trotting gait. They should be well bred along Morgan lines, but registration in the American Morgan Horse Register will not be necessary."

It is interesting to note that the government considered the over-15-hand horse more desirable in the proposed breeding program despite the fact that many of the best examples of the early Morgans were under this height. This was soon to be a sore point with some of the old Vermont breeders, and they criticized the Department of Agriculture for what they considered failure to produce the true or "ancient" (as it was sometimes called) type.

Of the mares purchased in Vermont only three were not registered

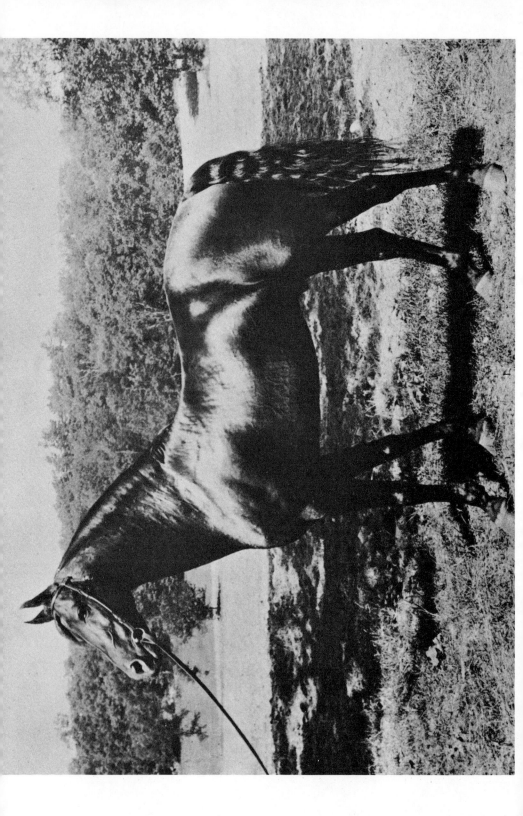

or eligible to be recorded in the Morgan *Register*. But the real trouble came when the Department of Animal Industry brought back from Kentucky two mares sired by the illustrious Harrison Chief, a registered American Saddlebred. Both mares through their dams traced to Morgan blood, however, and their purchase was an experiment to determine whether or not a careful outcross to the blood of Harrison Chief would produce the desired increase in size and the quality without loss of the Morgan type.

The uproar among Morgan breeders caused by the Kentucky purchase brought down upon the heads of the department much acid criticism. One comment was that the department was attempting to restore the Morgan by the same method that had been used to destroy it, namely the outcrossing to other blood. The department retaliated by pointing out that the bloodlines of the Kentucky mares were established from Morgan foundation stock brought to Kentucky from New England farms. They also argued that the outcross to Saddleblood was far different from the crossing to the Standardbred which was done earlier when speed was the sole objective and type was lightly considered, if at all. However, the department was content to let the Kentucky experiment stand as planned.

The Move to Weybridge

In 1907, through the great generosity of Colonel Joseph Battell, the United States Government was presented with his 400-acre Breadloaf Farm in Weybridge (near Middlebury), Vermont, for the perpetuation and improvement of the Morgan horse. The stock from the Vermont Experimental Station at Burlington was taken to the Battell farm in the latter part of 1907, and at the donor's request Breadloaf Farm became officially known as The United States Morgan Horse Farm. In 1908 Colonel Battell donated another tract of land adjoining the farm, and in 1917 nearly 500 adjoining acres were purchased. Today the farm consists of 942.5 acres, divided into meadows, pastureland and woods. There are thirty-five buildings on the land and a half-million feet of timber.

General Gates and His Get

The foundation stud of the government farm was General Gates 666, foaled May 6, 1894, and bred by Colonel Battell. A black without any white markings, General Gates stood 14.3 hands, weighed 1,000 pounds and was a fine, impressive horse. He was sired by Denning Allen 74, a son of Honest Allen and a grandson of the great Ethan Allen 50.

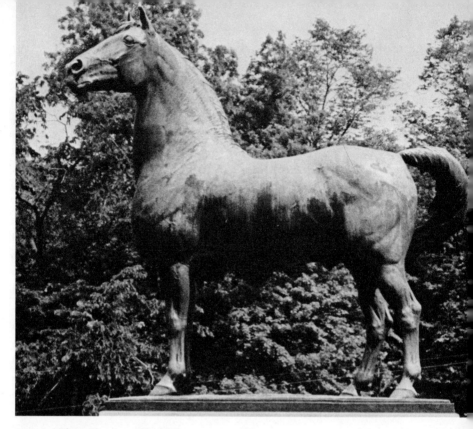

Statue of Justin Morgan at Weybridge.

His dam was Fanny Scott, who was by the noted Thoroughbred Revenue, Jr., and out of a mare by the old Morgan Copperbottom. A full brother to Lord Clinton, whose trotting record was 2:10¼, General Gates was the head of the government farm until he died in 1920.

Although admitted to be an excellent horse, General Gates was the object of much criticism because of his other-than-Morgan blood, the more vitriolic calling him a mongrel and no more than a half-bred Morgan. This reaction may have had some justification, but men of the time who were well acquainted with old Black Hawk 20 declared that General Gates resembled the famous son of Sherman Morgan to a remarkable degree. As far as the Thoroughbred cross in General Gates' pedigree is concerned, it needs little defense when you consider that, according to the best information available, Justin Morgan himself had much more Thoroughbred blood than General Gates and that even old Black Hawk's dam, as far as can be determined, was a "half-bred" mare.

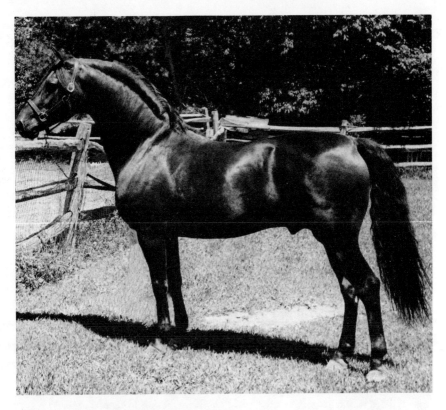

Modern Morgan's resemblance to Justin Morgan.

The purchase of General Gates to head the government stud, despite the disparaging remarks made at the time, has proved to be a successful venture and few can deny at this later date that the work of The United States Morgan Horse Farm has been the backbone of Morgan horse production since the breeding program's inception. General Gates was purchased after much careful consideration and the selection was made not only because he himself was a fine individual of the modern Morgan type but also because his offspring possessed his outstanding conformation and were easily recognized as being sired by him. He epitomized the type of Morgan that the government felt would best suit the modern markets, where the demand had shifted somewhat from the harness to the saddle horse.

Some of the early Morgans had a tendency toward coarseness, with round withers and low backs. Unfortunately, there also was in evidence a choppiness and irregularity of gait and occasionally a tendency to pace and mix gaits. The aim of the government farm was to attempt to eliminate these unfavorable characteristics of the breed while keeping its splendid conformation, spirit and endurance.

BENNINGTON

Probably General Gate's best-known son as far as today's breeders are concerned was Bennington 5693—although his sons Red Oak 5249 and Linsley 7233 also figure prominently in Western Morgan pedigrees, as the former went to Texas under the ownership of Richard Sellman, and the latter stood in Kansas.

Bennington, a bay foaled in 1908, was to become one of the most important factors in the government's line-breeding program. By General Gates and out of Mrs. Culvers (one of the mares purchased in Kentucky), he had his disparagers, because feeling was still much against the use of the Harrison Chief mare.

Harrison Chief was by Clark Chief 2993 (foaled 1861, bay, 16 hands) and was registered as a Trotting horse. However, because he

Bennington.

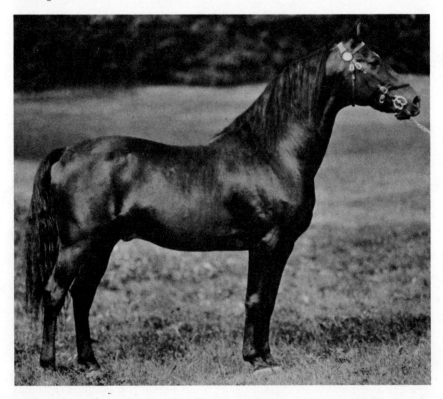

showed tremendous quality, he subsequently became a star of the show rings of the time. His dam, Lute Boyd, was a fine little show mare and a great-great-granddaughter of the famous Sir Archy, one of the finest Thoroughbreds ever imported to this country. She was one of Kentucky's best show mares, winning many championships even at an early age. Lute Boyd was bred to Clark Chief three times: the first resulting in a rather disappointing bay stud foal and the second in a bay filly which became one of the great Saddlebred foundation mares; her third foal was Harrison Chief. This stallion, a beautiful blood-bay, had eight brilliant seasons in the ring shown always in harness; it is said that it was unlikely that he ever wore a saddle in his life.

Harrison Chief had an exceedingly successful record at stud, siring some of the best Saddlebreds of that or any time. As mentioned earlier, the well-known Bourbon Chief and the great show mare Lou Chief were among the countless names to bring fame to their sire. Mrs. Culvers, therefore, combining the blood of Harrison Chief and that of Cabell's Lexington (sired by Gist's Black Hawk, a son of Black Hawk 20, and registered both as a Morgan and as an American Saddlebred) through her dam brought to the Morgan breed a generous share of beauty and show ability. It was pointed out by those furthering the cause of the government's breeding program that much of the blood that produced Justin Morgan himself flowed richly in the veins of these Kentucky-bred horses. Even many of their critics who had found such fault with government ideas on breeding Morgans soon came around and later were known to have referred to the government Morgans as "the proper type."

MANSFIELD AND ETHAN ALLEN 3RD

Bennington was not used extensively at the government farm until 1925, having been used mainly in the military horse breeding program for twelve to fifteen years. It was after he stood at stud at the farm that many felt much valuable time was lost by not using this horse sooner. His first foals at Weybridge came up to expectations and were to be the foundation of the line-breeding program carried on by the government there for almost thirty years. Bennington and his outstanding son Mansfield 7255 were both used extensively until the mid-'30s, when Mansfield carried on alone as the leading sire. This great chestnut headed the stud for twenty years and won championships virtually every time he was shown, as well as siring some of the most outstanding Morgans ever produced there.

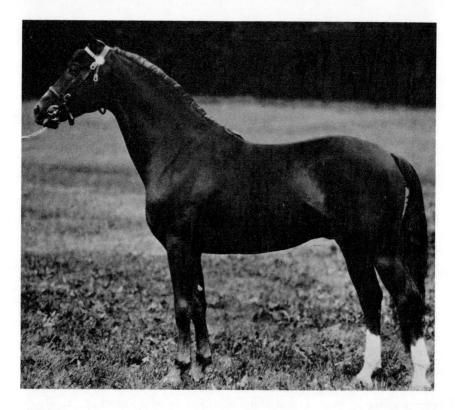

Mansfield.

Mansfield was foaled in 1920. One of the Morgan horse farm's most highly esteemed stallions in the opinion of just about everyone, he was out of Artemisia (chestnut, foaled 1909) who was by Ethan Allen 3rd. His dam's bloodlines show old Vermont breeding at its best, for she traced in male line to Hale's Green Mountain Morgan and Gifford Morgan, and her dam was by Bob Morgan (by Ethan Allen 2nd), a stallion of excellent type and breeding. Ethan Allen 3rd (Borden's) was by Ethan Allen 2nd and out of a granddaughter of old Green Mountain Morgan. He was described by one of his owners as having a remarkably gentle disposition and his style and action were likened to a Hackney. This same style and action have come down through this line of breeding to the present day. A son of Ethan Allen 3rd, Sir Ethan Allen 6537, was twice Grand Champion Morgan Stallion at the Vermont State Fair, and his son Sealect was reserve to him there in 1922. Cornwallis, a son of Sealect, displayed the same high-headed, sprightly action of this line.

Bennington

General Gates
- Denning Allen
  - Honest Allen
    - Ethan Allen 50 by Black Hawk by Sherman
    - chestnut mare, s.t.b.* by Brooks Horse by Sherman
  - Rena, s.t.b.* by Ward's Flying Cloud by Black Hawk by Sherman
- Fanny Scott
  - Revenue Jr.
  - mare by Copperbottom

Mrs. Culvers
- Harrison Chief
  - Clark Chief by Mambrino Chief
  - Lute Boyd
- Billie
  - Cabell's Lexington
    - Gist's Black Hawk by Blood's Black Hawk
    - dam, s.t.b.* by Tom Hal by Sorrel Tom
  - mare by Copperbottom

*said to be

QUERIDO, ULYSSES AND CANFIELD

Mansfield's full brothers, Querido 7370, Ulysses 7565 and Canfield 7788, went on to make names for themselves as well, and their get were in great demand the country over, such was their excellence. Querido, foaled in 1923, went to California and has gone down in Morgan history as the sire of qualified stock horses. He was used for many years by Roland Hill on his Horse-Shoe Cattle Company Ranch; and Sonfield, by Mansfield out of Quietude by Troubadour of Willowmoor, followed Querido in producing working stock horses for ranch use.

Ulysses, foaled in 1927 and Grand Champion in 1932 and 1939, if he had done nothing more than sire the great Ulendon 7831, would still have his niche in the Morgan Hall of Fame. Ulendon, the black stallion foaled in 1933, has been a champion himself and the sire and grandsire of champion after champion down to the present day. Orcland Leader, out of Vigilda Burkland, and his full brother Orcland Vigildon—Grand Champions in their own right—are two of Ulendon's outstanding sons. One could go on to great lengths describing the show records chalked up by the sons and daughters of old Ulendon.

Canfield was foaled in 1932 and although not the sire of so lengthy a list of champions, had the Grand Champion Stallion Panfield to his credit, who in turn sired the Grand Champion Mare Symphonee. Panfield was used in the breeding program of the University of Connecticut. Many of Canfield's progeny have been noted for their fine gaits and endurance.

Results Achieved

The Morgans bred at the government farm have repeatedly met the demands of breeders and single buyers alike. Their varied abilities have proved the worth of their background and pedigree. Almost every important breeder of Morgans in the country has horses of government farm bloodlines and it is certainly safe to say that, whether pro or con, General Gates, Bennington, Mansfield and their get are stallions who have had a marked effect on the Morgan of today.

On the bridle path and trail, government-farm-bred Morgans have racked up impressive records through the years. In the records of the old 300-Mile Endurance Rides and the 100-Mile Trail Ride (see Chapter 11) in Woodstock, Vermont, the names of farm-bred Morgans appear frequently. Old Castor 5833, an 800-pound son of Gen-

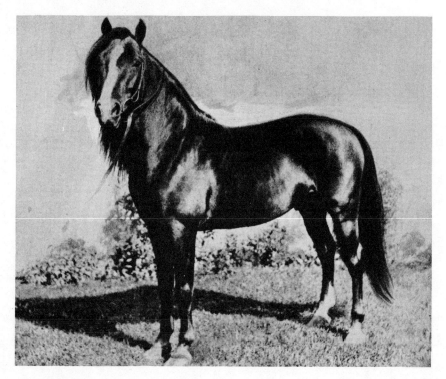

Ethan Allen 3rd.

eral Gates, made quite a reputation for himself in the early '20s on the endurance rides, as did the gelding Gladstone 6922, his paternal half-brother.

Mansfield's get in later years also carried high the government farm banner: Friendly, by Mansfield out of a Bennington mare, won the Lightweight Division of the 100-Mile Trail Ride in 1942 and '43; and Lippitt Morman, out of the well-known mare Lippitt Kate Moro, became the first stallion to win a division of the ride: he won the Heavyweight in 1945 and the following year the Sweepstakes. Cassandra, another mare by Mansfield, also was an outstanding trail-ride contestant.

In the show ring the records of government farm Morgans are too numerous to list here, for all through the years the Weybridge-bred horses have showered the farm with honors. It is easy to see from the many winnings of Troubadour of Willowmoor 6459 to the Morgans that carried on, Panfield, Mentor, Tutor and Trophy—to

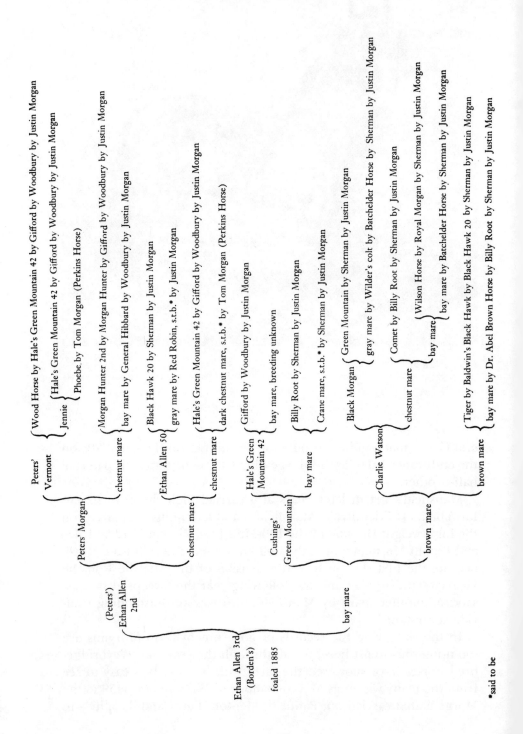

Ethan Allen 3rd (Borden's) foaled 1885

(Peters') Ethan Allen 2nd

Peters' Morgan
— Peters' Vermont
  — Wood Horse by Hale's Green Mountain 42 by Gifford by Woodbury by Justin Morgan
  — Jennie
    — Hale's Green Mountain 42 by Gifford by Woodbury by Justin Morgan
    — Phoebe by Tom Morgan (Perkins Horse)
— chestnut mare
  — Morgan Hunter 2nd by Morgan Hunter by Gifford by Woodbury by Justin Morgan
  — bay mare by General Hibbard by Woodbury by Justin Morgan

chestnut mare
— Ethan Allen 50
  — Black Hawk 20 by Sherman by Justin Morgan
  — gray mare by Red Robin, s.t.b.* by Justin Morgan
— chestnut mare
  — Hale's Green Mountain 42 by Gifford by Woodbury by Justin Morgan
  — dark chestnut mare, s.t.b.* by Tom Morgan (Perkins Horse)

bay mare
— Cushings' Green Mountain
  — Hale's Green Mountain 42
    — Gifford by Woodbury by Justin Morgan
    — bay mare, breeding unknown
  — bay mare
    — Billy Root by Sherman by Justin Morgan
    — Crane mare, s.t.b.* by Sherman by Justin Morgan
— brown mare
  — Charlie Watson
    — Black Morgan
      — Green Mountain by Sherman by Justin Morgan
      — gray mare by Wilder's colt by Batchelder Horse by Sherman by Justin Morgan
    — chestnut mare
      — Comet by Billy Root by Sherman by Justin Morgan
      — bay mare
        — Wilson Horse by Royal Morgan by Sherman by Justin Morgan
        — bay mare by Batchelder Horse by Sherman by Justin Morgan
  — brown mare
    — Tiger by Baldwin's Black Hawk by Black Hawk 20 by Sherman by Justin Morgan
    — bay mare by Dr. Abel Brown Horse by Billy Root by Sherman by Justin Morgan

*said to be

mention only a few—that the government farm blood has perpetuated outstanding Morgans and so has kindled the public's interest in a breed that had come dangerously close to disappearing.

Earl Krantz as Superintendent

The superintendent of the government farm for a great many years until his retirement in June 1951 was Earl B. Krantz, a veteran horseman of the United States Department of Agriculture. A native of Nebraska, Mr. Krantz was graduated from Iowa State College in 1915 with a degree in animal husbandry and received a Master of Science degree in this subject from Washington State College the following year. Research work with horses in Washington, D.C.; Laramie, Wyoming; and Miles City, Montana, culminated in his taking the post at the Morgan farm in April 1928.

He was recognized as a national authority on horses, especially the light breeds, and managed the Weybridge farm so capably that it was brought to a point of international recognition, attracting widespread interest among Morgan breeders. Always maintaining that the modern Morgan must be bred for the saddle to be suitable for present-day demands, Mr. Krantz spent his years on the farm developing the breeding program which has successfully produced Morgans with size, ability and endurance while preserving type. That this breeding program has had a dominant influence on Morgan horse production throughout the country can be seen by the number of Morgans of government farm breeding which are carrying on in the show ring, on the trail and at stud.

In 1941 under Mr. Krantz's direction, the Bureau of Animal Industry began conducting performance tests on three-year-old Morgans for the purpose of determining the characteristics associated with performance, and whether these characteristics are inherited and can therefore be used in the selection of breeding stock. The object of the experiment, carried on for ten years, was to correlate the horse's physique with its ability to do useful work.

The three types of performance studied were speed, endurance and ease of riding. Many characteristics were measured or scored for each horse so that associations between them and performance could be determined. Under his direction, sixty-eight 3-year-old Morgans, raised and trained on the farm, were used in this experiment. They were sired by eight different stallions and ranged from two to twenty-five offspring per sire. Included among these were six stallions, twenty geldings and forty-two mares.

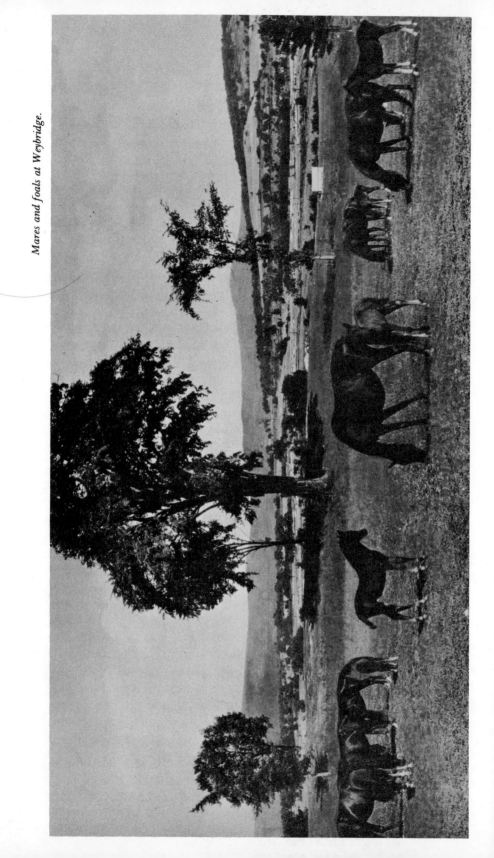

Mares and foals at Weybridge.

Fascinating results were obtained from these tests, which were scored on general conformation, style and beauty, quality and other characteristics; action at the walk and trot, as well as endurance, recuperative powers and comfort to the rider at various gaits. The relationship between conformation and various other desirable characteristics was measured and recorded under Mr. Krantz's direction. The results were valuable to all light-horse breeds.

VERMONT TAKES OVER

Despite all the good work accomplished by The United States Morgan Horse Farm, the government in December 1950 voted to discontinue funds for the farm's operation at the end of the fiscal year. Funds were offered and provided by private sources until the legislature of the state of Vermont could consider a proposal for the state to take over the farm.

In January 1951, after the General Assembly of Vermont had decided in favor of continuing the operation, a dispersal was ordered because the state did not choose to maintain the complete herd. Reserving twenty mares and four stallions to be used on the farm, which was to be run by the University of Vermont and the State College of Agriculture, the other stock—eleven mares and sixteen stallions—were offered to the public for sale by sealed bid. However, four Eastern universities were granted horses to aid in their respective Morgan breeding programs. They were: University of Massachusetts, eleven mares and fillies and two stallions; University of Connecticut, four mares and one stallion; University of New Hampshire, two mares; University of Pennsylvania, two mares.

When the 398 bids were opened on January 3, 1951, it was obvious that the public was well impressed by Morgans of government farm breeding, if the prices these horses brought were any indication. The top-priced horse of the sale was the good three-year-old mare Riviera, a daughter of Mentor, who went to Nelson White for $2,525. Another daughter of Mentor, a four-year-old named Quakerlady, brought $1,751, and went to Pennsylvania State College. Panfield, among the stallions, went to Kansas for the price of $1,600. These prices, for the time, were impressive.

The United States Government officially turned over the farm to the University of Vermont on July 1, 1951, and this institution has successfully continued the work to which Mr. Krantz devoted so much of his life and talents.

Students at UVM—as the university is called—work with, feed, fit and show the Morgans. In addition, annual Morgan Horse Judging Schools have been held at Weybridge since 1954, for the benefit of horse lovers, breeders and professional judges. Riding clubs and 4-H light-horse groups also come for information to the farm, whose demonstrations have proved of great value to the area. Besides all those dyed-in-the-wool fanciers, many thousands of people from all over the country have visited the farm to see the Morgans.

More Records

With UVM management the farm has continued its winning ways at the shows as well as in the production of fine Morgans. From the days of Ulysses, Mentor, Tutor and Cantor to today's stars, UVM has continued the traditions of producing outstanding Morgans. Under the direction of Dr. Donald J. Balch, the UVM farm has had many winners at the shows and provided highly regarded breeding stock throughout the country. Most notable of the farm's stars has been UVM Promise. A fantastic show horse himself, Promise has sired an extremely large number of winners. UVM Flash, UVM Watchman

Mentor.

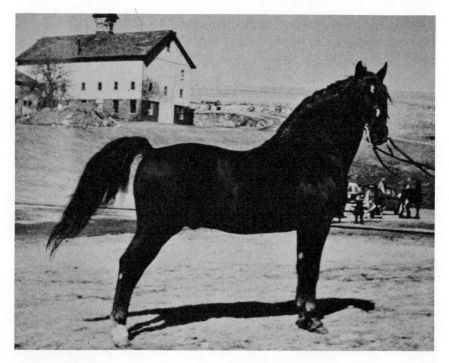

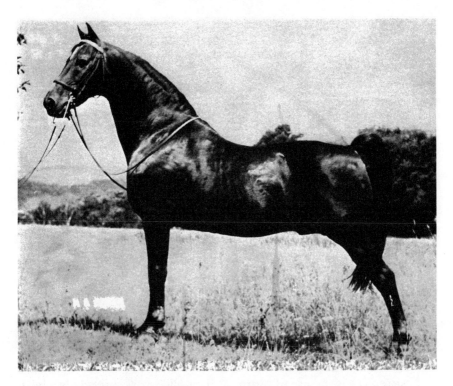

Trophy, the government-bred sire of distinction, a son of Mentor.

and UVM Elite are a few other familiar stallion names from the Vermont farm. And UVM mares figure in successful pedigrees everywhere!

More Interest

Although the show records and the scores of ribbons hanging in the barn office indicate the farm's avid interest in the exhibition of their stock, nevertheless the production of Pleasure horses is equally important. The Morgan endurance and disposition is evidently known on a world-wide scale among horsemen, as buyers from as far afield as Peru, China, Puerto Rico and Israel have had Morgans shipped to their respective countries. In 1947 Magellen, a government-farm stallion, headed a group of twenty-five Morgans to be shipped across the sea to Nationalist China to bolster the cavalry stock there. What became of the horses after the fall of the mainland to the Communists is anybody's guess, but it is reported that two of the Morgans were recognized during the Korean War—and that one of them was Magellen, being ridden by a Chinese Communist general: a strange fate for a Yankee stallion from New England!

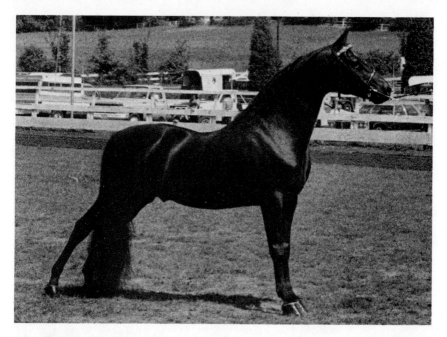

UVM Promise.

Less remote is the use of Morgans for police work, especially where mounted officers are "on show." This equable, competent and striking breed is represented on several metropolitan police forces, including the United States Park Police in the nation's capital.

The demands for Morgans pour into the office of the farm at Weybridge in increasing numbers as the years go by, valid proof that the work of the federal government in perpetuating the breed and the continuing efforts of the University of Vermont have been greatly appreciated and highly successful. To quote Dr. Donald Balch, "We cannot begin to satisfy the calls for Morgans, though we raise from twelve to fifteen foals a year, and the demand for mature animals which are trained or even partially trained is tremendous."

Professor Balch is optimistic about the farm's future, although at times recently it looked as if the state of Vermont would vote to discontinue the farm. Letters of encouragement and enthusiasm for the farm's value to the College of Agriculture as well as to the Morgan breed poured in from all parts of the country in hopes to dissuade the legislators from abandoning the operation of the farm. It is fervently hoped that soon continuation will be definitely and permanently assured—especially since the 1961 General Assembly voted to make the Morgan horse Vermont's official state animal.

Meanwhile, the heroic statue of Justin Morgan, symbol of years of

Morgan horse breeding at Weybridge, stands above the sweeping green fields where foals in its image play beside their dams. The neat white barn, which rang with the hoofbeats of General Gates and Bennington and Mansfield, bears on its worn wooden floors the imprints of newer champions. And it is the earnest wish of Morgan admirers everywhere that the sound of horses' feet will never cease to echo in the shadow of their patriarch, Justin Morgan.

A rare photograph gives today's Morgan enthusiasts a glimpse of Ethan Allen 3rd 3987 in action.

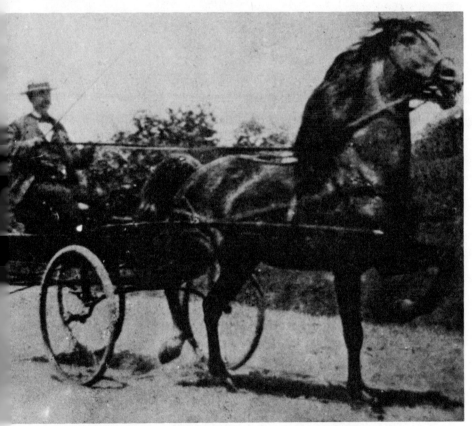

5

Growing Pains
and Breeders' Guidelines

W HEN JUSTIN Morgan trod the earth in the early 1800s, folks found him able to handle just about any task despite his diminutive size. Yet many even in that day voiced the opinion that he and his descendants were too small and that they would be even more valuable if, with their other qualities, they "came in a larger size."

Of course, there was a decided variation in size in the early Morgans, as can be noted by a short perusal of the Morgan *Register*. Still, the best-type Morgans of the time were those which were not too large. An increase in size brought about by the use of outside blood from the mid-1800s to the present century proved to be detrimental to the Morgan, as many breeders were to learn. But since they were probably not so concerned with Morgan type as with Morgan aptitude, they outcrossed to cold blood for farm teams and to Messenger blood for trotting speed. The practice may have been frowned upon or not, but it continued nevertheless. It is a wonder that the Morgan breed ever survived during the days of the establishment of the Standardbred, for the demand for size as well as for trotting speed nearly proved the undoing of the Morgan.

Here would be a good place to pause for a quick rundown of the rules for admission to the Morgan *Register*. In Volume I (1894) "any animal in either of the following classes" were eligible for registry: "RULE I—Any meritorious stallion or mare that traces in direct male line to the original Justin Morgan Horse, and has at least *one sixty-fourth* of his blood [italics mine]"; and "RULE II—The produce of a sire and dam both registered in The Morgan Register."

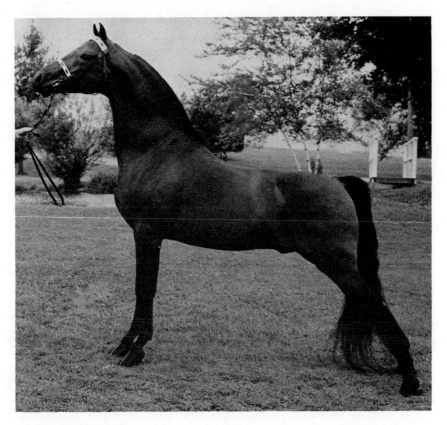

Morgan stallion of today.

However, by 1905, when Volume II came out and breeders had had a decade to reconsider the leniency allowed in the matter of outside blood, the regulations were tightened somewhat: Rule I allowed registry to "any meritorious stallion, mare or gelding that traces in direct male line to Justin Morgan, and has at least one sixty-fourth of his blood: provided the dam and sire's dam were bred in approved speed or roadster lines."

Rule II granted eligibility to "any meritorious stallion, mare or gelding having *one thirty-second or more* [italics mine] of the blood of Justin Morgan: provided the sire and dam were bred in approved speed or roadster lines." Rule III repeated the second criterion laid down in 1894, i.e., that the produce of a sire and dam both carried in the *Register* was eligible.

The 1905 Rule II was rescinded as of January 1, 1948. Since then an X preceding a number in the *Register* indicates an inclusion prior to 1948 under this old rule, which allowed some animals to be registered although one parent was not itself registered in the AMHR. As can be seen readily, this rescinding really "closed the books," for subsequently only foals of registered Morgan sires and out of registered Morgan dams have been eligible for the AMHR.

In the darkest days of the breed—the early 1900s—with the appearance of the automobile and the subsequent disappearance of the harness road horse, the Morgan again was dealt a serious setback. Only the efforts of a few dedicated breeders and the U.S. Department of Agriculture's Morgan farm in Vermont saved the breed at all.

Older breeders of the Morgan objected heatedly to the government farm's use of Saddleblood, saying that the harm done outweighed the fact that Morgans were increasing in both popularity and numbers. The farm retaliated with the declaration that the Morgan was improved by the controlled quantity of outside blood. They felt that Morgan character was being retained in a modified form and that the twentieth-century markets were no longer dictating the raising of speedy road horses or harness-race horses—the automobile quelled the one and the Standardbred the other.

As mentioned earlier, it was the differences of opinion over the outcrossing to Saddleblood that caused the first split in Morgan ranks, the proponents of the old type objecting to Saddleblood, the backers of the so-called new type accusing them, in turn, of being unrealistic.

This situation has come down to the present day with varying intensity. With the rescinding in 1948 of Rule II (which, as we have seen, allowed horses of unknown or other than Morgan blood to be included in the *Register*), it seemed that the situation would smooth itself out, as no further outside blood could legally be introduced into the breed. But many felt that irreparable damage had already been done.

As for the matter of size, it would seem that, all things considered, any Morgan which fit the description in the Standard of Perfection (see pages 147–148) and was within the 14.1 to 15.2 height would not be too highly criticized, yet often there are great objections to Morgans which stand over 15.3 hands. The reason for this, possibly, is the fact that many individuals which are way over 15 hands lack the other characteristics of the breed as well. From this the trouble stems, and the ideal in height was set within 14.1 to 15.2. The majority of breeders feel that 14.3 is the ideal height and many have a tendency to lean more toward the 15-hand mark rather than the 14. Many

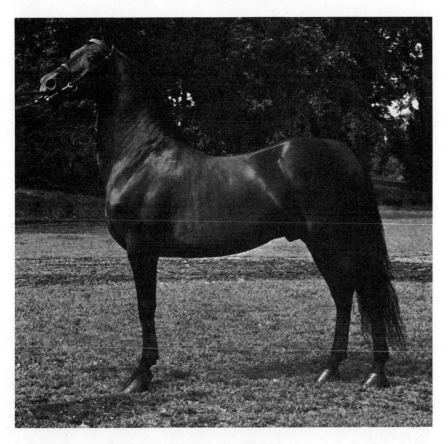

Morgan stallion showing high head carriage and refinement.

excellent-type individuals have been produced in recent years, however, which stand over 15 hands and still retain the best Morgan
characteristics.

On the touchy subject of type, it is best to say that most breeders
of Morgans, despite some variation, are aiming for the best possible
Morgans which are closest to the ideal in type as described in the
Standard of Perfection. That this is being accomplished by conscientious breeders can be seen at the horse shows where Morgans are
exhibited, and on the stock farms, too.

With all outside blood now ruled out, Morgans bred *with thought
and care* cannot help but return to the basic type of old Justin, with
modern-day variations necessary for today's markets. Even in the last
few years since Rule II was rescinded, Morgans are being raised that
are superior in a great many ways to some of the early ones. They
have quality and refinement as well as the character of the old type,

and the best individuals show a successful blending of the old and the new.

Conformation, as any horseman knows, is at least as important as type in any breed. Good conformation is essential. If a horse—any horse of any breed—has a definite weakness in conformation, he should be overlooked as a breeding animal, regardless of whether he is "typy" or "showy." Breeding animals with *glaring* conformation faults is just ordering trouble no matter the pedigree. Never be sold on a stallion or mare that you wish to use for breeding before carefully going over its conformation, and even if the pedigree shows the highest percentage of Justin's blood, beware if conformation faults are in evidence.

If a horse is structurally sound and shows no serious weakness he is a much better bet in a breeding program than one with type and a number of obvious weaknesses which he is likely to transmit. Too

Morgan mare of today.

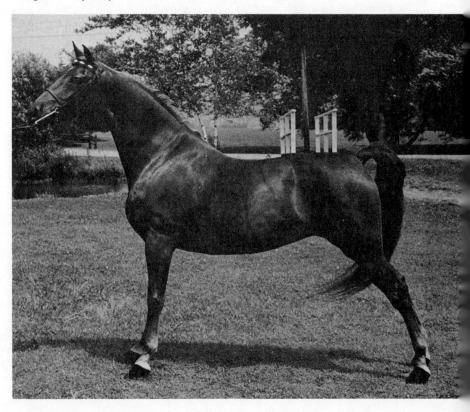

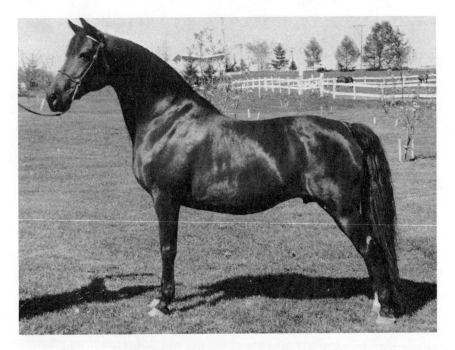

Morgan broodmare of excellent type.

much stress on pedigree and surface beauty without careful consideration of conformation will undermine many a breeding program.

Most Morgans of today can be said to have just about 10 percent of the blood of Justin Morgan. A few may have 12 percent, but anything over 14 percent is very rare indeed. Yet there are breeders who insist that a high percentage of Justin Morgan blood is a virtual guarantee that the animal *must* be superior to one less endowed. High-percentage Morgans descend from only one early strain: that of Hale's Green Mountain, carried via Ethan Allen 3rd, whose hey-day was the 1890s and among whose ancestors—not including Justin, Sherman and Woodbury—were Gifford, Hale's Green Mountain, Peters' Vermont, Black Hawk, Ethan Allen I (50), Billy Root, Royal Morgan and Vermont Morgan Champion. With such a record it's perfectly safe to say that the best individuals come from this strain. However, it is most important not to discount the other strains, because it is entirely possible—indeed it has been accomplished—to get fine individuals from less royally bred lines.

It is a paradox, though, that occasionally the high-percentage Morgan can exhibit the certain coarseness in the head and throttle that is becoming more and more undesirable in modern Morgans. The animal is often comparatively small and, although possibly possessing type to a marked degree, is quite likely to lack the quality and refinement which is so sought-after nowadays. It is advisable to examine thoroughly any horse before purchasing him and there is no need to keep stressing the point here. But keeping in mind that it takes more than high percentage and pedigree to make a fine horse, look at the horse *first* and the papers afterwards! Pedigrees *are* important: certainly there is no argument there. But always bear in mind that it is a grave mistake to fall for the "percentage line" if the horse doesn't measure up to the true Morgan type promised by his papers.

Although of relatively small importance now, thirty-five years ago much had been discussed pertaining to the so-called X in modern Morgan pedigrees. As mentioned, the X beside a horse's name in a pedigree means that either one or both of its parents was of other than Morgan blood, i.e., either the blood of another registered breed or that of an unknown or a grade. Many horses were admitted into the *American Morgan Horse Register* that were of outside blood when Rule II was introduced. After 1948, when it was rescinded, the horses bred with this outside blood were given Xs by their names to denote that they were products of this outcrossing. An X can also be the result of a horse's being eligible for registration during this period but one whose owner failed to register.

Unless a few unscrupulous breeders, or those who fail to study the bloodlines of animals they employ for breeding, misuse the X in producing Morgans, it would seem that little harm can be done by the X at this time. Of course any concentration of the blood of animals which carry Xs is going to result in a loss of type and Morgan characteristics. In other words, if a breeder has several mares in his herd which have Xs in their pedigrees, and he keeps breeding them to stallions with a fair amount of outside blood, then it has to follow that loss of type will be the result. This did happen to some extent in certain strains and much of that intangible something that is known as the "Morgan look" was lost.

It is probably safe to say that the majority of breeders would prefer their Morgans to be of high-percentage blood, for they realize that true Morgan characteristics are produced through the concentration of this blood; but it is the wise breeder who selects carefully when mating animals of high-percentage pedigree because it is quite pos-

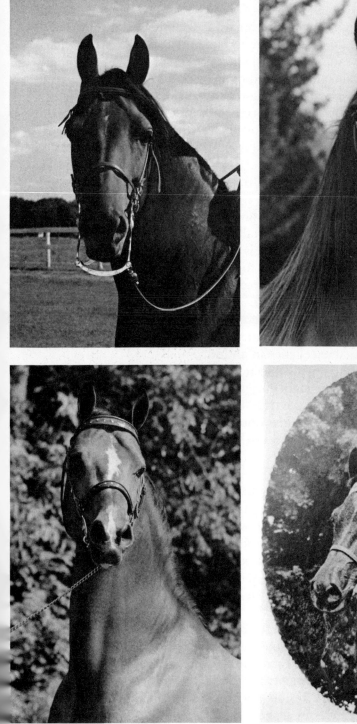

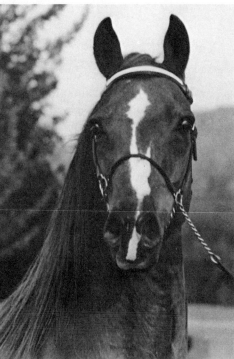

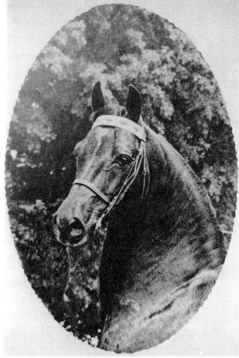

sible that even high-percentage horses have inherited a number of significant faults along with a generous measure of Morgan characteristics. As an example of this, say there is a fine high-percentage Morgan mare available for breeding. You like her looks in general but perhaps wish she had smaller ears and her bone was slightly flatter. She is basically a good Morgan, however, despite some coarseness about the head. Then you study her pedigree and find that there are several ancestors which have non-Morgan and unknown blood behind them. Perhaps the coarser characteristics the mare displays have been transmitted to her through her grandparents or great-grandparents, a few of which were grades. Realizing that she is likely to transmit some of these undesirable characteristics to her offspring, you would wisely breed her to a stallion dominantly excellent in these points—regardless of whether he is high percentage himself. It would be only folly to breed your mare to another high-percentage stallion merely because he was high percentage, if that stallion lacks, in a similar way, the refinement you wish to see in the foal. And yet it is surprising how often this has been done in the breeding of modern Morgans by people to whom fancy bloodlines on paper are more enticing than actual excellence in an individual.

In all breeds of horses in all sections of the country, there are some breeders who put their main emphasis on pedigree. The breeder of Thoroughbreds for the race track breeds speed to speed, as it were; and if the results look like greyhounds instead of horses, what does it matter so long as they are fast? Type and breed characteristics matter little. For many years the Palomino was bred strictly for color, with conformation secondary; likewise the Appaloosa. Other stockmen concentrate on breeding their horses for a special use: for working stock horses, for example, and the pedigree is secondary.

The best practice with Morgans would seem to be a practical blending of importance placed on pedigree, type, conformation and the future use the resulting foal will be put to.

Returning for a moment to the subject of the X in a Morgan pedigree, there is one well-known case where a whole strain of fine Morgans was virtually built around an X pedigree. The X in this particular example designated the blood of registered American Saddlebreds tracing to Morgan lineage. It is interesting to note that not all individuals in this particular family were ideal in Morgan type, and many resembled Morgans not at all; yet with certain crosses to other Morgan blood the results were horses which became consistent winners in Morgan classes at the shows. Careful selection, using this

Saddleblood judiciously, produced fine Morgan individuals which were winners in the ring under Morgan judges. A few members of this family lacked Morgan characteristics to a marked degree, while others were considered true in type. But in general the strain was, and is, noted for the quality and refinement it displays. A crossing of this blood with old Morgan blood seemed to have produced the best type for modern demands. A clear understanding of the reason for, and the meaning of, an X in a Morgan pedigree should result in Morgans of the modern type who will be good breeding prospects for the future despite their outside blood.

On the other hand, when dealing with Xs which designate unknown or grade blood (of no established breed), the controlling of its influence will be more difficult and often unsuccessful, because the breeder has no knowledge as to what traits might be recessive and could crop up in his foals from unknown ancestry. It is far easier to plan a breeding program when dealing with known factors than it is by using guesswork where the inheritance is doubtful. However, here again there are groups within the Morgan ranks who actually prefer to have any Xs which might be found in a Morgan pedigree designate a grade or unknown rather than have the so-called taint of Saddleblood there. This group has a dedicated following among some Morgan breeders, but the Morgans they produce are not necessarily any better than the ones produced by breeders who have wisely used the outcrossing to other recognized blood.

To sum up: Remember that high percentage is no *guarantee* of the excellence of an individual Morgan; that outside blood of a known breed (allowed by Rule II) has not "ruined" the breed and will **not** if handled wisely, and that the best rule to follow is to be selective and keep to the middle of the road and not veer off on a tangent either way!

STANDARD OF PERFECTION OF THE MORGAN HORSE

HEIGHT: 14.1 to 15.2 with 14.3 considered the ideal by many.

WEIGHT: 900 to 1,100 pounds.

GENERAL CONFORMATION: Good saddle conformation. In general, the Morgan should be compact, of medium length, well muscled, smooth and stylish in appearance.

QUALITY: The Morgan should have clean, dense bone with sufficient substance; well-developed joints and tendons, and a fine coat.

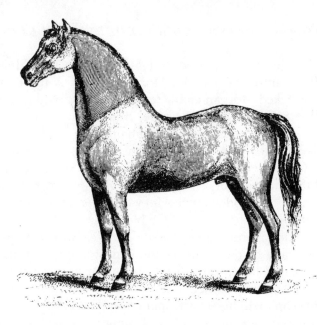

Peters' Vermont by Gifford, out of mare by Green Mountain 2nd, one of the purest lines from Justin Morgan.

TEMPERAMENT: The Morgan should be tractable but with good spirit.

HEAD AND NECK: *Head*—Medium size, clean-cut and tapering from the jaw to the muzzle. It should be wide between the eyes, long from ear to eye, short from eye to nostril. The profile can be straight or slightly dished but *never* Roman-nosed. The lower jaw should be wide and clean-cut and the muzzle fine with small, firm lips and large nostrils. The eyes should be large, dark and prominent, set well out on the sides of the head. The ears should be small, fine-pointed, set wide apart and always carried alertly. *Neck*—Medium in length, well crested on top, straight on the bottom line; clean-cut at the throat-latch. It should be smoothly joined to the shoulder and deep at the point of the shoulder. The crest should form a smooth curve from poll to withers. The mane and foretop should be full.

FOREHAND: *Shoulders*—Long, with good angulation. They should blend smoothly with the neck into well-defined but medium-high withers. The withers should be slightly higher than the point of the hip. *Forelegs*—Fairly short, squarely set, well apart, with short muscular arms. Viewed from the front, the legs should be thin and must be straight; viewed from the side should be wide and sinewy. *Forearm*—Wide, flat and muscular. Knees should be wide and flat. *Cannon*—Wide from the side, thin from the front and relatively short.

Fetlock joints—Rather wide but not round. *Pasterns*—Clean and strong, of medium length, the slope to correlate with the slope of the shoulder. *Feet*—Medium size, nearly round, open at the heel, smooth and dense but not brittle.

BODY: The body conformation of the Morgan is distinctive, with *chest* of good depth and width; with the *back* short, broad and well muscled. The *loin* should be wide and muscular and closely coupled. The *barrel* should be large and rather round, with well-sprung, closely joined ribs and deep full flank.

HINDQUARTERS: *Hind legs*—Squarely set and so placed that he turns on his hindquarters with legs well under him. *Hips*—Well rounded; hip bones should never show. *Croup*—Rounded gently with a fairly high-set tail, well carried. *Tail*—Long and full. *Quarters and thighs*— Deep and well muscled with strong stifles and medium-length, wide, muscular gaskins. *Hocks*—Wide, deep and clean; viewed from the rear, the hind legs should be perpendicular, with the hocks neither closer together nor wider apart than the fetlocks. *Cannons*—Short, wide and flat, with the tendons standing well out from the bone and well defined. *Pasterns*—Strong, medium length and not too sloping. *Hind feet*—Resembling the forefeet and round, medium in size, smooth and dense.

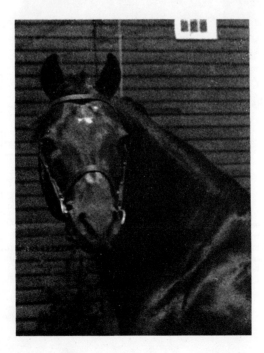

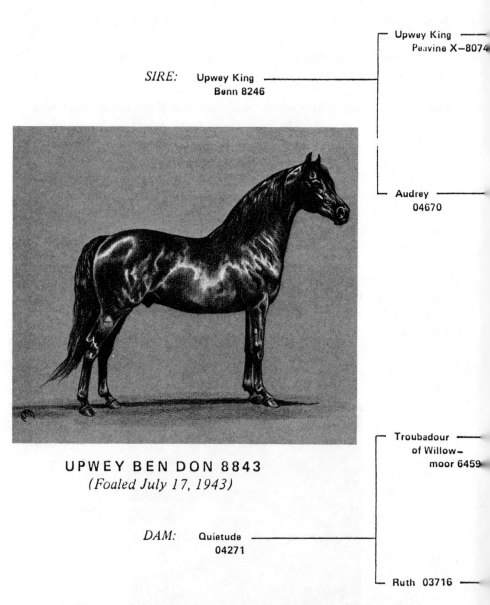

SIRE: Upwey King
Benn 8246

┌─ Upwey King
│ Peavine X—8074

└─ Audrey
   04670

UPWEY BEN DON 8843
(Foaled July 17, 1943)

DAM: Quietude
04271

┌─ Troubadour
│ of Willow—
│ moor 6459

└─ Ruth 03716

* X in the number in a horse's Morgan pedigree denotes that it was registered under AMHR Rule II (rescinded 1948), which allowed to be registered, upon application to the AMHR, an animal that traced to Morgan blood but was not the offspring of a registered sire *and* dam; since 1948 no horse may be registered unless both its sire and dam are registered.   † American Saddle Horse Register.   ‡ Said to be by.

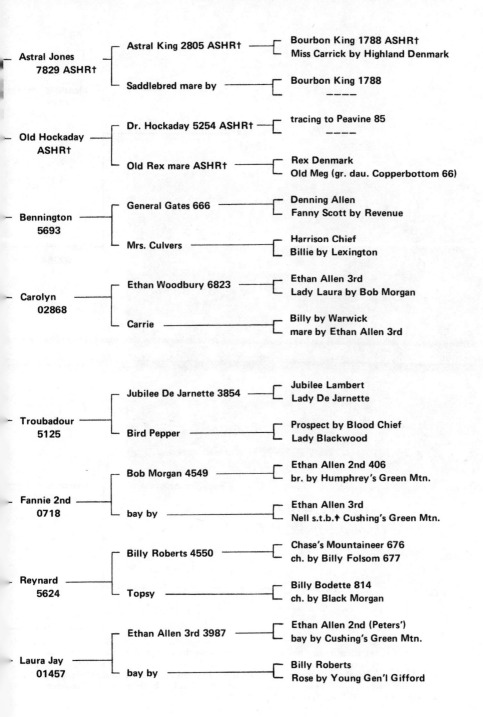

Astral Jones
7829 ASHR†
├─ Astral King 2805 ASHR†
│   ├─ Bourbon King 1788 ASHR†
│   └─ Miss Carrick by Highland Denmark
└─ Saddlebred mare by
    ├─ Bourbon King 1788
    └─ ————

Old Hockaday
ASHR†
├─ Dr. Hockaday 5254 ASHR†
│   ├─ tracing to Peavine 85
│   └─ ————
└─ Old Rex mare ASHR†
    ├─ Rex Denmark
    └─ Old Meg (gr. dau. Copperbottom 66)

Bennington
5693
├─ General Gates 666
│   ├─ Denning Allen
│   └─ Fanny Scott by Revenue
└─ Mrs. Culvers
    ├─ Harrison Chief
    └─ Billie by Lexington

Carolyn
02868
├─ Ethan Woodbury 6823
│   ├─ Ethan Allen 3rd
│   └─ Lady Laura by Bob Morgan
└─ Carrie
    ├─ Billy by Warwick
    └─ mare by Ethan Allen 3rd

Troubadour
5125
├─ Jubilee De Jarnette 3854
│   ├─ Jubilee Lambert
│   └─ Lady De Jarnette
└─ Bird Pepper
    ├─ Prospect by Blood Chief
    └─ Lady Blackwood

Fannie 2nd
0718
├─ Bob Morgan 4549
│   ├─ Ethan Allen 2nd 406
│   └─ br. by Humphrey's Green Mtn.
└─ bay by
    ├─ Ethan Allen 3rd
    └─ Nell s.t.b.† Cushing's Green Mtn.

Reynard
5624
├─ Billy Roberts 4550
│   ├─ Chase's Mountaineer 676
│   └─ ch. by Billy Folsom 677
└─ Topsy
    ├─ Billy Bodette 814
    └─ ch. by Black Morgan

Laura Jay
01457
├─ Ethan Allen 3rd 3987
│   ├─ Ethan Allen 2nd (Peters')
│   └─ bay by Cushing's Green Mtn.
└─ bay by
    ├─ Billy Roberts
    └─ Rose by Young Gen'l Gifford

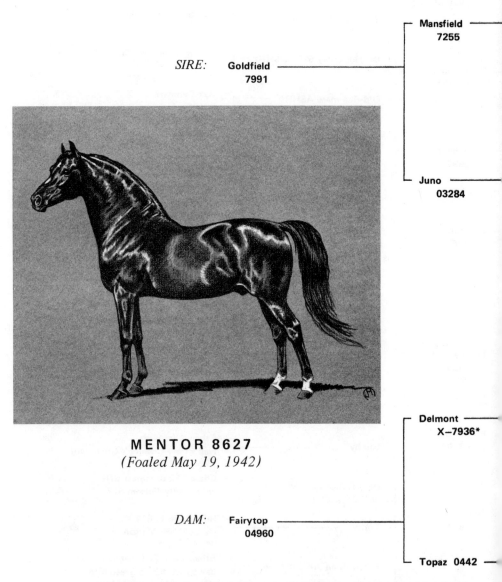

SIRE: **Goldfield**
7991

┌─ **Mansfield** ─
│ **7255**

└─ **Juno** ─
   03284

MENTOR 8627
(Foaled May 19, 1942)

DAM: **Fairytop**
04960

┌─ **Delmont** ─
│ **X–7936***

└─ **Topaz 0442** ─

* **X** in the number in a horse's Morgan pedigree denotes that it was registered under AMHR Rule II (rescinded 1948), which allowed to be registered, upon application to the AMHR, an animal that traced to Morgan blood but was not the offspring of a registered sire *and* dam; since 1948 no horse may be registered unless both its sire and dam are registered.   † American Saddle Horse Register.

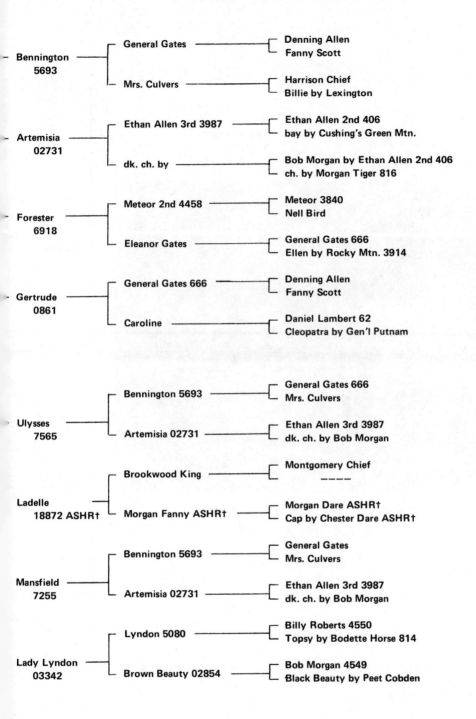

Bennington
5693
- General Gates
  - Denning Allen
  - Fanny Scott
- Mrs. Culvers
  - Harrison Chief
  - Billie by Lexington

Artemisia
02731
- Ethan Allen 3rd 3987
  - Ethan Allen 2nd 406
  - bay by Cushing's Green Mtn.
- dk. ch. by
  - Bob Morgan by Ethan Allen 2nd 406
  - ch. by Morgan Tiger 816

Forester
6918
- Meteor 2nd 4458
  - Meteor 3840
  - Nell Bird
- Eleanor Gates
  - General Gates 666
  - Ellen by Rocky Mtn. 3914

Gertrude
0861
- General Gates 666
  - Denning Allen
  - Fanny Scott
- Caroline
  - Daniel Lambert 62
  - Cleopatra by Gen'l Putnam

Ulysses
7565
- Bennington 5693
  - General Gates 666
  - Mrs. Culvers
- Artemisia 02731
  - Ethan Allen 3rd 3987
  - dk. ch. by Bob Morgan

Ladelle
18872 ASHR†
- Brookwood King
  - Montgomery Chief
  - ____
- Morgan Fanny ASHR†
  - Morgan Dare ASHR†
  - Cap by Chester Dare ASHR†

Mansfield
7255
- Bennington 5693
  - General Gates
  - Mrs. Culvers
- Artemisia 02731
  - Ethan Allen 3rd 3987
  - dk. ch. by Bob Morgan

Lady Lyndon
03342
- Lyndon 5080
  - Billy Roberts 4550
  - Topsy by Bodette Horse 814
- Brown Beauty 02854
  - Bob Morgan 4549
  - Black Beauty by Peet Cobden

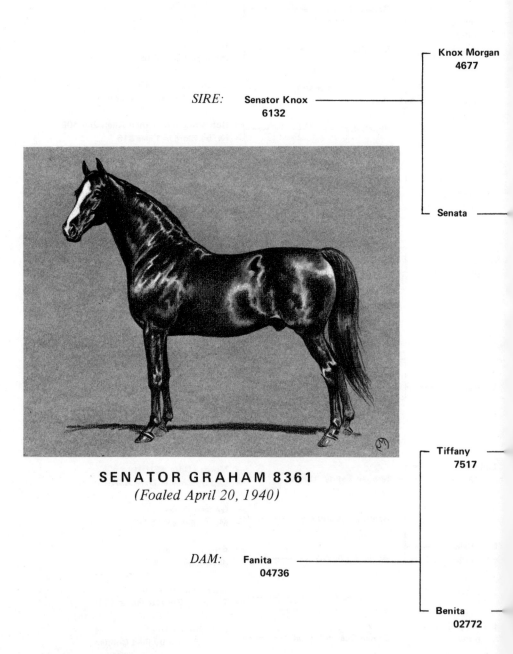

SIRE: Senator Knox ─────── Knox Morgan
          6132   4677

                                        Senata ─────

                                        Tiffany ─────
                                        7517

DAM: Fanita ───────
         04736

                                        Benita ─────
                                        02772

SENATOR GRAHAM 8361
(Foaled April 20, 1940)

✝ Said to be by.

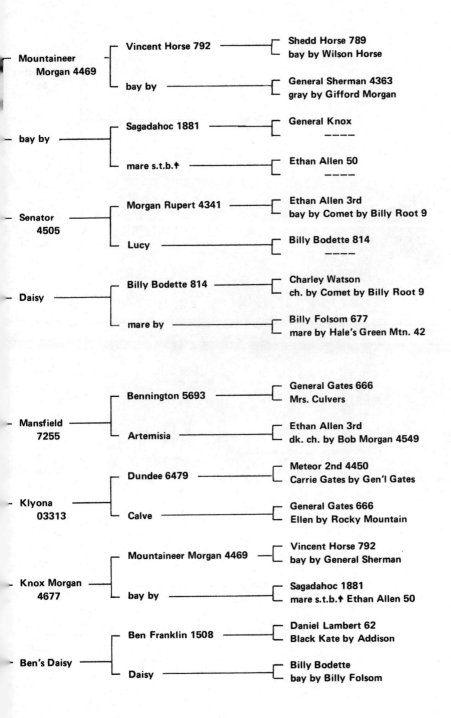

Mountaineer Morgan 4469
- Vincent Horse 792
  - Shedd Horse 789 — bay by Wilson Horse
  - General Sherman 4363 — gray by Gifford Morgan
- bay by

bay by
- Sagadahoc 1881
  - General Knox ————
- mare s.t.b.✝
  - Ethan Allen 50 ————

Senator 4505
- Morgan Rupert 4341
  - Ethan Allen 3rd — bay by Comet by Billy Root 9
- Lucy
  - Billy Bodette 814 ————

Daisy
- Billy Bodette 814
  - Charley Watson — ch. by Comet by Billy Root 9
- mare by
  - Billy Folsom 677 — mare by Hale's Green Mtn. 42

Mansfield 7255
- Bennington 5693
  - General Gates 666
  - Mrs. Culvers
- Artemisia
  - Ethan Allen 3rd — dk. ch. by Bob Morgan 4549

Klyona 03313
- Dundee 6479
  - Meteor 2nd 4450
  - Carrie Gates by Gen'l Gates
- Calve
  - General Gates 666
  - Ellen by Rocky Mountain

Knox Morgan 4677
- Mountaineer Morgan 4469
  - Vincent Horse 792 — bay by General Sherman
- bay by
  - Sagadahoc 1881 — mare s.t.b.✝ Ethan Allen 50

Ben's Daisy
- Ben Franklin 1508
  - Daniel Lambert 62
  - Black Kate by Addison
- Daisy
  - Billy Bodette
  - bay by Billy Folsom

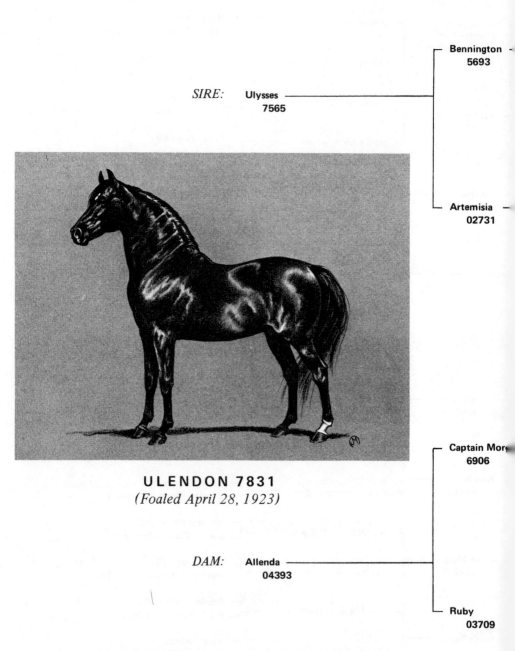

SIRE: **Ulysses**
7565

┌─ **Bennington**
5693

└─ **Artemisia**
02731

ULENDON 7831
(Foaled April 28, 1923)

DAM: **Allenda**
04393

┌─ **Captain Morg**
6906

└─ **Ruby**
03709

† American Saddle Horse Register.

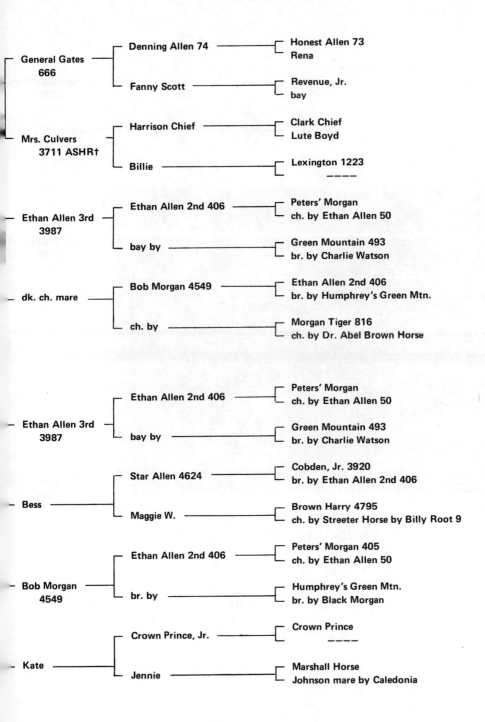

SIRE: Sealect
7266

Sir Ethan Allen
6537

Bell Marea
0189

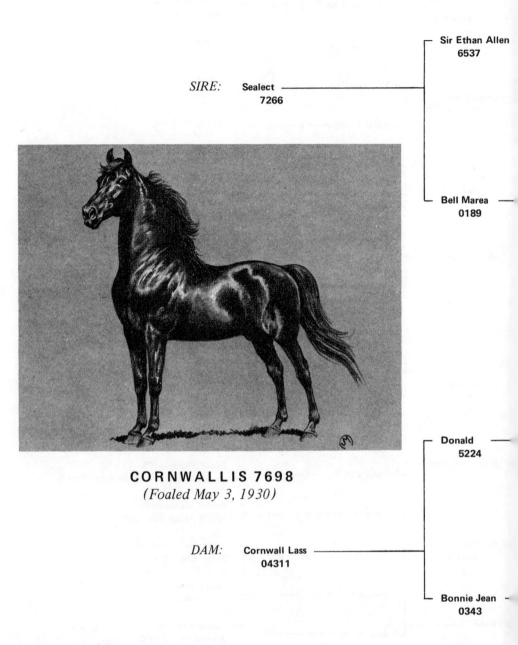

CORNWALLIS 7698
(Foaled May 3, 1930)

Donald
5224

DAM: Cornwall Lass
04311

Bonnie Jean
0343

✝ Said to be by.

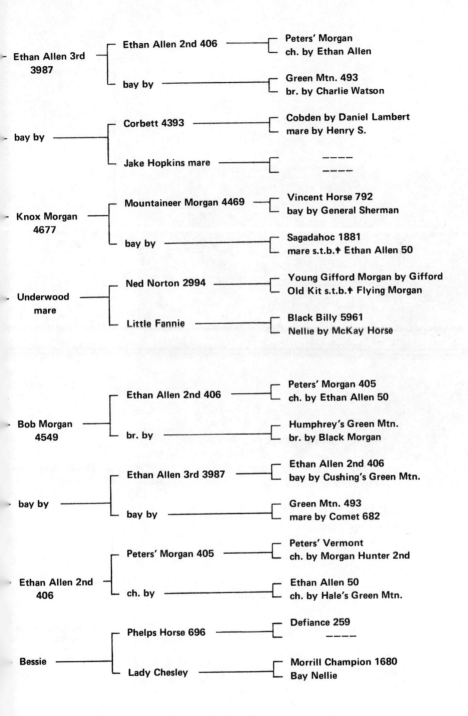

- Ethan Allen 3rd
  3987
  - Ethan Allen 2nd 406
    - Peters' Morgan
    - ch. by Ethan Allen
  - bay by
    - Green Mtn. 493
    - br. by Charlie Watson
- bay by
  - Corbett 4393
    - Cobden by Daniel Lambert
    - mare by Henry S.
  - Jake Hopkins mare
    - _ _ _ _
    - _ _ _ _
- Knox Morgan
  4677
  - Mountaineer Morgan 4469
    - Vincent Horse 792
    - bay by General Sherman
  - bay by
    - Sagadahoc 1881
    - mare s.t.b.✝ Ethan Allen 50
- Underwood
  mare
  - Ned Norton 2994
    - Young Gifford Morgan by Gifford
    - Old Kit s.t.b.✝ Flying Morgan
  - Little Fannie
    - Black Billy 5961
    - Nellie by McKay Horse

- Bob Morgan
  4549
  - Ethan Allen 2nd 406
    - Peters' Morgan 405
    - ch. by Ethan Allen 50
  - br. by
    - Humphrey's Green Mtn.
    - br. by Black Morgan
- bay by
  - Ethan Allen 3rd 3987
    - Ethan Allen 2nd 406
    - bay by Cushing's Green Mtn.
  - bay by
    - Green Mtn. 493
    - mare by Comet 682
- Ethan Allen 2nd
  406
  - Peters' Morgan 405
    - Peters' Vermont
    - ch. by Morgan Hunter 2nd
  - ch. by
    - Ethan Allen 50
    - ch. by Hale's Green Mtn.
- Bessie
  - Phelps Horse 696
    - Defiance 259
    - _ _ _ _
  - Lady Chesley
    - Morrill Champion 1680
    - Bay Nellie

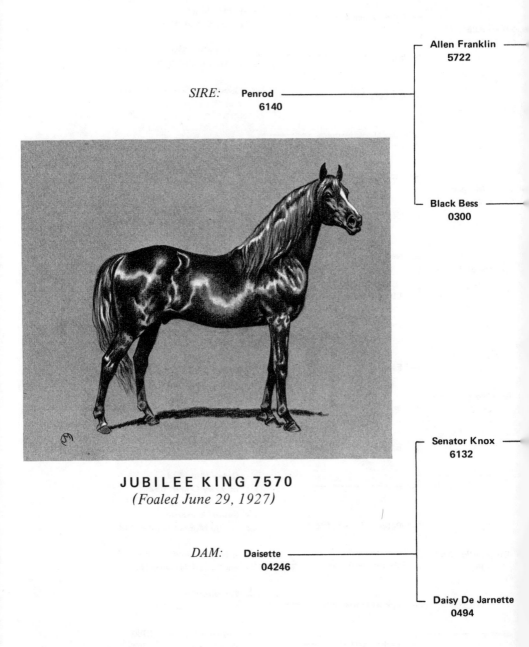

SIRE: Penrod
6140

↳ Allen Franklin ──────
5722

↳ Black Bess ──────
0300

JUBILEE KING 7570
(Foaled June 29, 1927)

↳ Senator Knox ──────
6132

DAM: Daisette ──────
04246

↳ Daisy De Jarnette
0494

✝ Said to be by.

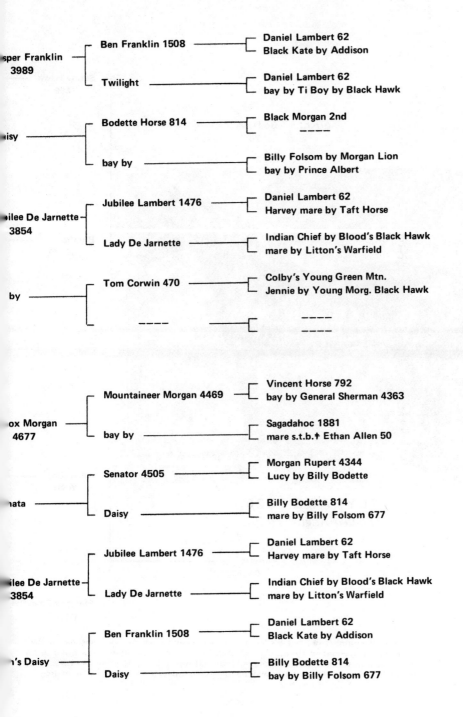

sper Franklin 3989
- Ben Franklin 1508
  - Daniel Lambert 62
  - Black Kate by Addison
- Twilight
  - Daniel Lambert 62
  - bay by Ti Boy by Black Hawk

aisy
- Bodette Horse 814
  - Black Morgan 2nd
  - ————
- bay by
  - Billy Folsom by Morgan Lion
  - bay by Prince Albert

ilee De Jarnette 3854
- Jubilee Lambert 1476
  - Daniel Lambert 62
  - Harvey mare by Taft Horse
- Lady De Jarnette
  - Indian Chief by Blood's Black Hawk
  - mare by Litton's Warfield

by
- Tom Corwin 470
  - Colby's Young Green Mtn.
  - Jennie by Young Morg. Black Hawk
- ————
  - ————
  - ————

ox Morgan 4677
- Mountaineer Morgan 4469
  - Vincent Horse 792
  - bay by General Sherman 4363
- bay by
  - Sagadahoc 1881
  - mare s.t.b.† Ethan Allen 50

ata
- Senator 4505
  - Morgan Rupert 4344
  - Lucy by Billy Bodette
- Daisy
  - Billy Bodette 814
  - mare by Billy Folsom 677

ilee De Jarnette 3854
- Jubilee Lambert 1476
  - Daniel Lambert 62
  - Harvey mare by Taft Horse
- Lady De Jarnette
  - Indian Chief by Blood's Black Hawk
  - mare by Litton's Warfield

n's Daisy
- Ben Franklin 1508
  - Daniel Lambert 62
  - Black Kate by Addison
- Daisy
  - Billy Bodette 814
  - bay by Billy Folsom 677

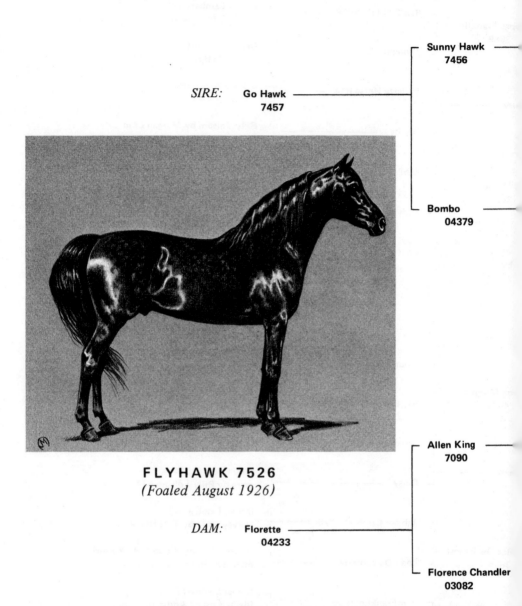

SIRE: Go Hawk
7457

— Sunny Hawk
7456

— Bombo
04379

FLYHAWK 7526
(Foaled August 1926)

DAM: Florette
04233

— Allen King
7090

— Florence Chandler
03082

* **X** in the number in a horse's Morgan pedigree denotes that it was registered under AMHR Rule II (rescinded 1948), which allowed to be registered, upon application to the AMHR, an animal that traced to Morgan blood but was not the offspring of a registered sire *and* dam; since 1948 no horse may be registered unless both its sire and dam are registered.   † Said to be by.

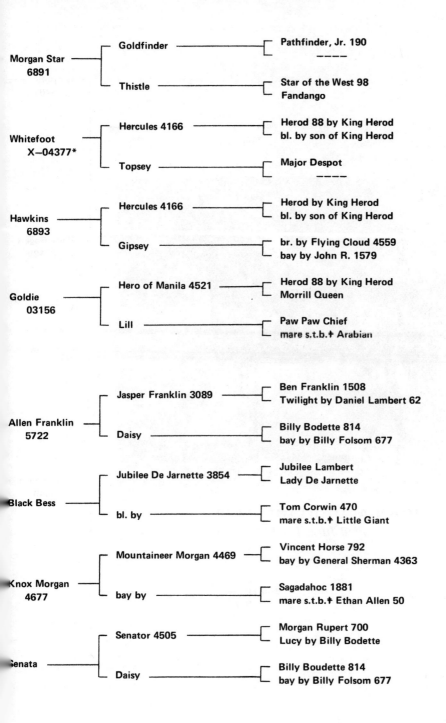

Morgan Star
6891
├─ Goldfinder ──────── ┌─ Pathfinder, Jr. 190
│   └─ ────
└─ Thistle ──────── ┌─ Star of the West 98
                    └─ Fandango

Whitefoot
X–04377*
├─ Hercules 4166 ──────── ┌─ Herod 88 by King Herod
│   └─ bl. by son of King Herod
└─ Topsey ──────── ┌─ Major Despot
                   └─ ────

Hawkins
6893
├─ Hercules 4166 ──────── ┌─ Herod by King Herod
│   └─ bl. by son of King Herod
└─ Gipsey ──────── ┌─ br. by Flying Cloud 4559
                   └─ bay by John R. 1579

Goldie
03156
├─ Hero of Manila 4521 ──────── ┌─ Herod 88 by King Herod
│   └─ Morrill Queen
└─ Lill ──────── ┌─ Paw Paw Chief
                 └─ mare s.t.b.✝ Arabian

Allen Franklin
5722
├─ Jasper Franklin 3089 ──────── ┌─ Ben Franklin 1508
│   └─ Twilight by Daniel Lambert 62
└─ Daisy ──────── ┌─ Billy Bodette 814
                  └─ bay by Billy Folsom 677

Black Bess
├─ Jubilee De Jarnette 3854 ──────── ┌─ Jubilee Lambert
│   └─ Lady De Jarnette
└─ bl. by ──────── ┌─ Tom Corwin 470
                   └─ mare s.t.b.✝ Little Giant

Knox Morgan
4677
├─ Mountaineer Morgan 4469 ──────── ┌─ Vincent Horse 792
│   └─ bay by General Sherman 4363
└─ bay by ──────── ┌─ Sagadahoc 1881
                   └─ mare s.t.b.✝ Ethan Allen 50

Senata
├─ Senator 4505 ──────── ┌─ Morgan Rupert 700
│   └─ Lucy by Billy Bodette
└─ Daisy ──────── ┌─ Billy Boudette 814
                  └─ bay by Billy Folsom 677

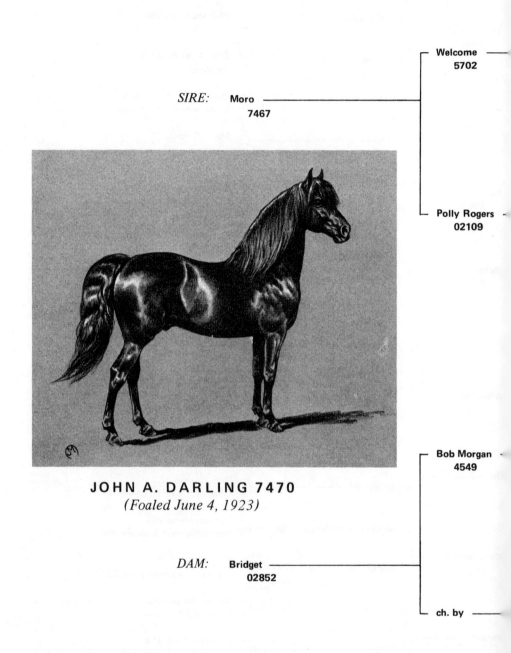

SIRE: Moro ──────────────┬── Welcome ──────
        7467   5702
                                    └── Polly Rogers ─
                                         02109

JOHN A. DARLING 7470
(Foaled June 4, 1923)

DAM: Bridget ──────────────┬── Bob Morgan ─
        02852   4549
                                    └── ch. by ───────

✝ Said to be by.

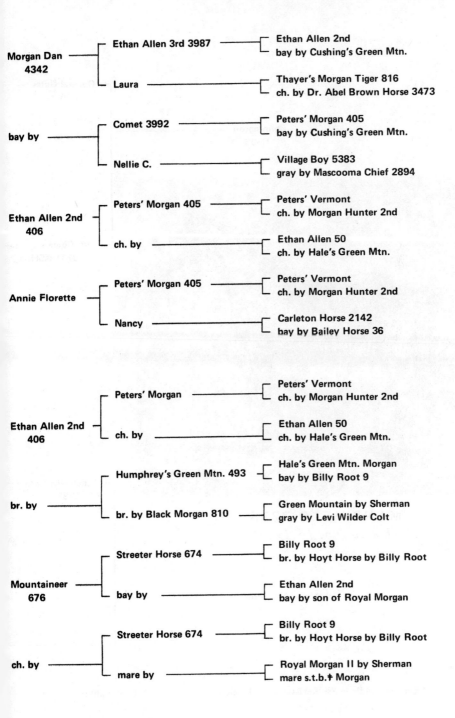

Morgan Dan 4342
├─ **Ethan Allen 3rd 3987**
│   ├─ Ethan Allen 2nd
│   └─ bay by Cushing's Green Mtn.
└─ **Laura**
    ├─ Thayer's Morgan Tiger 816
    └─ ch. by Dr. Abel Brown Horse 3473

bay by
├─ **Comet 3992**
│   ├─ Peters' Morgan 405
│   └─ bay by Cushing's Green Mtn.
└─ **Nellie C.**
    ├─ Village Boy 5383
    └─ gray by Mascooma Chief 2894

Ethan Allen 2nd 406
├─ **Peters' Morgan 405**
│   ├─ Peters' Vermont
│   └─ ch. by Morgan Hunter 2nd
└─ **ch. by**
    ├─ Ethan Allen 50
    └─ ch. by Hale's Green Mtn.

Annie Florette
├─ **Peters' Morgan 405**
│   ├─ Peters' Vermont
│   └─ ch. by Morgan Hunter 2nd
└─ **Nancy**
    ├─ Carleton Horse 2142
    └─ bay by Bailey Horse 36

Ethan Allen 2nd 406
├─ **Peters' Morgan**
│   ├─ Peters' Vermont
│   └─ ch. by Morgan Hunter 2nd
└─ **ch. by**
    ├─ Ethan Allen 50
    └─ ch. by Hale's Green Mtn.

br. by
├─ **Humphrey's Green Mtn. 493**
│   ├─ Hale's Green Mtn. Morgan
│   └─ bay by Billy Root 9
└─ **br. by Black Morgan 810**
    ├─ Green Mountain by Sherman
    └─ gray by Levi Wilder Colt

Mountaineer 676
├─ **Streeter Horse 674**
│   ├─ Billy Root 9
│   └─ br. by Hoyt Horse by Billy Root
└─ **bay by**
    ├─ Ethan Allen 2nd
    └─ bay by son of Royal Morgan

ch. by
├─ **Streeter Horse 674**
│   ├─ Billy Root 9
│   └─ br. by Hoyt Horse by Billy Root
└─ **mare by**
    ├─ Royal Morgan II by Sherman
    └─ mare s.t.b.✝ Morgan

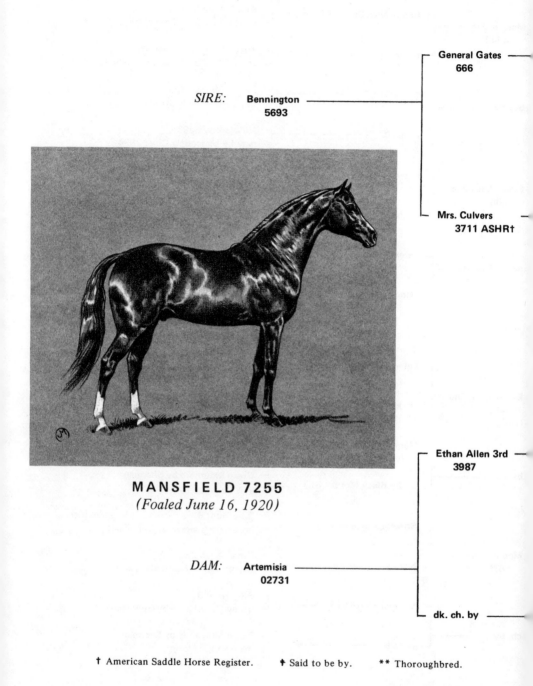

MANSFIELD 7255
(Foaled June 16, 1920)

SIRE: Bennington
5693

General Gates
666

Mrs. Culvers
3711 ASHR†

DAM: Artemisia
02731

Ethan Allen 3rd
3987

dk. ch. by

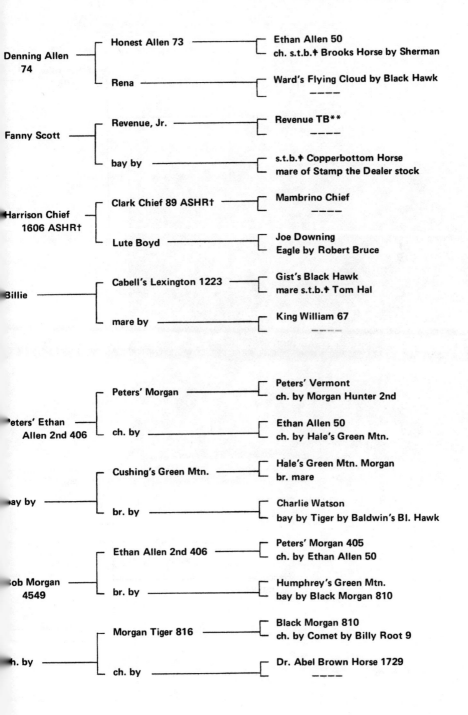

Denning Allen 74
- Honest Allen 73
  - Ethan Allen 50
  - ch. s.t.b.✝ Brooks Horse by Sherman
- Rena
  - Ward's Flying Cloud by Black Hawk
  - – – – –

Fanny Scott
- Revenue, Jr.
  - Revenue TB**
  - – – – –
- bay by
  - s.t.b.✝ Copperbottom Horse
  - mare of Stamp the Dealer stock

Harrison Chief 1606 ASHR†
- Clark Chief 89 ASHR†
  - Mambrino Chief
  - – – – –
- Lute Boyd
  - Joe Downing
  - Eagle by Robert Bruce

Billie
- Cabell's Lexington 1223
  - Gist's Black Hawk
  - mare s.t.b.✝ Tom Hal
- mare by
  - King William 67
  - – – – –

Peters' Ethan Allen 2nd 406
- Peters' Morgan
  - Peters' Vermont
  - ch. by Morgan Hunter 2nd
- ch. by
  - Ethan Allen 50
  - ch. by Hale's Green Mtn.

bay by
- Cushing's Green Mtn.
  - Hale's Green Mtn. Morgan
  - br. mare
- br. by
  - Charlie Watson
  - bay by Tiger by Baldwin's Bl. Hawk

Bob Morgan 4549
- Ethan Allen 2nd 406
  - Peters' Morgan 405
  - ch. by Ethan Allen 50
- br. by
  - Humphrey's Green Mtn.
  - bay by Black Morgan 810

ch. by
- Morgan Tiger 816
  - Black Morgan 810
  - ch. by Comet by Billy Root 9
- ch. by
  - Dr. Abel Brown Horse 1729
  - – – – –

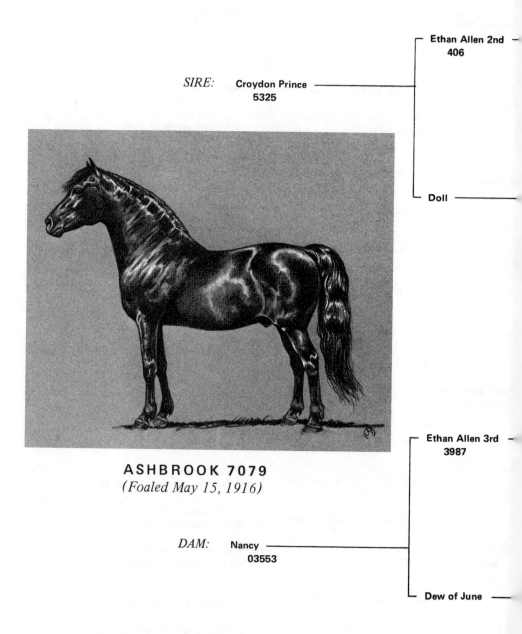

SIRE: **Croydon Prince**
5325

┌─ **Ethan Allen 2nd** ─
│ **406**

└─ **Doll** ─────

ASHBROOK 7079
(Foaled May 15, 1916)

┌─ **Ethan Allen 3rd** ─
│ **3987**

DAM: **Nancy** ──────

└─ **Dew of June** ───

✛ Said to be by.

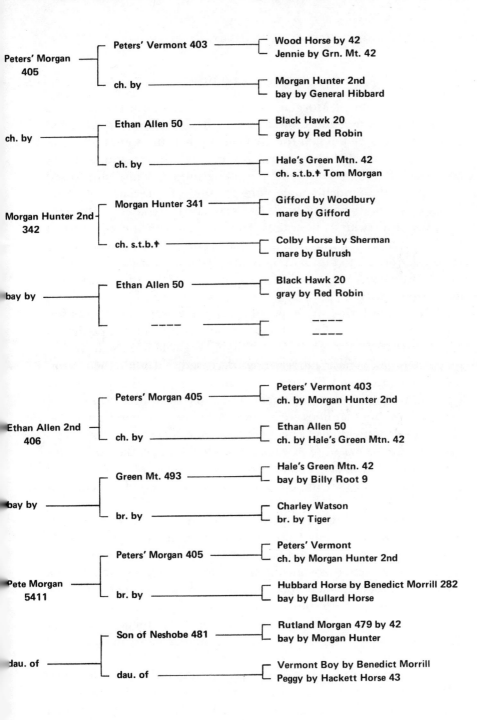

Peters' Morgan
405
├─ Peters' Vermont 403 ────┬─ Wood Horse by 42
│   └─ Jennie by Grn. Mt. 42
└─ ch. by ─────────────────┬─ Morgan Hunter 2nd
                           └─ bay by General Hibbard

ch. by
├─ Ethan Allen 50 ─────────┬─ Black Hawk 20
│   └─ gray by Red Robin
└─ ch. by ─────────────────┬─ Hale's Green Mtn. 42
                           └─ ch. s.t.b.✝ Tom Morgan

Morgan Hunter 2nd
342
├─ Morgan Hunter 341 ──────┬─ Gifford by Woodbury
│   └─ mare by Gifford
└─ ch. s.t.b.✝ ────────────┬─ Colby Horse by Sherman
                           └─ mare by Bulrush

bay by
├─ Ethan Allen 50 ─────────┬─ Black Hawk 20
│   └─ gray by Red Robin
└─ ──── ───────────────────┬─ ────
                           └─ ────

Ethan Allen 2nd
406
├─ Peters' Morgan 405 ─────┬─ Peters' Vermont 403
│   └─ ch. by Morgan Hunter 2nd
└─ ch. by ─────────────────┬─ Ethan Allen 50
                           └─ ch. by Hale's Green Mtn. 42

bay by
├─ Green Mt. 493 ──────────┬─ Hale's Green Mtn. 42
│   └─ bay by Billy Root 9
└─ br. by ─────────────────┬─ Charley Watson
                           └─ br. by Tiger

Pete Morgan
5411
├─ Peters' Morgan 405 ─────┬─ Peters' Vermont
│   └─ ch. by Morgan Hunter 2nd
└─ br. by ─────────────────┬─ Hubbard Horse by Benedict Morrill 282
                           └─ bay by Bullard Horse

dau. of
├─ Son of Neshobe 481 ─────┬─ Rutland Morgan 479 by 42
│   └─ bay by Morgan Hunter
└─ dau. of ────────────────┬─ Vermont Boy by Benedict Morrill
                           └─ Peggy by Hackett Horse 43

POINTS ON BREEDING

In any discussion of Morgans, sooner or later one will arrive at a point in time when the topic turns to the bloodlines of the great horses in the breed. Then the air heats up and the sound of voices is raised a few decibels as each participant in the conversation delivers opinions, oftentimes with table-pounding fervor. Names are tossed back and forth, staunchly championed by some, depreciated by others and met with indifference by still others. The newcomer to Morgans feels his head swim as he listens. He wonders if he'll ever acquaint himself with the seemingly endless names that almost crackle in the air. And it occurs to him that there must be a right track somewhere in this breeding thing, because certainly the caliber of the horses is increasing yearly.

Before considering the basic guidelines that serious breeders follow, the novice might find helpful the somewhat extended pedigrees of ten of the best-known and most highly regarded Morgan sires in modern times. These horses, now deceased, through their sons, daughters and grandchildren still influence greatly the quality and type of Morgans foaled today from coast to coast. Successful crosses to these most popular lines are producing today's—and tomorrow's— outstanding individuals. The pedigrees here reproduced are verbatim from the *American Morgan Horse Register,* and therefore they contain the spelling discrepancies and the occasional ellipses inherent in material furnished in the more casual manner of nineteenth-century owners.

Theories on breeding and bloodlines are apparently very personal to some folks, and firmly held convictions are not easily toppled. It is best to remain silent if you have any theories of your own in mind when someone else is advancing his! So listen and learn, and shuffle through it all later when you are alone: it does no good to argue unless you can back up your arguments with facts. Therefore, if you are a newcomer, you are well advised to commit to memory as many opinions and bloodlines as possible, and to learn all you can about the characteristics of each modern family. You needn't be overly concerned, no matter what some may say, about the possible effect a "black sheep" that lived seventy-five years ago might have on the foal your mare is carrying. But look sharply at the *sire* of that foal and the general qualities of the lines which produced him.

And it is important for the novice breeder to have a goal in mind, a goal based on sound breeding principles and careful study of individual animals. Breeding Morgans should never be haphazard. This random approach can lead swiftly to disappointment and disillusionment—and be a disservice to the breed.

GUIDELINES FOR NOVICE BREEDERS

If breeding Morgans is to be your pleasure, here are some points to keep in mind.

1. *Be sure your own personal preference in a horse coincides with the typical characteristics of the Morgan.* If you like a horse to be over 16 hands and which will, for example, be a notable Three-Day Event competitor (cross-country jumping, stadium jumping, and dressage) perhaps the Morgan isn't really big enough for you. Morgans are relatively small horses, with their Standard of Perfection recommending that they be between 14.1 and 15.2 hands, with *individuals* occasionally over or under. If you decide to breed Morgans a hand taller for a specific purpose of your own, it is feared that you will soon lose the breed type.
2. *Line-breeding or inbreeding generally "fixes" the family characteristics—both good and bad.* You must be very selective and extremely objective if you plan to embark on this line of thought. To line-breed or inbreed successfully, the breeding animals must be outstanding in conformation and way-of-going. You will note by looking over the pedigrees just given that a tremendous amount of inbreeding and line-breeding was practiced by the early Morgan fanciers.
3. *Breed animals of similar type and characteristics, if not similar bloodlines, to strengthen these points in future foals.* Going to a good outcross where the other characteristics are similar is recommended. Like begets like (hopefully). If you have a mare that is just about your ideal, breed her to a stallion of the same type whose bloodlines have been known to cross well with hers.
4. *A stallion or mare with a top pedigree will usually prevail over the lesser animal in a given cross, and the foal should be superior to the lesser individual in the mating.* Remember that a horse with a hodgepodge pedigree will not generally "breed true" even if he is a good individual himself. Stay with the lines with *known* characteristics.

We often see grade Morgans (half-breds, etc.) which seem to have an abundance of Morgan type. The reason for this is that the purebred, in this case the Morgan, has characteristics which have been fixed over generations, while the grade is, in essence, a mongrel without strong family traits. Thus, the better-bred animal prevails.

5. *Learn the qualities and attributes of the different families—as to type, disposition and action—which you feel are important to the horses you wish to produce.* If disposition is paramount in your mind, look for the family which most consistently seems to have produced individuals with good dispositions. Although handling does have a great deal to do with a horse's manners, those individuals foaled with naturally pleasant ways are not readily changed by handling except in extreme cases.

6. *An old theory is to breed the sire to the best lines found in his dam.* This principle dates way back, and has worked well in many breeds of livestock; certainly it is one highly regarded among horsemen.

7. *Horses with the quality and refinement to make them top individuals will almost always improve on the poorer animal.* You may not get exact perfection, but you will have a better horse in the foal than you had in the lesser parent. Quality and refinement will almost always prevail in a cross of this type.

8. *When breeding a Morgan horse which will be registered, remember that you do owe a responsibility to the breed as a whole.* You do the entire breed a marked injury if you do not at least strive for the best possible individuals from your breeding program. Breeding to the stallion down the road simply "because he is there" is not the way to be successful in a horse-breeding venture!

9. *And lastly, be aware that though Nature really has the final say on how your foals will turn out, if you breed horses with the goal of quality and type in mind, you will come out ahead a good percentage of the time.*

APPLYING THE GUIDELINES

Most experienced Morgan breeders have a clear-cut idea of the characteristics and traits of certain bloodlines, and, depending on their own requirements, establish programs based on judicious crosses of the most highly regarded lines. With Morgan excellence as a goal, they strive to produce animals which will be in demand by other breeders as well as by newcomers to the ranks of Morgan owners.

It cannot be overemphasized that hit-or-miss breeding usually produces, year after year, culls which no one wants or needs, and which are a definite detriment to the breed they unfortunately represent. Only a careful study of bloodlines and the individuals produced therein

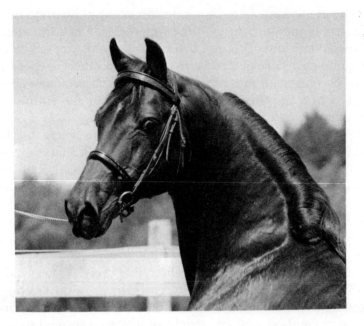

can lead to a sound breeding program and the production of Morgans really worthy to be issued registration papers. Granted, not every animal foaled will meet all expectations and the requirements of his breed, but the odds of producing inferior stock are greatly reduced when a thorough knowledge of bloodlines and an objective outlook is the basis for your breeding operation.

To be aware of the requirements of excellence and to be objective and not "stable blind" when some of your foals don't measure up are very necessary to achieve success over the long course. Make geldings out of stallions which, though good average individuals, are not stud material. In the long run they will be more valuable as good-using horses than they would ever have been as inferior breeding stock. It isn't easy to train yourself to take a long, cold look, grit your teeth, and admit that the young horse you see doesn't quite make it. But it really is a necessary part of improving next year's crop—be it one or twenty.

If you are interested in becoming a serious breeder of Morgans, visit established farms—as many as you can. Talk with other breeders; learn all you are able to about the fundamentals of their programs.

And be sure to keep an open mind while doing it! Learn to recognize a successful operation beyond the superficials. Look for uniformity and disposition and of course, basically, *type*. See if you can determine why some farms are obviously successful and others are less so. Try not to become sold on a certain bloodline because someone recommends it as being the "only one": it may be for the enthusiast who is speaking, but perhaps it may not be for you.

Make definite decisions as to what your aims are in the field of breeding Morgans. It has always been widely felt that if one breeds for type, disposition, athletic ability and soundness, one will have animals which will be in great demand and which will promote their breed as well.

THE OBLIGATION TO THE BREED

Breeders must be alert to the possibility that breeding too assiduously for excellence in a single field of performance—with resulting over-concern for extreme refinement of bone and skeletal structure, and too much emphasis on, say, height of action—can tend to produce so many "off type" individuals that there could be loss of the basic conformation that makes the Morgan horse uniquely himself. This sadly misplaced zeal was responsible for the near loss of the Morgan's characteristics in the 1920s and subjected him to an uphill climb to preserve his breed type above and beyond his abilities as a performer in the show ring.

While acknowledging that of course there are always likely to be found some variations on type within so versatile a breed, those people who are dedicated to the Morgan *per se* realize their obligation to perpetuate, intact, his basic character and disposition. No matter

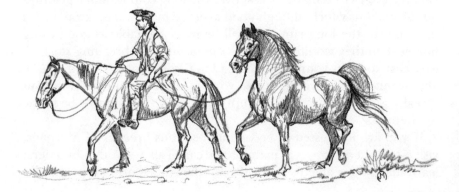

how much we applaud him as a high-going, sparkling Park horse or as a quick-thinking and agile cutting horse, when he is stripped and judged for type and conformation he must possess the characteristics that identify him immediately as a good representative of the breed as a whole. Without this adherence to basic type, he would soon be pulling further and further away from the very thing that sets the Morgan apart from all other horses: the unique qualities possessed by Justin and passed on so richly by his sons.

6

The Morgan Stallion, Mare and Gelding

THE STALLION

Proud and lofty of bearing, the Morgan stallion has always exhibited the true Morgan type with the greatest definition. His symmetry, in the ideal, is at once apparent. The high-held head, the great depth and angulation of shoulder, the placement of the neck upon the shoulder—these are the best-known and most easily recognized characteristics of the breed. In short, they comprise the Morgan trademark, which, while exemplified in the stallion, is the sought-after stamp—slightly modified—for mares and geldings as well.

Even to the eye of the most casual observer, the breeding stallion must possess these characteristics of type. Of course, he must have good general conformation too, with straight legs and good feet. But type is still the most important factor in selecting a stallion to buy or to serve your mare. No matter how excellent his conformation, without type he would be just another good horse. Without type we really *have* no breed, no standard to strive for. That a horse should have good conformation is elementary. That each succeeding generation has more firmly fixed the Morgan type toward its ideal can be seen by a perusal of the early volumes of the *Morgan Horse Register* and by comparing the *Register* with photos of Morgan horses today. More beautiful and with more quality and refinement than their predecessors while still maintaining the general description of Justin Morgan, today's top Morgans again present a picture of their progenitor, with perhaps a bit more size and quality which is needed in today's competitive horse world.

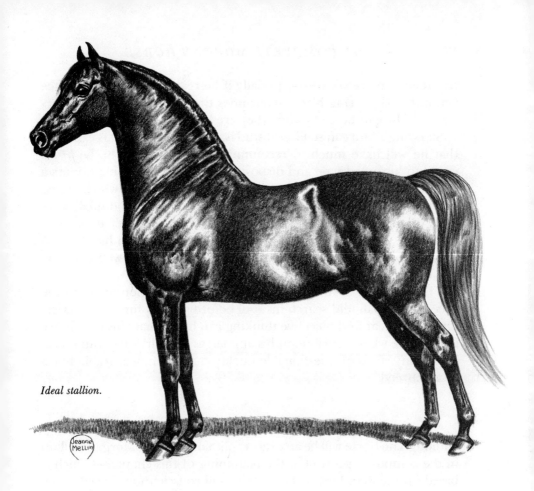

Ideal stallion.

If Morgan type and conformation are lacking in an individual, many believe that, regardless of his other attributes, he is really a Morgan in name only. He most certainly shouldn't be considered a breeding animal. Also, there is little market for the individual with show-ring action but with no type to share the same hide.

On the other hand, the individual which possesses *both* type and action becomes the most sought-after stallion, and is almost priceless to his owner. However, it is wise to remember that all individuals with the Morgan characteristics of type and disposition will always find a ready market, whether they have extremely high action or not. The demand for top-quality Pleasure Morgans with type and disposition far exceeds the supply today.

Type is necessary in any Morgan that is bound for the show circuit, so a prospective first-time owner can easily become familiar with the requirements for type by noting the qualities evidenced by consistent winners during a season. Then he can go off on his horse-buying trip feeling more secure—especially if he realizes that what they see win in the show ring often determines the selection made by experienced Morgan fanciers when they are buying a horse of their own.

Standing a Morgan stallion at stud is a serious matter. It is expected that he will have much to recommend him, and that he be *first* a credit to his breed type and disposition, with his show-ring honors a secondary consideration. Does he possess a pedigree which shows every indication of his being prepotent for his own good qualities— or is he merely an unusual individual from a lackluster line? Does he have a good disposition which he will pass along to his foals, so they can be easily handled and trained by amateurs as well as by the professional horseman?

The owner of a Morgan stallion owes a real responsibility to the breed and he should search his soul before putting him into service. Only with clear and objective thinking can he evaluate his own horse and decide what contribution his animal, as an individual, can make. Too many studs of questionable quality can do immeasurable harm to any breed.

CONFORMATION

Although no horse will be an exact replica of the ideal Morgan stallion in the composite portrait at the beginning of this chapter—which is based on the Standard of Perfection—all conscientious breeders set themselves the task of producing Morgans which at least approach the model. By setting an ideal, they then have something specific toward which to aim their breeding programs: such is the reason for having a Standard of Perfection in any breed of livestock.

So study this ideal Morgan point for point, and become familiar with the silhouette and substance of the model. Compare the stallions you see in the flesh with the firmly fixed mental picture of the ideal, and you will be able personally to score them on points of conformation and type.

The Head
Many enthusiasts consider the head of the Morgan horse to be his most outstanding feature. A saying you will often hear around the stables or show ring is, "If you can't get beyond the head, forget the rest!" Perhaps this is a bit extreme, since you certainly must consider other attributes; but nevertheless an attractive, expressive head is one of the Morgan's best features.

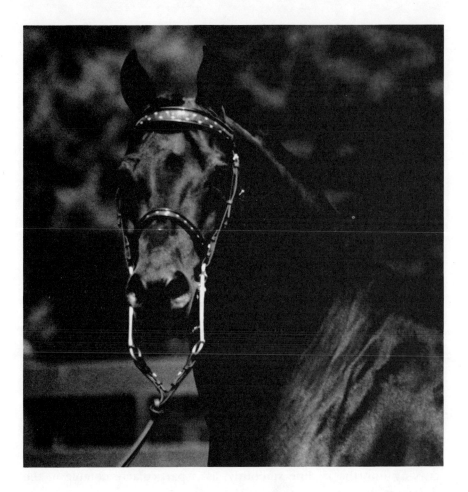

EXPRESSION: We all, upon seeing a horse for the first time, have an eye for what we call the "Morgan look." It is a bright, proud expression, at once intelligent, mischievous, a bit defiant and—totally irresistible! It is usually coupled with a snorty attitude, a tossing mane and an abundance of nervous animation, and it can be found in mares and geldings as well as in stallions. This look or expression just seems to say *Morgan!* Yet in spite of the pronounced appearance of inner fires and smoldering energy, the Morgan is noted for his tractability and exceptionally pleasant disposition.

QUALITY: The structure of the head of the stallion is as distinctive as his expression. Fundamentally, quality should be paramount in the list of requirements. To be specific: quality is the clean lines of the bone structure, the fineness of the skin and the refinement of the muzzle and jaw.

The head of the stallion should show masculine depth and breadth and yet still exhibit the chiseled lines in the bone structure which denote quality. There should be no tendency toward coarseness. The muzzle is small with firm lips, the nostrils slightly flared even in repose. The eyes must be prominent, large and bright. The Morgan's ears should be small, nicely shaped, and set fairly wide at the poll. In profile, the line of the face should be straight or slightly dished; never, *never* convex or Roman-nosed. A convex profile in a Morgan immediately denotes coarseness, and very often is coupled with a mulish disposition.

The prominent eyes—set low in the head with a wide forehead between—should be dark and expessive, with no white showing at the back edge. Much can be determined from the size and expression of the eyes. A horse with a small, white-rimmed eye is very often untrustworthy. Width between the eyes is also important not only aesthetically but practically: a horse must have "brain space." And the Morgan as a breed is characteristically broad between the eyes.

From the side the Morgan stallion's head should be wedge-shaped, with the line of the jaw tapering into the small muzzle. A shallow jaw—especially when coupled with a heavy muzzle—gives a horse a coarse, common look not typical of the Morgan.

THE THROTTLE: Although the jaw should be prominent, it should not be too heavily muscled or overly thick. It should be free of meatiness where it connects with the neck, and the throttle should be fine, curving into the jawline smoothly, as is particularly notable in the drawings showing variations of the neck.

Very often stallions coarsen in the throttle as they mature. This is the reason for preferring a young stallion without too much depth of neck or crest, because such conformation is some insurance against the tendency to thicken with age in this area. Sometimes the use of a jowl-hood or -wrap will help to prevent thickening by causing the horse to sweat off the excess tissue beneath the wrap.

A coarse-necked, heavily crested stallion will very often have difficulty flexing his neck to the bridle. This can lead to the noisy breathing often in evidence when an overly flexed horse is especially coarse in the throat: as he flexes to give in to the bits, he partially cuts off the air passages in his throttle, thus causing the gagging sound often noticed with mature stallions. This same horse when not "set up" in the bridle will breathe quite normally. However, it is far more desirable to insist on correct conformation in the first place than it is to try to cope with this problem as the horse gets older.

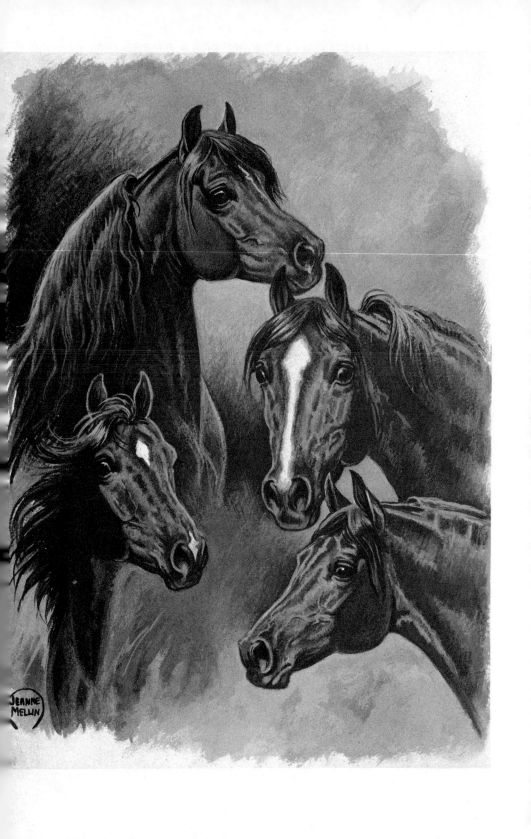

The Neck

The smoothly crested neck blending into oblique shoulders is a basic characteristic of the Morgan stallion. The line from the poll to the withers should be one continuous curve, with the neck blending into *and on top of* extremely sloping shoulders.

IDEAL NECK: There should be no evidence of lumpiness, nor should there be any hollows in the neck or where it attaches to the shoulder. As you run your hand down the horse's neck and shoulder, you should be able to feel the smooth blending of the muscles of the neck in a hard but not "cordy" manner: you are not aware of every muscle and tendon—there is just a continuous blending of them all under the skin.

The withers should be of medium height and they too should blend smoothly into the line of the neck. There should never be a dip in front of the withers to spoil the continuous curve of the neck from poll to back. Ideally, the withers should be neither sharp nor too round, the latter ("mutton-withered") usually being more of a problem with Morgans.

The drawings indicate how simple it is to learn to distinguish the ideal neck from the variations. A good neck in the mature stallion is neither too heavy nor too fine. It has the smooth curve from the poll

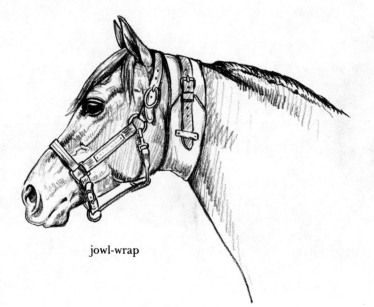

jowl-wrap

to the withers, with a graceful arch, and blends into the shoulders correctly. It has enough length to be in symmetry with the horse's length of body.

VARIATIONS IN THE NECK: Also shown is a neck too short, too coarse and too lumpy. The throttle of this horse is meaty and wrinkled, allowing for very little flexion in the neck. The topline from the poll lacks the ideal curve, while the bottom line of the neck is convex: this is an example of what is often called an "upside-down neck."

A stallion with a neck of this sort not only cannot flex properly but also will not, probably, be very supple in his movements, and he is seldom light on the bit. Regardless of the use to which you might wish to put him, he would be prone to clumsiness. A neck of this type also very often is found in a horse which is coarse in every respect: short pasterns, bone, etc., and totally lacking in grace of form or movement.

The angle at which the neck is joined to the shoulders is also of primary importance. For here again we notice a typical Morgan characteristic. The illustrations show the ideal and its variations. The neck of the Morgan is set *on* the shoulders, not in front of them. In other breeds, for example the Thoroughbred, the neck comes out at a much different angle: it is set low, with correspondingly low head carriage; the structure is altogether opposite to that of the Morgan. Many breeds tracing to Morgan blood also show some of this high neck-set—the Saddlebred and the Walking Horse particularly.

Other variations seen in Morgan stallions' necks are one that is too fine and that lacks the graceful curve from poll to withers; one that is too short and wedge-shaped, and is not masculine in character; and one set on poor shoulders and in front of, not on top of, them.

With the ideal in mind, and a number of examples noted for comparison, the newcomer to the Morgan breed will learn quickly to distinguish the components of good Morgan type from the variations.

The Body

As mentioned above, the shoulders should be long and well sloped from the withers to the point, thus placing the withers well back of the forelegs—also a Morgan characteristic.

The body of the Morgan stallion should be relatively deep and compact, with well-sprung ribs, and rounded and well-muscled hindquarters. It should be close-coupled, with a short back, the topline giving the appearance of being short while the bottom line is com-

The Morgan Stallion Neck
Ideal and Variations

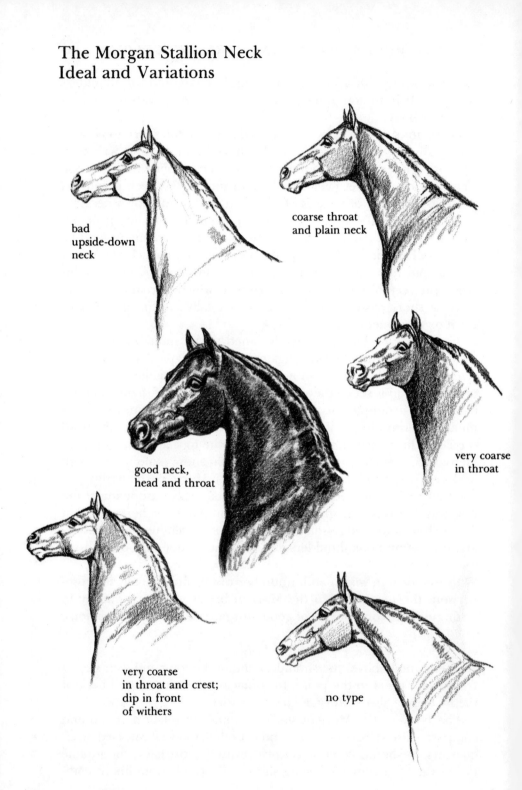

bad
upside-down
neck

coarse throat
and plain neck

good neck,
head and throat

very coarse
in throat

very coarse
in throat and crest;
dip in front
of withers

no type

paratively long due to the shoulder angulation and the depth of the quarters from the point of the hip to the buttock.

The chest should be well muscled but neither too narrow nor too wide and "beefy."

Tail-set and Croup

The croup should be fairly long and well muscled, with very little downward slope. The tail should be set high and carried gracefully when the horse is in motion.

A short, steep croup is a decided fault in the Morgan, as is a low, "drafty" tail carriage. Many a prospective horse-buyer's face falls with disappointment at this undesirable characteristic, for it spoils the entire picture of an otherwise likable animal. Some slight degree of slope must be permissible, however, as few horses are perfect in this area. A croup that is short in the extreme is also not typical of the Morgan and should be faulted.

Legs and Feet

Sound, correctly conformed legs and feet are essential to any breed of horse. Since the usefulness of any horse is dependent upon the soundness and form of his underpinnings, it is all-important to become familiar with correct and faulty conformation in this area.

The Morgan has legs of medium length, with strong forearms and gaskins. His cannons should be short, the bone being flat and dense with well-defined tendons. His feet should be round and open at the heel.

THE FORELEGS: The illustrations show ideal forelegs and chest width from the front. A narrow-chested horse very often exhibits other related faults, such as toeing-out and knock-knees; he also can appear "weedy" and generally lacking in substance.

From the side, the forelegs should be straight, with a well-muscled arm and short cannon bones. The pastern should be of medium length, with enough slope to make the horse's step springy and smooth. Short, steep pasterns make a horse subject to unsoundness, and also are a sign that he will be a very uncomfortable ride.

HIND LEGS: The ideal hind legs are shown in the illustrations. The gaskins should be well muscled; the hocks wide and deep and clean, without any evidence of swellings. The cannon bones should be clean and perpendicular to the ground. From the rear, the hocks are parallel—as are the cannons—and straight to the ground.

Tail-set and Variations of the Croup

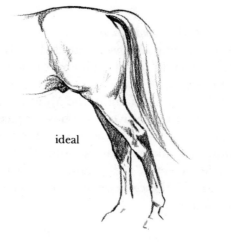

ideal

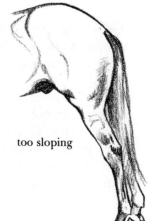

too sloping

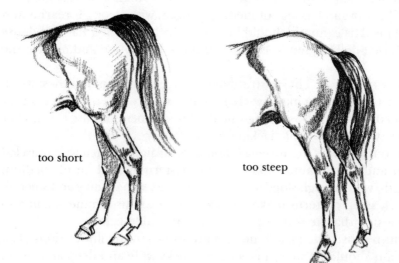

too short

too steep

Faults include weak gaskins, sickle hocks, thoroughpins, spavins, curbs and cow hocks.

To sum up: The legs of the Morgan should show quality, be flat-boned and free from blemishes. They should be straight and of medium length, corresponding to the symmetry of the body. It is best to remember that it is the quality of the bone rather than the size of it that determines a horse's soundness. Heavy, round bone is not necessarily going to be stronger than bone with good refinement.

It might be desired that a horse which is going to be put in heavy work with stock or extensive trail- and endurance-riding be somewhat heavier in the bone than the show-ring performer; but again, the quality of the bone really determines the soundness of the horse. Variations could reasonably occur, depending on the breeder and the uses he plans for his horses.

MOVING IN HAND

The Walk

The walk should be rapid, elastic and free-moving. The horse should move straight, going away, with no sideways motion. It is important that when you're showing your horse in hand either to a group of folks at the farm or in the show ring, he should be alert and up in the bridle. Brightness and animation are basic to the Morgan stallion. But he should be under control and not fighting you. This is a matter of training and discipline. Excessive head-tossing and going off-gait make it difficult to know whether an animal *can* move correctly.

A "pacey" walk is a definite fault, usually resulting in elimination in the show ring. Here the horse's cadence is two-beat rather than the correct four beats of the flat-footed walk. It is an unattractive, sloppy gait, often resulting from laziness and the horse's tendency to hang back on the lead. Have someone working behind the horse to wake him up and get him on his feet and up in the bridle. If this doesn't help, perhaps he is a confirmed pacer—in which case his problem is serious.

Another fault is the tendency to "go wide behind" (if it looks as though you can roll a barrel between his hind legs when he is moving away from you, that's going wide behind!).

Conversely, a horse can "go too close behind" (where he is quite likely to interfere, striking his fetlock joints with the opposite foot as he moves).

The Morgan Stallion

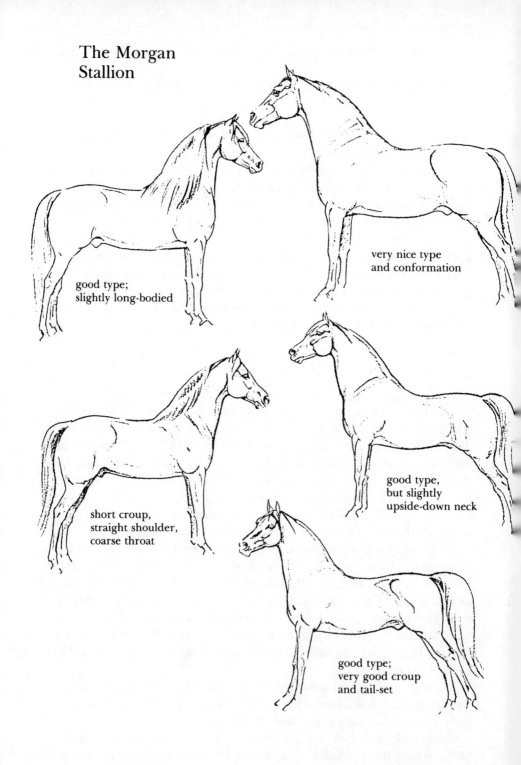

very nice type
and conformation

good type;
slightly long-bodied

short croup,
straight shoulder,
coarse throat

good type,
but slightly
upside-down neck

good type;
very good croup
and tail-set

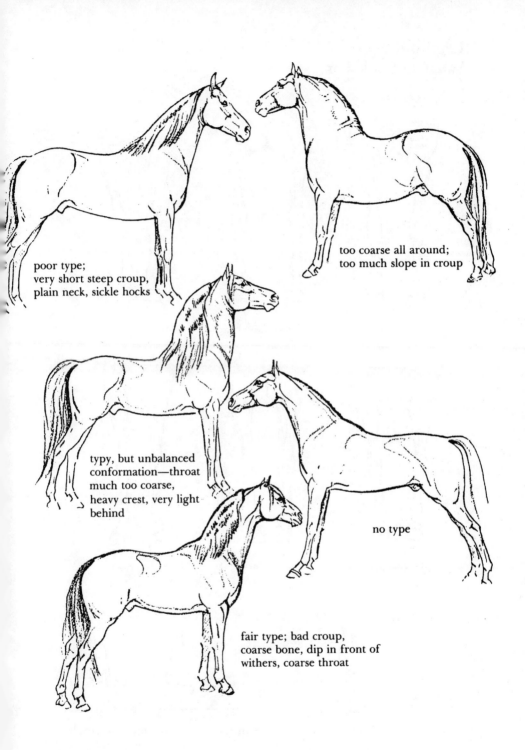

poor type;
very short steep croup,
plain neck, sickle hocks

too coarse all around;
too much slope in croup

typy, but unbalanced
conformation—throat
much too coarse,
heavy crest, very light
behind

no type

fair type; bad croup,
coarse bone, dip in front of
withers, coarse throat

Legs and Feet:
What to Look For

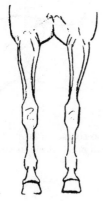
good front end

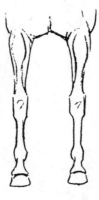
too wide

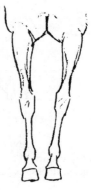
base narrow

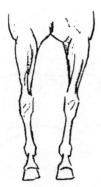
bow-legged

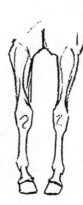
toeing in

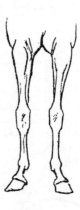
toeing out

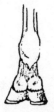
good open heel

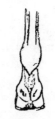
contracted heel

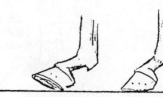
hitting on the heel   hitting correctly

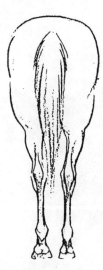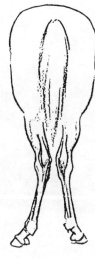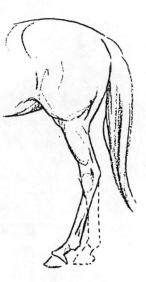

good hind legs   cow-hocked   sickle-hocked

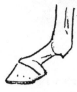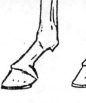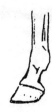

weak and sloping   short and steep   too long   good   too short

Blemishes, faults and unsoundness

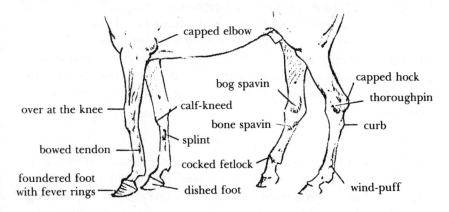

capped elbow

over at the knee

bowed tendon

foundered foot
with fever rings

bog spavin

calf-kneed

bone spavin

splint

cocked fetlock

dished foot

capped hock

thoroughpin

curb

wind-puff

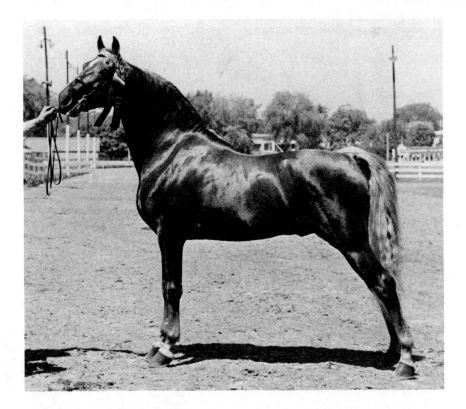

Winging and paddling in front are also faults in evidence when a horse walks or trots. Watching a horse move away from you will show you whether he is braiding his forelegs out and in—which is "paddling"—or flipping his lower legs to the outside—which is "winging."

While not entirely overlooking the importance of a horse moving correctly at the walk, some judges in the show ring will occasionally allow an animal some leeway in deportment as long as a few strides demonstrate that the animal appears to have no obvious defects. However, another judge may demand a flat-footed walk all the way down the rail—and he means *walk!* Letting your horse break into a jog before such a judge could mean a penalty. It is wise to know in advance what a particular judge will be looking for when you are showing a horse in front of him.

The Trot

Basically, the Morgan stallion's trot should be square, free-going, collected and balanced when moving in hand. He should move straight along the rail and, as in the walk, should show no evidence of paddling or winging. He should be loose and free-moving in the shoulders.

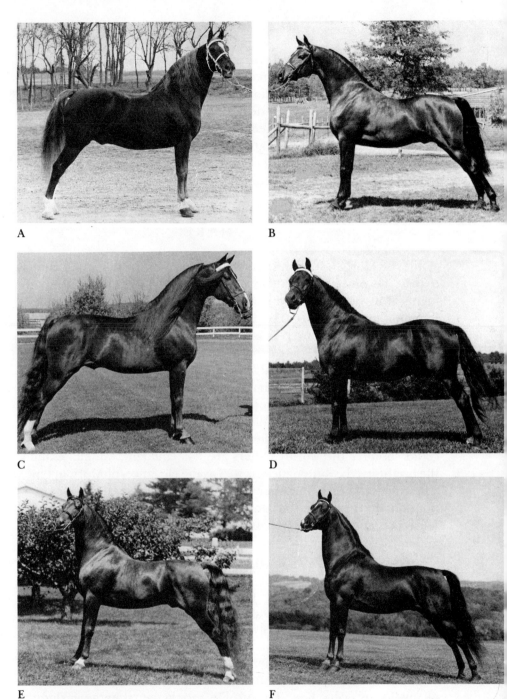

A

B

C

D

E

F

How Do *You* Judge Them?

Give first place through sixth to these stallions on the basis of type, conformation and presentation—strictly as you see them in the photographs. Then check your placing against the author's, on pages 361–362.

His head should be up and correctly set, without his fighting the bit, to give him a totally co-ordinated appearance.

In the show ring the stallion should not only move correctly but should also exhibit to a high degree the alertness and sparkling presence typical of his breed. Keep him on his feet, however: don't let him leap and do sidepasses all the way down the rail. If your horse has an abundance of natural motion and presence, fine. But this will not take precedence over a correct way-of-moving—so say the rules.

THE MARE

While the Morgan stallion should always possess the bold masculinity that is the outstanding attribute of the breed, the mare—though identical in symmetry and excellence of type—should be strikingly feminine in appearance. Her lines are modified, as it were, with less depth in the crest, more refinement through the throttle, and a lovely and expressive head.

There are many beautiful Morgan mares that are as showy and high-headed as any stud, with the same impudent boldness and seemingly boundless energy. These individuals make outstanding show horses because they are usually highly competitive and will flag their tails at the slightest provocation, blowing and snorting as though they could conquer the world! Others are less ebullient, but still exhibit the bright-eyed countenance, as well as the elegance, of Morgan type. These are our ideals, and they usually make the greatest broodmares: not only do they have the Morgan characteristics, but they have intelligence, spirit and personality as well.

CONFORMATION

The Head

A beautiful, refined and feminine head is the hallmark of the ideal Morgan mare: large expressive eyes, prominent and with width between them; alert, well-shaped ears; a well-defined jaw that is not as heavily muscled as the stallion's; a small muzzle with firm lips and large nostrils. The head should be smoothly chiseled with evidence of quality in every line. The profile should be straight or slightly dished. She should have a clean-cut throttle blending smoothly into a graceful, lightly crested neck.

As mentioned earlier, of all the points considered in horses, heads

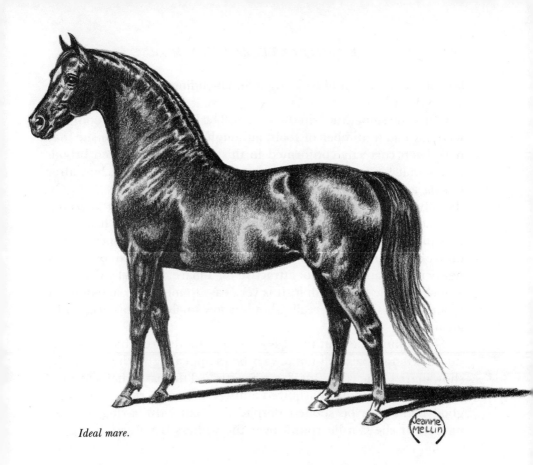

Ideal mare.

always seem to make the greatest impression. Thus, if a mare has a really poor head, it is often difficult for a person to look beyond it. Even if her general conformation is good and she is really not a bad all-around individual, we often tend to pass her by if her head doesn't measure up to expectations. The old saying, "You can't ride the head!" has some pithy truth in it when you consider how we are all guilty sometimes of placing too much emphasis on a beautiful head when some other characteristics are faulty. Being able to judge a mare objectively for her total appearance rather than for one or two features is essential.

The Neck

Although the neck of the mare should show greater refinement in the crest than the stallion's does, it should possess the same smooth curve from the poll to the withers. It should be of good length and set on the shoulders in a similar way. The crest should be finer when viewed from the top and not contain the heavy muscling of the stallion's. There should be no dip in front of the withers; the bottom line of the neck should be straight and blending into a smooth curve at the throttle.

Often the smoothness in the neck will be lacking in the broodmare who has had a number of foals, although as a young mare she may have been correctly conformed in this regard. I have seen broodmares that have quite cresty and shapely necks as fillies, but, after raising a few foals, they lost the ideal smoothness in the neck. On the other hand, I have also seen mares which never seem to go out of condition regardless of the number of foals they have had.

Some Morgan mares, as they mature, tend to develop crests not unlike the stallion's. To some extent this can be tolerated, but a very heavy muscular crest is not attractive on a mare, especially if she has a thick throttle to go with it. It is very easy to mistake coarseness for typiness, but the mare really should show quality in this area to be ideal.

The point to bear in mind is that the broodmare which has produced several foals will not always be as appealing to the eye as the show mare in the ring. But if one has studied the basic characteristics of the Morgan and has acquired a discerning and critical eye, these good points can be spotted despite the "old lady having lost her figure." If she is a bit round over the withers from easy living, or

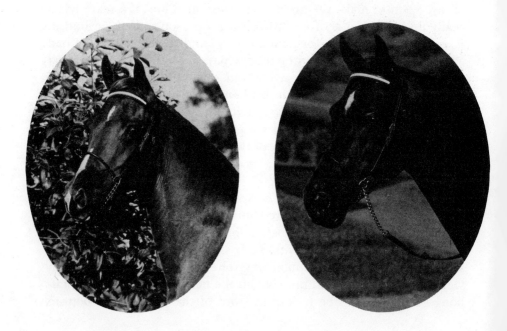

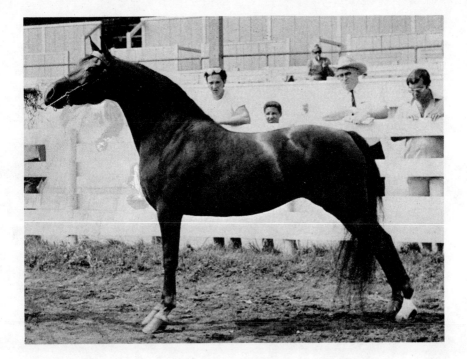

thin in the neck from giving too much of herself to her foals, take these things into consideration when judging her. Experience will help you see beyond the superficials.

The Body

Basically, the mare should be conformed similarly to the stallion in regard to Morgan type and conformation. She may be allowed a bit more length of body, but she should have well-sprung ribs and depth of barrel. She may not be quite so deep in the flanks nor so heavily muscled over the croup. Her tail-set should be relatively high, but the croup should not be too short and horizontal; neither should it be "dippy," though.

Study the two pages of drawings of mares to clarify this in your mind. They show several variations in conformation and type from the ideal to the very poor. Your study of them will give you a better understanding of the points of the Morgan mare than a thousand words could do.

Legs and Feet

Since most mares eventually end up in the broodmare band, it is certainly advisable that they have sound conformation in the legs and

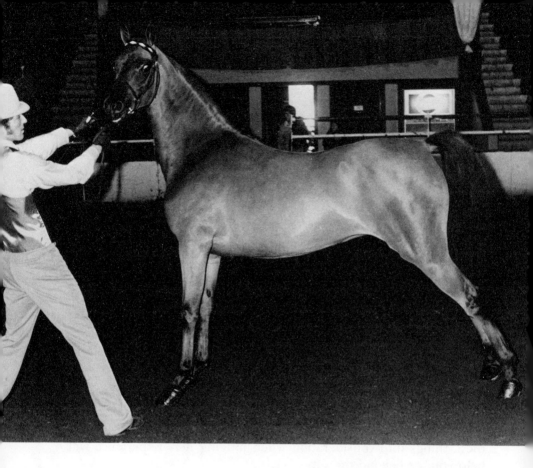

feet. (Take another look at the illustrations in the preceding section on stallions; the same factors hold true for mares.) Many novice breeders will use a mare that has a rather severe fault—extreme sickle hocks are one example—hoping that the stallion they choose might counteract this fault in the foal. Very often the foal may be free of the fault, but still there is a chance that the fault will be passed along. Using breeding animals that are free of very obvious faults is the only way to eliminate undesirable characteristics. Minor faults, such as splints and thoroughpins, are not usually hereditary—although sometimes a susceptibility to them can be.

The feet of the mare should be round with open heels. If they are dished and/or ringed, quite possibly the mare has had some trouble, such as laminitis or a very high fever from another illness. She may still travel sound, however, depending upon the severity of the indisposition and the care she received in the interim. If she is to be used as a broodmare only, this should present no problem. But having once been foundered, she is likely to suffer the ailment again, and lameness could recur should the animal be put back to regular work. However, I have seen horses that have been badly foundered, returned to normal usefulness with care and proper handling during the indisposition and afterward.

Good, sound feet and legs are essential to a horse which is to receive heavy usage. So if you have a hectic show schedule planned, or endurance trail-riding as your goal, be sure to select a mare—or any horse—with extremely good underpinnings.

Overall Symmetry

A word about symmetry is appropriate to sum up this section. When all the points of the mare have been appraised, how do they all add up? Is she a well-balanced, symmetrical animal with enough length of neck to balance the length of her body? Are her legs in the right proportion to her total length? Symmetry is a salient point when judging Morgans, in my opinion. Without it, one or two nice features just don't add up to perfection, no matter how you look at it. If a mare has a lovely head, say, but her neck is far too short to be in proportion to the rest of her, she is lacking in symmetry. If an animal has legs that are too long—or too short—to go with the length of the body, the total picture is spoiled.

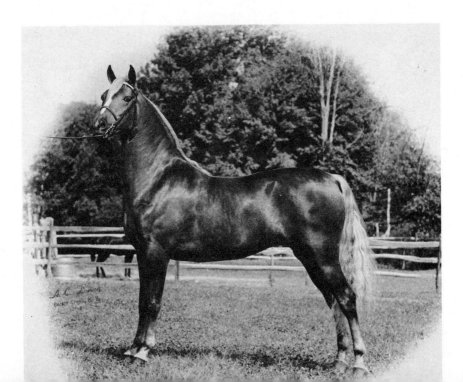

The Morgan Mare

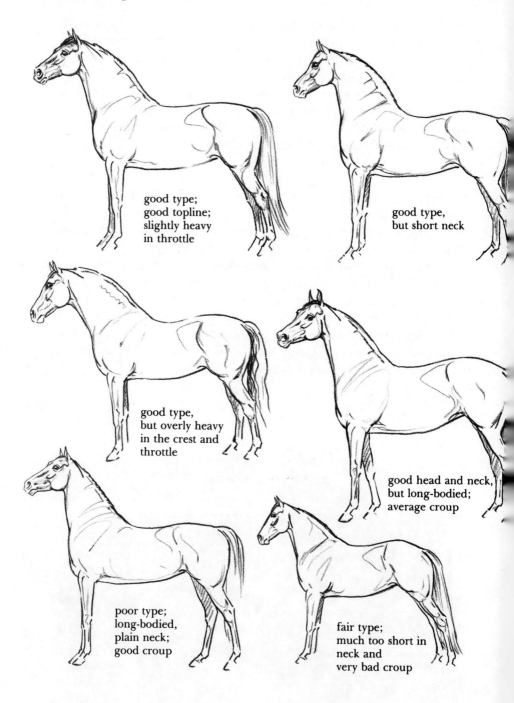

good type;
good topline;
slightly heavy
in throttle

good type,
but short neck

good type,
but overly heavy
in the crest and
throttle

good head and neck,
but long-bodied;
average croup

poor type;
long-bodied,
plain neck;
good croup

fair type;
much too short in
neck and
very bad croup

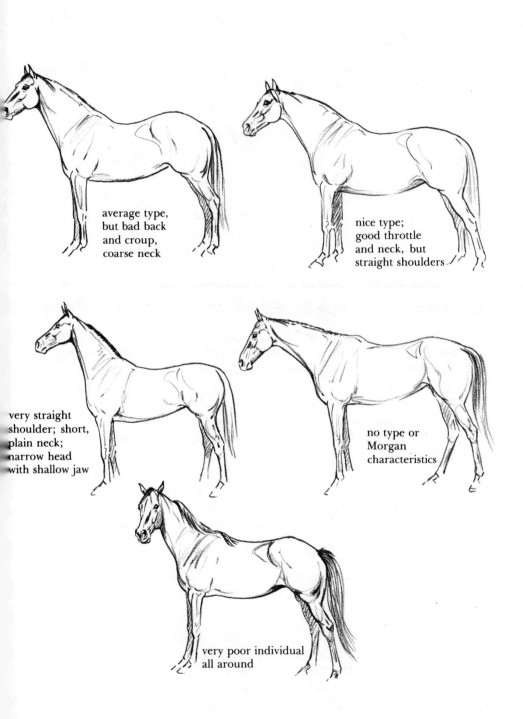

average type,
but bad back
and croup,
coarse neck

nice type;
good throttle
and neck, but
straight shoulders

very straight
shoulder; short,
plain neck;
narrow head
with shallow jaw

no type or
Morgan
characteristics

very poor individual
all around

Try to see a horse as a profile silhouette. If something is out of proportion, it will show up then. A smooth, curve-into-curve contour is Morgan type exemplified. Awkwardness is not, and should not be anywhere in evidence in the ideal Morgan, whether mare, stallion or gelding.

MOVING IN HAND

There will always be a little controversy about the requirements for the way a Morgan should be moved in hand, as long as there are horses which have high action and horses which do not. The Rules say that in the show ring, a horse must move *correctly* (this was discussed in the section earlier on the stallion in hand). They also state that height of action will not take precedence over the correct way-of-moving. This is how it should be. But there will always be mares which have a great deal of natural motion, as, conversely, there will be those with little knee and hock action but which move alertly and correctly.

The pinnings generally depend upon a judge's personal preference in the show ring. If a judge happens to like a contestant with "show horse" ways, and two individuals come before him which are tied in their conformation and type, he will undoubtedly give the nod to the one that is a bit more of a show horse. This is not to say that both individuals are not equal in excellence to type; it is simply that in the show ring, the showier horse will have an edge over the other, thereby breaking the tie in the most obvious way (to the spectators, especially). Since a show is, as its name implies, an entertainment of sorts, who is to say why this should not be agreeable? Another judge may see it differently next time out. But woe to the judge who sees *only* the showy motion and fails to give consideration to the type and conformation of the individual who possesses it!

The walk and trot in hand are subject to similar requirements whether in the stallion, mare or gelding divisions.

The Walk

The same elastic, flat-footed walk (a four-beat gait) is required of the mare. She should also move straight and behave herself on the line. Since most mares are a bit more subdued that stallions this deportment usually is achieved without undo effort. Alertness is desirable, however, so you should keep her up in the bridle even at the walk.

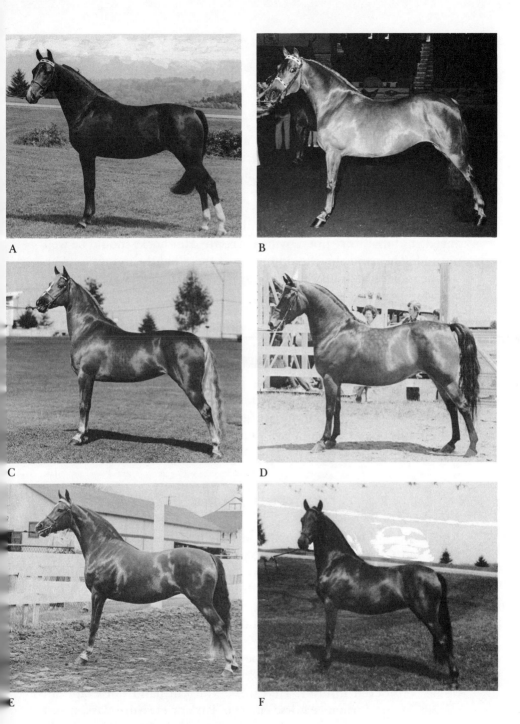

A

B

C

D

E

F

How Do *You* Judge Them?

Give first through sixth place to these mares on the basis of type, conformation and presentation—strictly as you see them in the photographs. Then check your placing against the author's, on pages 361–362.

She shouldn't be allowed to move sideways or break gait. And of course pacing is really taboo!

The Trot

As mentioned above, some mares are just born hams and will move with every bit as much height of action and presence as any stallion, and, also as noted, this can't help but be a definite asset in the show ring.

A balanced trot is essential, though. A mare who has an abundance of action up front and merely scuffs the ground behind is *not* balanced, and therefore not moving correctly. Her hocks should be well up under her and she should move off them lightly and airily. The two-beat cadence should always be apparent. Skipping or mixing gaits is always penalized.

When discussing ideals, it must be realized that not every horse will be perfect in every point, but should approach perfection in as many ways as possible before being considered for the show ring. Bear this in mind when looking for a show prospect. Excellence in type and conformation as well as performance should be given great consideration. When we are putting Morgans before the public, it avails us little if the horses we show, though they may perform well, carry little breed type: for, what then have we promoted? Food for thought?

THE GELDING

Appealing and with a personality all his own, the Morgan gelding is more and more coming into his own with fanciers of the breed. He is useful in the extreme, he doesn't have to be laid off to raise a foal, and his life is not complicated with breeding schedules and bothersome stabling considerations. The gelding is the delight of children and amateurs who do their own stable work and want a pet they can enjoy 365 days a year.

Possessed of as much type and personality as the mare or stallion—perhaps more!—the gelding needn't have a lesser role, nor should he be considered inferior. He can be a top in hand horse and an equally top performance horse either in Park or Pleasure classes; and on the trail he can be superb. Generally, he is the same steady, reliable horse every day of the week, with all the cleverness you might wish to develop in him. He can be a friendly companion who doesn't need the restrictions of the stallion or the enforced confinement of the pregnant mare.

CONFORMATION

In conformation the gelding ideally should resemble the stallion, with some modification of the masculine characteristics, the main ones being a slightly less-crested neck and a well-defined throttle. Whereas the stallion often becomes "staggy" as he matures, the gelding should remain relatively fine in the neck and throttle.

Since Morgan type was discussed at length in the stallion and mare sections, and the ideal gelding should also possess the basic Morgan conformation, there is no need for repetition here on general points. The portrait shows a gelding with the ideal type, and the drawings depict a few departures from the ideal. As will be seen below, a gelding can be as beautiful, in every way, as a stallion or mare.

Morgan geldings make excellent equitation horses too, so many

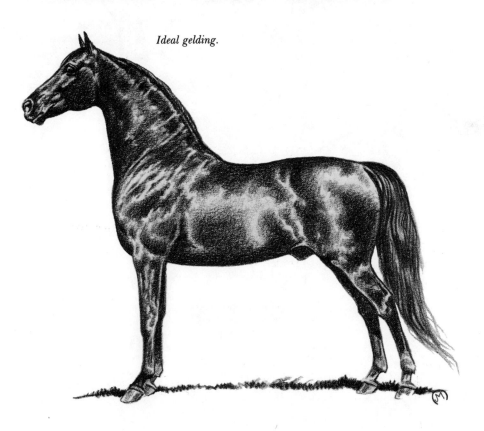

Ideal gelding.

The Morgan Gelding

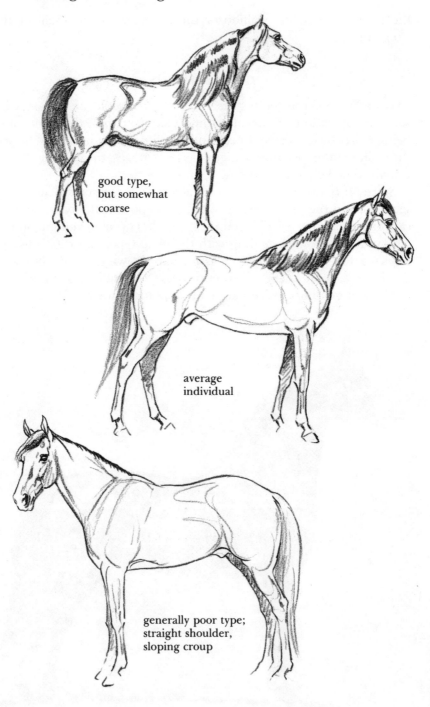

good type,
but somewhat
coarse

average
individual

generally poor type;
straight shoulder,
sloping croup

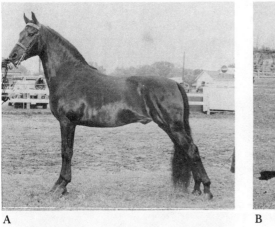

A

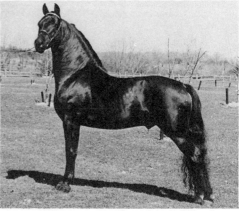

B

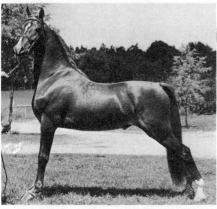

C

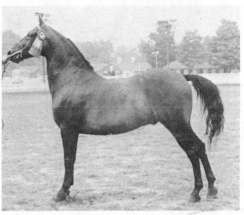

D

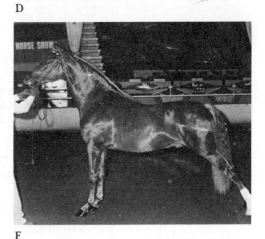

E

F

How Do *You* Judge Them?

Give first through sixth place to these geldings on the basis of type, conformation and presentation—and strictly as you see them in the photographs. Then check your placing against the author's, on pages 361–362.

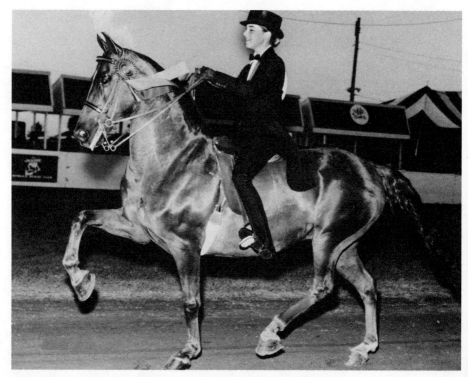

A Saddle Seat Equitation Champion on her very suitable Morgan gelding.

young riders have won ASHA medals on reliable Morgan geldings. When seeking a gelding, remember that he should have type and good conformation too. And *soundness is essential.* If you are a new horse-owner (and for you, the gelding is ideal), it is best to purchase a trained horse, if possible. He may make you dig a bit deeper into your pocketbook, but every dollar spent for a well-trained animal is money well invested. Green riders plus green horses often produce astonishing shades of black and blue.

The gelding can be every bit as affectionate as the mare, and he can have Morgan personality in abundance. Since personality is a matter of intelligence in the individual horse, with the love, patience and understanding of his owner to nurture it, you may make what you will of your horse. That you will have the raw material to mold into a beautiful friendship there is little doubt. Find a good-looking Morgan gelding and see!

7

Versatility and
the Show Ring

A T T H I S T I M E it would be well to talk about versatility, for, more than any other, this attribute has always been linked with the Morgan horse. Although every breed of light horse claims versatility as one of its merits, the Morgan was the earliest claimant to the term among all the American breeds. The old New England farmers knew and exploited it, and today we call versatility the Morgan's greatest stock in trade.

Much publicity has been given the versatile individual, the horse that "does everything," and the great numbers of really remarkably talented horses attest to the fact that the Morgan is a truly versatile horse—individually, and as a breed.

We see Morgans at the shows everywhere going from class to class, switching tack and appointments almost as fast as a photographer's model changes poses. From Western Pleasure to Pleasure Driving to English Pleasure, or from Road Hack to Trail Class: the transition between classes and their requirements is achieved as simply as the changing of tack. Some of these same horses have been schooled for jumping, and yet are also able to give a good account of themselves as working stock horses. This is the versatility that is such a tremendous selling point for the Morgan breed.

But even more spectacular is the versatility within the breed itself. Not only does the Morgan produce Pleasure horses with amazing abilities, but its Park horses are as brilliant and exciting as any animals bred specifically for the show ring. What other breed can produce the beautiful, high-going Park horse as well as his complete antithesis, the working stock horse on the ranch? From one end of the scale to

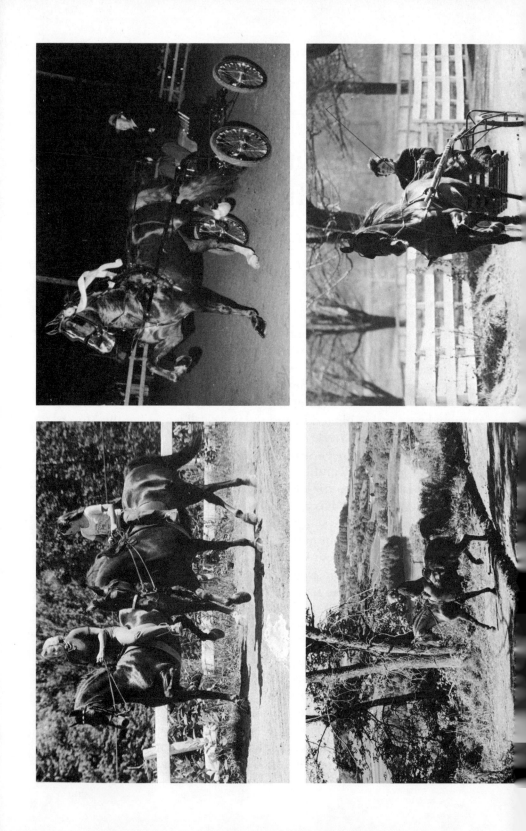

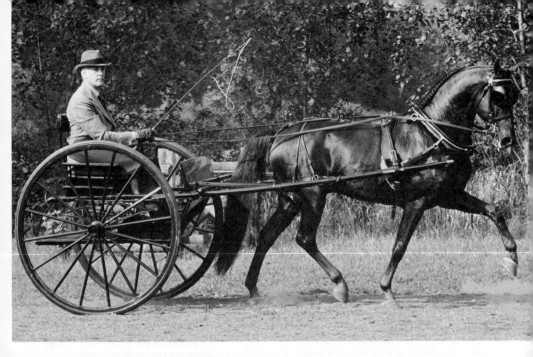

Carriage horse showing French braid in mane.

the other—one an animated, high-actioned show horse, the other a cool and agile cow horse. This is exceptional versatility within a breed, and proves that Morgan horses indeed have something to offer anyone and everyone. In everything but the racing scene, Morgans can compete successfully with other breeds on any terms.

Since versatility is so much a matter of training (always provided that the horse is talented this way to begin with), who can know how many Morgans with top potential have never been developed due to the dearth of trainers talented enough, and with the time, to put them into competition? The field of accomplishment is wide open here. Making a name for a versatile Morgan is a challenging and rewarding experience.

As far as the Morgan Park horse is concerned, he is indeed a specialist in his breed, just as the racing Quarter horse is different from the rodeo contender. While he is showing in this division, the Park Morgan has his activities limited to being as finely tuned as possible for his performance in the show ring. Why would it be any other way?

Here is where the term "versatility" sometimes tends to be misunderstood by the tyro. As was indicated earlier, the newcomer often has the mistaken notion that, because the Morgan is indeed a breed with diversified talents, *every* horse in the breed will be versatile to the same extent. This, of course, is not only unrealistic but is also impractical. While a top-winning Park horse might easily make a pleasurable Trail horse one day, during the time he is competing in the Park Division wouldn't it be wiser to keep him sharp and keen during the show season so he will be always at the peak of his performance in the ring? In today's top competition one must aim his horse at either the Pleasure Division *or* the Park Division according to the individual horse's talents, because realistically one should not plan to show the horse in both at the same time.

Besides—hypothetically—what if the horse were able to perform well in both divisions at a show; just how many classes in a show would one horse be able to handle?

And really, what would justify his being asked to?

The Morgan will always retain his tremendous versatility *as a breed* simply because individuals are foaled with distinct attitudes and abilities which, when properly channeled and developed, will make them

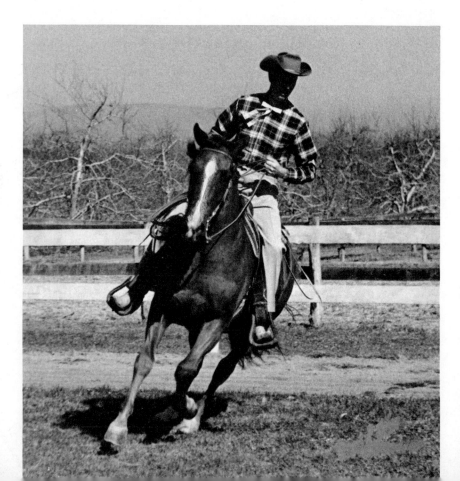

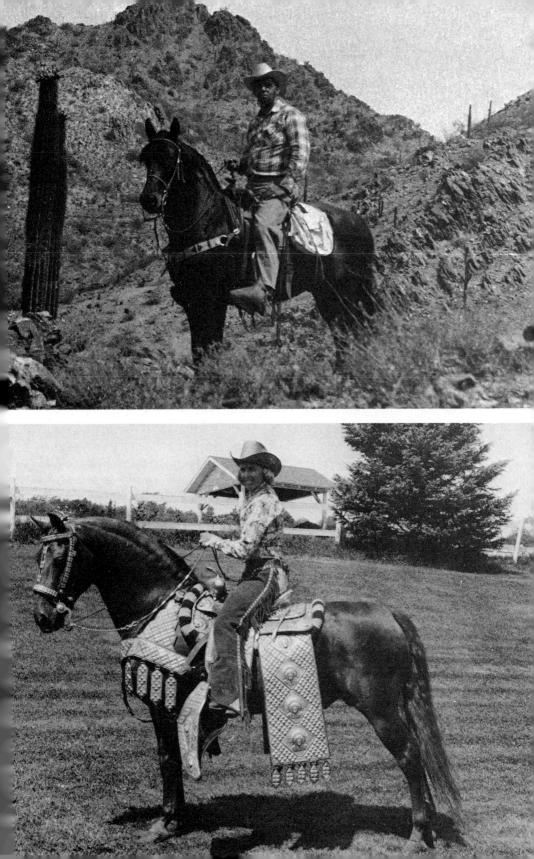

the outstanding Park horses, Pleasure horses, stock horses and sport horses of tomorrow.

AN INTRODUCTION TO THE SHOW RING

Although you may not have aimed your sights for the show ring at the outset of your Morgan ownership, sooner or later you are going to succumb to the magnetism of competition. And the better your horse, the sooner you will be drawn to the challenges offered there. In some capacity you will probably find yourself admitting that showing horses might be fun after all!

If you are an aspiring breeder, however, it is almost a necessity to become involved in showing. To make the horse-buying public aware of your horses and their excellence of type and performance, you must exhibit them at their best before prospective buyers, competing with other breeders on equal ground.

Competition is vital to any breeding program because it makes every breeder strive for excellence. One has to do only a bit of research to see how competition has improved the quality of the Morgan in areas where the breed was, at first, seldom seen. A case in point: one person acquires a rather outstanding animal and suddenly springs him on the local scene. Immediately, the horse's beauty and quality begin to be applauded (perhaps grudgingly by his competitors); and shortly a few other folks, determined not to be outdone, set out to find something good enough to beat the newcomer. Interest is increased, and soon three or four top animals are in competition in an area originally quite devoid of, or at least sparsely populated with, outstanding horses.

This is a healthy, progressive situation, and the snowballing effect is obvious: one good horse indeed generally leads to another and yet another, until the whole area may begin to emerge as a mecca for good Morgan horses. This may sound rather like a simplification of the situation, but I have seen it happen just that way. There have been many areas where Morgans were only slightly known at the outset but which have become important "Morgan country" because of show-ring activities.

The show ring has always been the show*case,* as it were, since earliest times to the present. Certainly, it was the Morgans which were exhibited and so much admired at the nineteenth-century fairs and expositions in the South and Midwest that prompted breeders to journey to the New England area to purchase top stock from

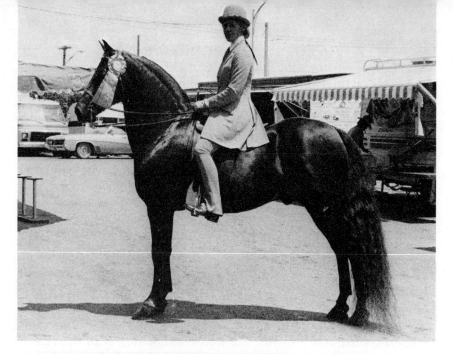

Correct tack and apparel to show English Pleasure or Park.

Morgan breeders there. The stallion Hale's Green Mountain Morgan 42, for example—one of the most widely shown Morgans of early times—was shipped by train many thousands of miles to be exhibited during the 1840s and 1850s. His success in the ring demonstrated the Morgan horse at his best. Green Mountain was a strikingly beautiful and typy Morgan, and his triumphs were so impressive that he alone was responsible for untold numbers of horsemen seeking out Morgans for breeding and show.

Where else but in the show ring can horse-conscious people see so many of the best individuals of the breed placed before them? Where else may a person more easily compare each horse on its own merit? The show ring has won new members to the Morgan cause in the past, and continues to do so. And at a very satisfying rate: for who can resist the best horses, turned out to perfection, performing with brilliance and precision? You would have to travel hundreds, perhaps thousands, of miles to see all the top horses which the show ring has gathered together for you under one roof. How better could you evaluate them all objectively than by seeing them together and comparing each to the other as they are shown in their respective classes? At the All Morgan shows one has an opportunity also to see the produce of dam and get of sire without the somewhat biased commentary often received at the stud farm—as well as seeing all the horses at their best: trimmed, groomed and performing as required.

Classes offered at the ever-increasing number of All Morgan shows attest to the fact that the Morgan is truly a most versatile breed. Almost anyone with an interest in horses can find Morgan classes that appeal to him, and a healthy variety of events it can be—ranging from all age groups in hand, to Western or English Pleasure, to Park, to Roadsters flying around the ring, and—at some All Morgan shows— the thrilling Justin Morgan Class, which is a continuing tribute to the founder of the breed.

If you are an amateur owner with a well-mannered Park horse, you will enjoy competing with your peers in the classes offered for amateur riders and drivers. Then, flushed with an exciting victory, you may welcome the challenge of competing with the pros in Open classes for Park Morgans.

The Pleasure-horse owner will find enough variety in the classes offered to make his horse begin to wonder if perhaps it might not be preferable to be a Park horse—for the average All Morgan show has at least eight classes in which a single horse could be entered!

Events for ladies and children in both Park and Pleasure divisions include classes in harness and under saddle. Ladies' Harness classes allow the exhibitor to get gussied up in her finery and startle friends who may have last seen her in jeans and sneakers, giving her horse a sudsy shampoo or grooming him with dust flying.

The young horse may be shown in his age group in harness or under saddle. In classes for junior horses (limited to four years and younger), the youngster need not be made to compete with horses of greater experience unless his owner feels that he is capable of doing so. Very often, though, the junior horses have the greatest zing, and can—and do!—compete successfully against their elders.

And though the amateur and the junior exhibitor (the latter under age eighteen) have classes especially for their respective groups, they often give the older campaigners and the pros a run for their money on any level.

But perhaps the most exciting event to lovers of the Morgan tradition has always been the Justin Morgan Class, a competition introduced at the New England Morgan Show. This event demands that the same horse be raced one-half mile at a trot in harness, one-half mile at a gallop under saddle, shown at walk, trot and canter in the ring, and then, as a final flourish, he is asked to don a work harness and willingly draw a stoneboat the required distance!

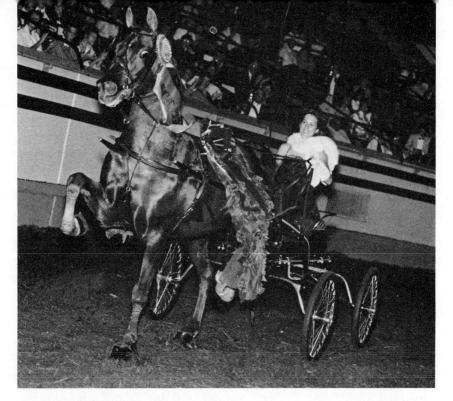

An Amateur Park Harness Morgan.

Open Park Harness.

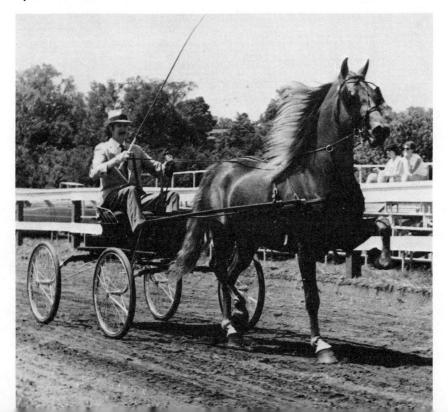

Also exciting, though in a different way, is the colorful American Heritage Class. Horse-drawn vehicles of another era delight the spectators as they circuit the ring, with the passengers in traditional costumes, smilingly acknowledging the crowd's appreciation for their entries—which required no small expenditure of time, effort and imagination.

The Championship Stakes

To qualify for competition in Championship Stakes in each division, horses must have been shown in at least one class offered in that division. For example, to qualify in a Park Saddle Championship Stake, an exhibitor must have shown—though not necessarily have been in the ribbons—in one of the Park Saddle classes earlier in the show. Championship classes include Park Saddle, Park Harness, Western Pleasure, English Pleasure, Junior Saddle, Junior Harness and Pleasure Driving.

Performance counts 50 percent, and type and conformation count 50 percent, so therefore the horses in all Saddle Championships are stripped for judging. Each horse is allowed one groom, who will enter the ring, when called, to help remove the saddle and to wipe the horse down. The reins are taken over the horse's head and he is

Pulling a stoneboat in a Justin Morgan Class.

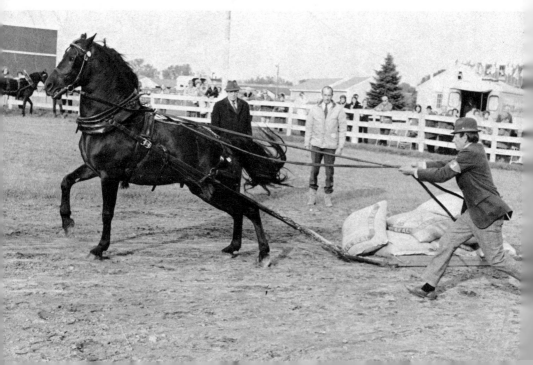

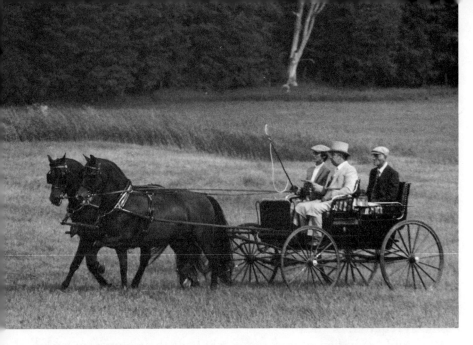

American Heritage Class entry.

asked to stand squarely to be judged individually.

All harness horses are also judged for type and conformation (but are not stripped), and the same 50/50 percentages are given in the judging.

In qualifying classes the percentages are 60 percent for performance and 40 percent for type and conformation.

Due to the 50/50 percentage basis in Championship classes, theoretically the Morgan horse with the best type as well as the best performance will be pinned champion. This is a rule heartily endorsed by all who value Morgan type so highly. A top performer should also be a typy Morgan if he is to be championship material; if he lacks type, he could be simply any well-schooled horse and thus not really be contributing to the Morgan breed. On the other side of the coin, a horse with excellent type should also be a top performer if he is to place high. A good judge knows how to evaluate his entrants and will give the proper percentages to the right horses. In the case of a tie performance, the horse with the best type of course should take the Tricolor.

On some occasions a judge will ask a few of his best horses to work again on the rail to break the tie after they have been judged for type. This workout may be required in both Park and Pleasure championships under saddle or in harness. Qualifying classes are also subject to a workout if the judge so desires one.

If a judge requires a workout, he must work all the horses *both ways* of the ring at either a walk and trot or a walk, trot and canter. If a good horse has made a slight mistake in the beginning of a class but performs well until the horses are asked to line up, a judge may ask that horse or horses to work again. This workout will cancel out any mistakes made in the earlier part of the class. And it will give, perhaps, the best horse a chance to redeem himself. Of course, this is at the judge's discretion, and an exhibitor doesn't always have that chance to have his horse's earlier indiscretions canceled out! Usually a judge will have his horses placed by the time the class is lined up the first time.

Some horses are at their best in a workout and really "get into it" when asked to work again. Others seem never to get into gear again and hang back and sulk, thinking that they have already done what has been required of them.

Many judges, in lieu of a workout, will have their horses go back into a trot again after the last canter to settle a tie among their contenders for high placings. Since the trot is the "show gait" of both Park and Pleasure horses, a tie can be settled quite often by this method. If it is more complicated than that, a full workout may be required, with two to four horses being asked to work again. Sometimes a judge will leave his winner in the line-up and work

Stripping for a Saddle Class Championship.

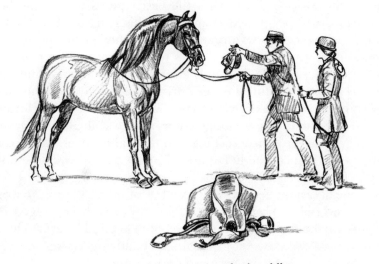

cut-back saddle

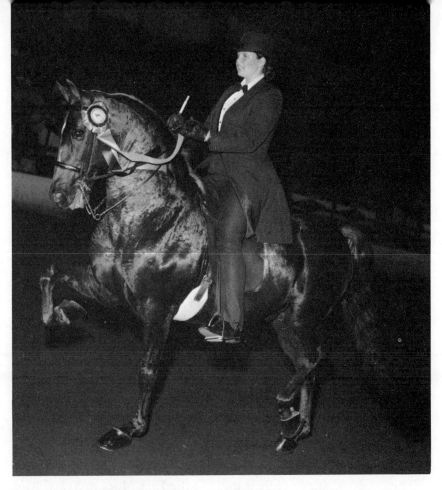

An Amateur Park Saddle Champion.

out for second ribbon and below. Each judge usually has his own method. Some highly experienced judges *never* call for workouts!

Suitable Equipment for English Pleasure and Park Saddle
The customary saddle for the Morgan "shown English" has become, through popular acceptance, the cut-back show saddle. A flat style with a low cantle and wide skirts, this saddle has a cut-back pommel as shown in the preceding drawing of a Park Saddle entry stripped for a Stake Class. It was developed first for the American saddle horse to accommodate his regally high head carriage. A saddle was needed to allow the high-headed horse more freedom to elevate his neck without the saddle's binding at the withers. The cut-back style of saddle solved the problem very well.

Since the high neck-set originated with the Morgan—who has deep, well-angulated shoulders and a neck which is set on high—the cut-

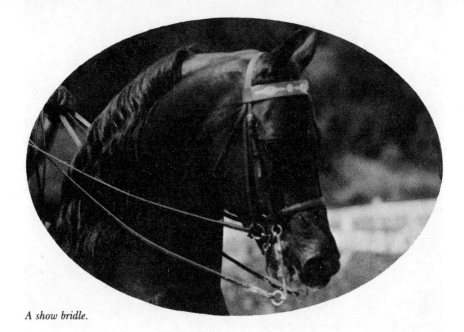

A show bridle.

back is a logical choice for him too. Placed well back on a horse, this style of saddle best reveals the beautiful shoulder and proud head carriage typical of our Morgans and allows for greater freedom of motion in the forehand.

The cut-back show saddle is used on the Park Morgan today. And most exhibitors showing in the English Pleasure classes prefer to use it also. It is a comfortable saddle, perfectly suitable for trail-riding as well as in the show ring. I have ridden many a mile in a show saddle and found it equal to any of the so-called "all-around pleasure saddles." Some riders like a dressage saddle for their Morgan Pleasure horses.

Obviously, then, one can use whatever style is comfortable in Pleasure classes. Caution is advised, however, on acquiring a saddle that has very heavy padding, which tends to raise it quite high off a horse's back. A heavily padded saddle is difficult to fit on a Morgan's broad back. Many agree that the cut-back saddle is still the best bet, since the great majority of exhibitors showing Morgans ride Saddle Seat, the most popular style.

A show bridle is a necessity if you are show-ring bound. This is a double bridle (also called a full bridle) of the Weymouth type, but with narrow leather cheekpieces and reins. Cavessons with colored nosebands that match the browband are a variation used by most exhibitors. On a horse whose nose is somewhat long from the eye to the muzzle, the use of a colored noseband sometimes seems to give the impression of shortening this distance, thus enhancing the horse's appearance.

Cavesson sets with stable colors and designs are very popular. Made in a wide variety and combinations of colors, not only do they enhance the head of your horse but they also identify your stable or your trainer's stable. These sets can be custom designed by a number of harness makers, so let your imagination go to work. But be conservative and don't go out in left field to be different—no fluorescents, etc.!

The bits include a show curb, which comes in a variety of lengths and mouth styles and widths, and a small snaffle or bridoon. Each horse should be fitted with the bits which are correct in width and length for him.

Care should be taken not to use a curb with a very long shank on a young horse. Indeed, the full bridle should be used with caution until the young horse has completely accepted it. Too many novices rush a horse into a show bridle before his training warrants it. Many sensitive mouths have been ruined by premature use of the full bridle in inexperienced hands.

While on the subject of bridles for Morgans, the illustration shows a useful training bridle for you to make up. It is an ideal arrangement to use on a green horse to ease him gradually into the action of the full bridle. As can be seen, it is a snaffle bridle with two reins and is used in conjunction with a running martingale. The action of the lower, or curb, rein will cause him to drop his nose and flex at the poll, while the top rein will elevate his head. The leverage comes from the martingale, instead of from a long-shanked curb bit. And while it is certainly less severe, it is very effective as a training bridle.

A colt that has been worked in the bitting harness (see Glossary) in a full bridle and then *ridden* in this rig will be soon ready to work willingly under saddle in the full bridle and adapt himself much more readily to it. This bridle is also useful for trail-riding, but should not be considered proper for the show ring.

Some exhibitors prefer to show their Pleasure horses in a Pelham bridle rather than with the two bits in the Weymouth bridle. This is permissible. But you should use the same show bridle, removing the entire snaffle section of the full bridle. A bit with loose rings and a 6¾-inch shank is the best Pelham, because it gives a similar appearance to the double bits in the complete show bridle.

Training Bridle and Martingale

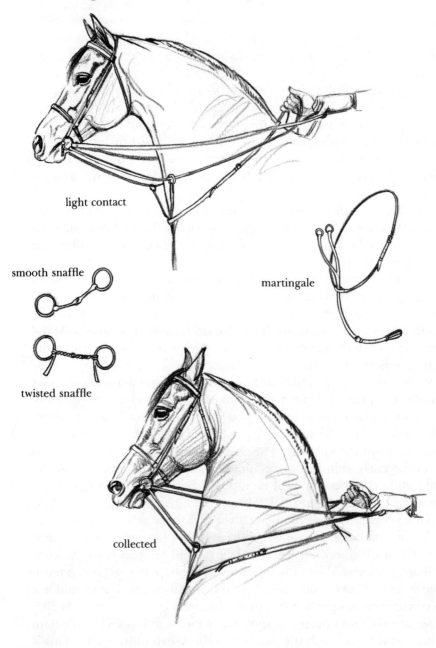

light contact

smooth snaffle

twisted snaffle

martingale

collected

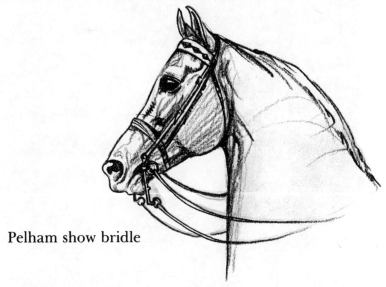

Pelham show bridle

Suitable Equipment for Western Pleasure

The first consideration when purchasing a Western, or stock, saddle is to be sure that it fits *you*. No matter how beautifully hand-carved and silvermounted it might be, if it doesn't fit you properly, it will surely spoil your ride completely. So before buying a Western saddle always *at least* sit in it—or, better yet, put it on a horse and try it. See if the stirrups are free-swinging, and if the seat is the right length and width for you and totally comfortable. There is no greater disappointment than buying a beautiful saddle and finding after a few miles on the trail that it is a torture to ride. Select one carefully!

The hundreds of makes and models in stock saddles today—as a result of the great popularity of this style of riding—can be confusing to the new horse-owner, to say the least. The various styles fall roughly into four categories: the cutting saddle, the roping saddle, the barrel racer, and the so-called all-around pleasure saddle. It is a matter of personal choice: but remember, *it should fit.*

Since the trees of most stock saddles are designed with the broad-backed horse in mind, there is usually little difficulty in fitting your saddle to your Morgan. Always use a thick Western-style saddle blanket with your stock saddle, because it protects both your horse's back and the sheepskin padding on your saddle. Blankets may be either single or double width. The double width is probably best if you plan to spend prolonged periods in the saddle. For show, many use a

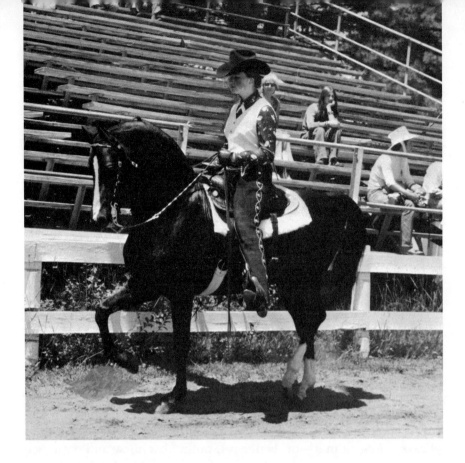

fleecy white, washable saddle blanket cut in the style of their saddle skirts: i.e., square or round.

In choosing your Western saddle, also bear in mind the conformation of your horse. If you have an extremely short-backed Morgan, then perhaps a round-skirted saddle would be best. It is also lighter to handle, which is a plus when putting it on your horse. Silver trimming has been popular in recent years. This can be either German silver or sterling plate or overlay. It won't necessarily get you a better ribbon in a Pleasure Class, but a nicely trimmed, well-designed saddle creates an image that you will feel proud to show. It is important to remember your correct appointments when showing Western. This *can* make a difference in your placing in the ring! The illustrations show the proper appointments for romal and split reins.

The array of Western bridles and headstalls at tack shops will leave your head spinning. For an everyday bridle, any style from the one-ear variety to the conventional browband headstall will do. For show, you may choose a fancier one with silver mountings. Bits also come in a variety of styles and types; select the length of shank and width

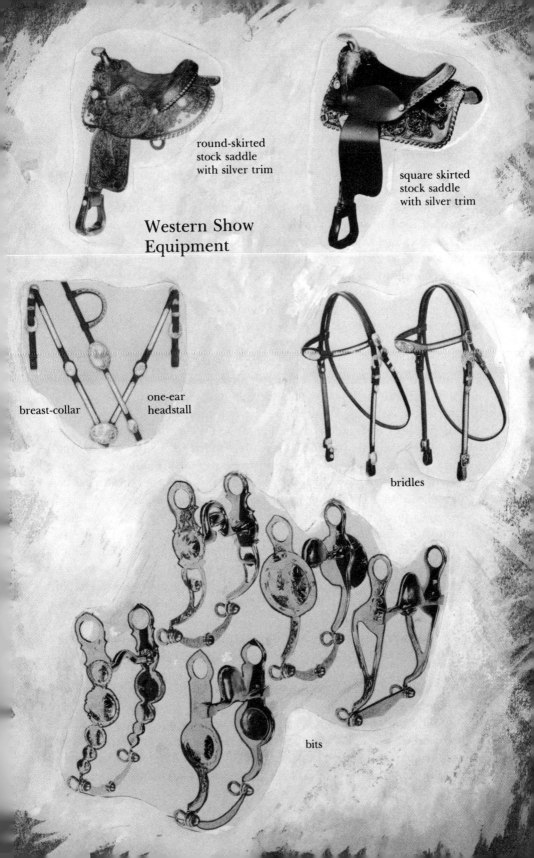

round-skirted
stock saddle
with silver trim

square skirted
stock saddle
with silver trim

Western Show
Equipment

breast-collar

one-ear
headstall

bridles

bits

of mouth that will fit your horse. Reins can be the romal style, or the split type.

If you like to use a breast-collar on your horse, there are several styles available. However, tie-downs, sometimes included with the collar, are not permissible in the show ring.

As noted, sterling-silver-mounted Western tack is extremely popular in many parts of the country now and, though it is very expensive, we see many horses shown nowadays with this beautiful equipment. People have always had a yen to adorn their horses with costly ornaments since men and horses first became partners, and thus it will always be, it seems. Silver equipment will not influence a judge, but it certainly does show that you take pride in your horse.

SHOWING IN HARNESS

Park Harness Equipment

There is only one correct harness and one correct vehicle for the Park Morgan in harness classes: the Fine (show) Harness and the four-wheeled Show Buggy. There was a time when cut-down Bailey buggies and ordinary road harness would do, but now these have long been relegated to the Cavalcade Americana Class. The Morgan Park Harness horse has all the distinction and brilliance of the Fine Harness horse today. And the elegant equipment he employs serves to enhance his appearance in the ring. He remains every bit a Morgan, but goes into the show ring second to none in his appointments and show-horse performance.

The Fine Harness is, as its name implies, beautifully made and super-quality with many show-ring refinements such as solid brass hardware, round leather traces, and patent-leather blinkers and trim. The illustration shows the Fine Harness correctly fitted to the Morgan.

The bridle shown is the traditional snaffle over-check Fine Harness style with cavesson. However, the Morgan also may be shown correctly in the combination bridle. This bridle has side-checks, rather than the over-check, round patent-leather blinkers, and is used with a Liverpool or Buxton bit. The illustration shows a correctly appointed combination bridle. It should be mentioned here that since a bridle of this type (used with the curb bit as shown) employs a certain amount of leverage, its use should be limited to those who are experienced horsemen fully aware of its functions. Greenhorns can get themselves into some really risky situations by misuse of the combination bridle.

The Show Buggy—or Fine Harness buggy, as it is sometimes called—was designed primarily for the show ring. It is a lightweight vehicle with a narrow body, suitable for one person, and has four wire wheels with inflatable tires. Although it is quite expensive to purchase new, with scrupulous care a Show Buggy loses little of its value over the years and has a "life expectancy" of several decades—barring accidents!

If you are bent on Morgan Park Harness classes the initial investment will seem slightly breathtaking, but you can console yourself with the knowledge that the best equipment will have very long usefulness, and used buggies and harness in top condition will bring almost as much on the market as the new.

In all harness classes it is advisable to carry a buggy whip. Never, never be guilty of slapping a horse with the reins to start him or urge him on: this immediately brands you as a novice in the ring.

Pleasure Driving Equipment

Although a Fine Harness may be used in a Pleasure Driving Class, a Pleasure harness that is neat and well-made will certainly be appropriate. It should have a cavesson and martingale, however, to be properly appointed. If the harness you purchase does not have a cavesson and driving martingale, these items may easily be purchased through a tack shop. Thimbles such as are seen on a training and jogging harness may be removed for the show ring, and the breeching is not used on the harness when showing in Pleasure classes.

The Pleasure Driving horse may be shown to a Fine Harness buggy, but the use of a two-wheeled jog cart has become more acceptable among exhibitors due to the tremendously large classes and the need for greater maneuverability.

There are a variety of suitable jog carts available for the Pleasure Driving exhibitor. They can be painted in stable colors or finished with a natural varnish. The boot (enclosed platform for the driver's feet) is always used on a jog cart in the show ring unless exhibiting in a Roadster Class, where instead, the driver uses the stirrups at each side of the shafts.

Because of the usual large numbers of entries in Pleasure Driving classes, it is inadvisable to use any antique vehicles, especially four-wheeled types, in these competitions. They are often too unwieldy and difficult to maneuver at the extended trot in a crowded ring and

Fine Harness

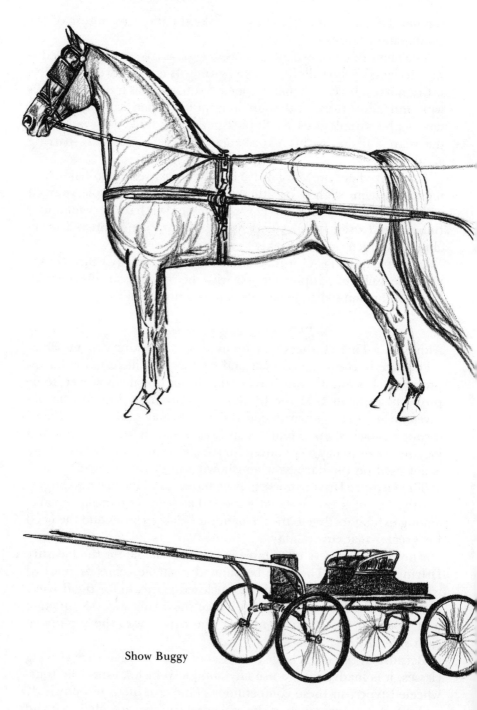

Show Buggy

Driving Bridles

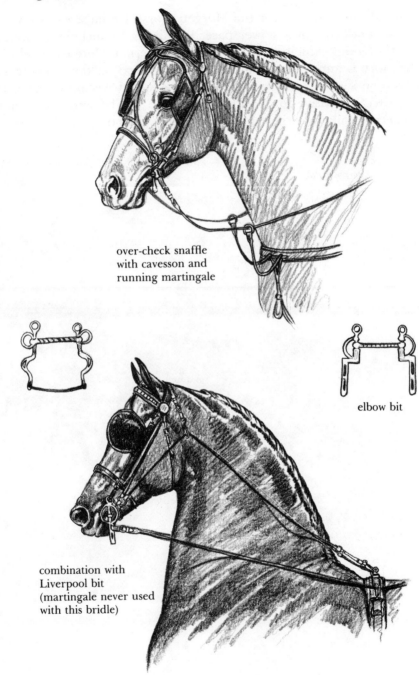

over-check snaffle
with cavesson and
running martingale

elbow bit

combination with
Liverpool bit
(martingale never used
with this bridle)

should be reserved for the Morgan Horse Heritage classes, which are conducted at a slower pace. Requirements include an antique vehicle and exhibitors costumed for its period. Here each vehicle's history is announced, and entries are judged on their beauty and authenticity. It is a class filled with color and nostalgia, and is the perfect showcase for the craftsman who has labored many hours methodically restoring an antique buggy to its original elegance.

Carriage Driving Pair.

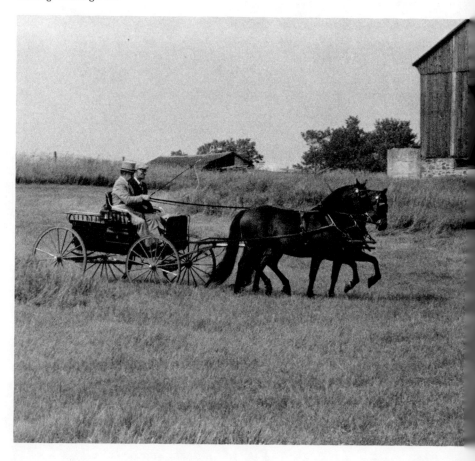

8

The Morgan Park Horse
and Pleasure Horse

BECAUSE SO many Morgans seem almost to be natural show horses at foaling, their early training is aimed at developing this potential. The young horse that possesses boldness and vivacity and innate show-off tendencies is far from unusual in this breed that has "personality plus." There are bloodlines which seem to produce individuals with this prevailing spirit as consistently as the Morgan itself has passed along its beautiful type. With careful nurturing, and skillful training, these sparkling animals become the stars of the show ring—and the shows draw new admirers into the Morgan ranks season after season.

To differentiate between the two divisions for Morgan horses in the show ring, the term "Park" horse was accepted by the American Morgan Horse Association and the American Horse Shows Association to designate Morgans with "high, natural action"; "Pleasure" horse, as the name indicates, is a good-using individual often having diversified talents.

THE PARK HORSE

Park classes are offered in harness and under saddle, with entries being shown in a manner to display all their brilliance and animation. The Park horses' forte is as high-stepping performers in the show ring, and most of them, seemingly, wouldn't have it any other way, being extremely competitive and apparently relishing the excitement of the ring and the zest of rivalry.

Ideally, the Park Morgan is the product of sensible training which has channeled his natural talent and developed him into a consistent and spectacular performer. The best ones do *not* require excessively heavy shoes or extremely long feet to "turn them into show horses." This erroneous opinion is one upon which the uninitiated observer has been known to expound at great length as he labors under the mistaken idea that all Park Morgans endure some mysterious and rigorous trial-by-fire to "make" them perform as they do in the show ring. But such is not the case: quite simply, the *best* horses perform well because they have the natural ability and are properly and thoroughly trained for their job.

To those whom the show ring offers endless challenges, the Morgan Park horse is the paragon of the breed. Admired for his exciting performance, he has sparked the interest of horsemen everywhere. The ability of some individuals in the ring never ceases to amaze people who see this performance for the first time. On how many occasions have we all heard people exclaim: "I didn't know Morgans could go like that!"

Well, they can. And they do.

However, it must be reiterated clearly that a really superior Park Morgan in today's competition must have two things going for him, and both are vital to his success: (1) he must be a born show horse, and (2) he must be the product of judicious and proficient training. Without both of these salient components he will be what the railbirds call a counterfeit. This appellation is often heard from the cluster of knowledgeable onlookers at the rail, and one has to admit that it is a concisely descriptive term.

Learning to recognize the counterfeit as opposed to the natural show horse is important to anyone considering the Park Division of the show ring. Go to the shows, watch classes closely. Do the top horses appear to be performing willingly and smoothly? Is their brilliance a matter of inborn enthusiasm and obvious training, or is it based on excessive artificiality—and, perhaps, on fear?

Brilliance and presence are basic to any Park horse, but you will find, upon observation, that he also seems to be performing fluidly and precisely—just as a dancer can make school maneuvers seem spontaneous. The same smooth precision must be evident in the Park horse, so that his total performance gives the impression of controlled fire and energy. The horse is an athlete and, like the professional dancer, must be in condition to perform correctly at his best. As in classical ballet, where each dancer has mastered his art to the degree

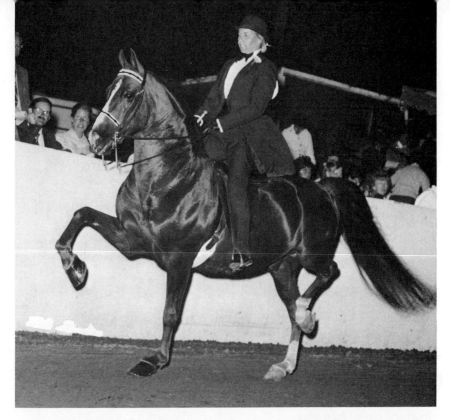

Two well-balanced Park horses.

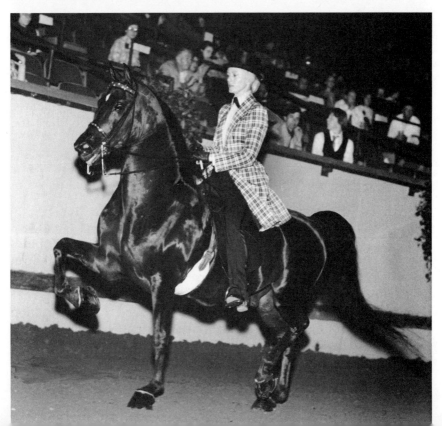

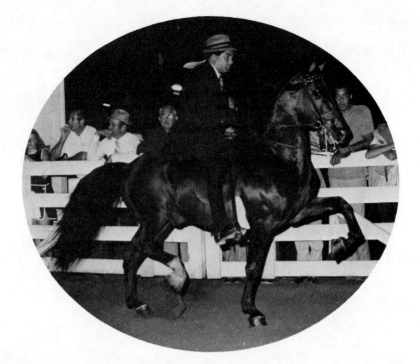

Another champion Park Saddle stallion.

where he can give a top performance each time on the stage, so should the Park horse be brought to perfection by his trainer in order that his performance will seem at once spontaneous *and* educated.

As in any sport, there are right ways to fulfill such a requirement—and definitely wrong ways too. A clear knowledge of both is the prerequisite for Park Morgans, and will be outlined here.

THE PARK HORSE UNDER SADDLE

The Walk

Alertness and a generous measure of bright-eyed presence are characteristic of the Park Morgan, and even at the walk these attributes must be apparent. A rapid, elastic step, performed in a collected yet free-moving manner, is correct. Horses that prance along sideways make judging difficult.

Generally, in the show ring the walk is judged at the transition between the trot and the canter, since the Park horses will enter the ring at their best sparkling trot and will be called back to the walk before being asked to canter. Some judges let their class make one or two initial circuits of the ring at a trot, noting each horse as it enters the gate. When the class is closed, they will call for a walk and, depending on their own individual preference, will then let the class walk a moment before asking again for a trot; they are likely to look hard at the walk at this time, making note of the horses that are fulfilling the requirements of an animated collected walk parallel to the rail.

Manners, also, are considered. A horse that jigs excessively, moves sideways, bumps into other horses, or misbehaves, is lacking in manners and is penalized accordingly. Head-tossing, fighting the bits and mixing gaits are other faults evidenced—and noted.

To sum up: The Park horse is expected to present an animated, collected, alert appearance at the walk. He minds his own business and stays on the rail.

The Trot

Coming into the ring, if you are really showing your horse, you will have him "up on the bits," well collected, and going his best at the outset. For here is where the judge's first impression of your horse is made, and often he will mark down or discount a horse on its first pass by him. If you are having a bad time of it at this point, you will have to make the second pass really right. Technically, a judge isn't judging the class until the entire class is present; nonetheless, he will be picking out the horses to watch when the gate closes. Many a high ribbon has been lost at these early stages, so it is advised that you have your horse in his best form at the start, if you can.

However, warm-up conditions on occasion can be less than favorable, and it will take a turn or two around the ring to get your horse on his feet and performing smoothly. An understanding judge, who keeps himself aware of conditions, will usually take this into consideration. If most of the class seems to need a bit of "loosening" time, he will let the horses have a moment to warm up. But as a general rule, if possible, try to have your horse performing well as he enters the ring.

THE IDEAL PARK TROT: The trot is, and should be, the Park Morgan's most exciting gait. First, it should be performed at the correct speed and with a definite two-beat cadence. Speed at the trot is not called for here—leave that to the Roadsters! The Park trot is, as its name

The Park Trot under Saddle

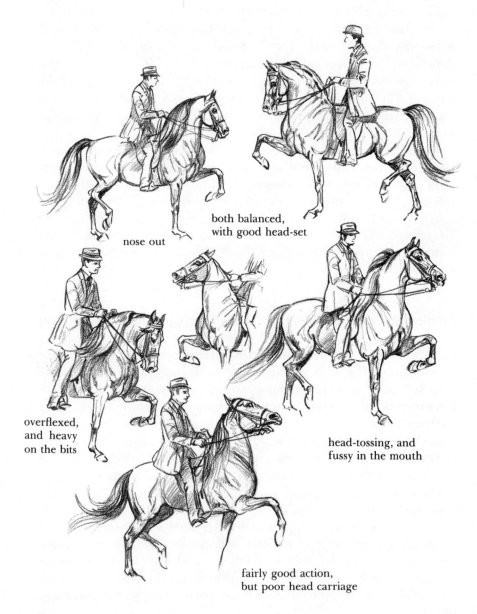

nose out

both balanced,
with good head-set

overflexed,
and heavy
on the bits

head-tossing, and
fussy in the mouth

fairly good action,
but poor head carriage

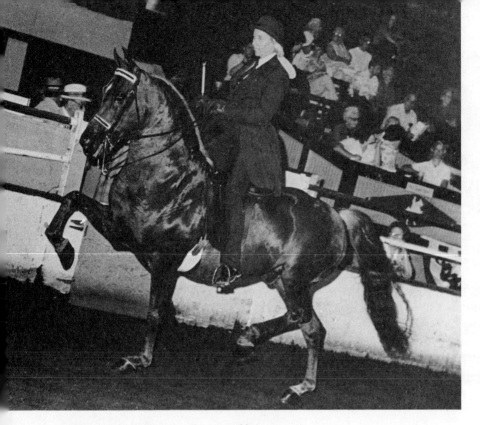

Park horse showing brilliance and a very athletic trot.

implies, a collected, balanced gait, with the horse in form at all times. Although high-headed, he should be flexed at the poll, without being overflexed or boring on the bits. Nor should he have his head high with his nose out, resisting the action of the curb. The illustrations show some of the faults seen in head carriage at the Park trot.

Once as we were watching a Park Class at the rail, someone remarked to me, "That horse has a real *oily* way of moving" (meaning that the horse was performing precisely and effortlessly for all its action and presence). Now, subconsciously, I think of that phrase whenever I watch Park horses at the trot. How many of them really have this "oily" way of moving, as though all parts were well lubricated and functioning smoothly? The word really applies to the ideal Park horse, if one thinks about it. A horse moving heavily or awkwardly or artificially certainly wouldn't fit this description. Or a horse working hard at his job ("laboring" is the term) would almost be expected to squeak and rattle by comparison. What's wrong? Is the horse uncoordinated, a poor mover all the way around? Generally, yes.

And the reasons why we see poor movers in the ring can be many and varied: poor conformation, bad training, overweighted shoes,

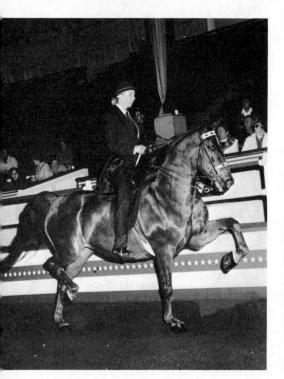

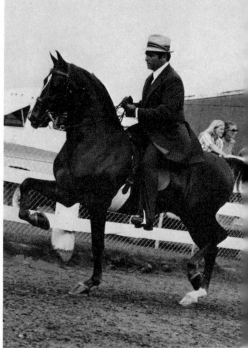

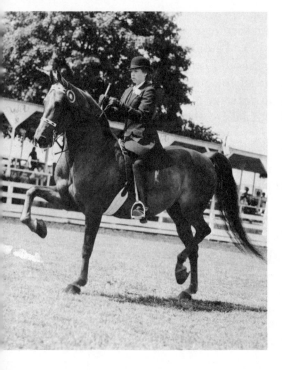

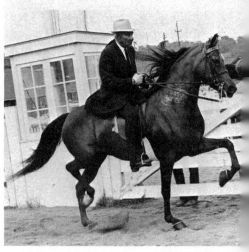

Park horse composite.

lack of natural ability and attitude, an unsoundness, a hereditary tendency to go off-gait. Where do we begin to analyze why they move poorly?

First, the ideal, or correctly moving, Park horse at the trot has his head properly set and is responsive to the bits. His ears are carried alertly forward most of the time. The horse should be light on both bits, so his front end moves freely, with his shoulders as well as his legs showing fluidity of motion. The height of his knee action should be in relation to the height of his action behind. In other words, the horse must be *balanced*. His hocks should be under him and well flexed at each stride. We often say of him that he "can use his front end and can get off his hocks too!" This is a simple and graphic description of the balanced trot.

FAULTS IN THE PARK TROT: Unfortunately, with more and more people who have little understanding of the requirements of the talented horse—the correct training, shoeing and presentation— showing Park Morgans, one sees animals in the ring which fall far short of the ideal. Sometimes a simple lack of knowledge of what is required is responsible for an exhibitor's putting an unqualified horse before the public; sometimes "shortcut" training is to blame; and sometimes the horse completely lacks any real potential as a Morgan Park competitor. Whatever the reason, following are the faults most found in the Park horse at the trot.

- *The "One-ended" Gait*

  Heading the list would seem to me to be the "one-ended" gait: everything up front, nothing behind. This horse seems to be "climbing" in front, with extremely high action in the knees while his hind legs appear to be simply striding along, almost unable to keep up. The horse lifts his forelegs so high that he can't get the hind ones co-ordinated. Very often he will hitch or skip a step or two to keep up with his front end—and then he is in real trouble. For no matter how brilliantly he is performing in front, the total impression is ruined by the antics of the rear parts. He is hopelessly failing as a correctly moving horse.

  A more balanced trot might be achieved with this horse were he shod in such a way as to give less encouragement to the front action. Thus, by getting him to use his front end less spectacularly, he might get his hocks in under him and start using them: that is, flexing them and springing off them, rather than just letting them follow along.

The Park Trot: A Comparison

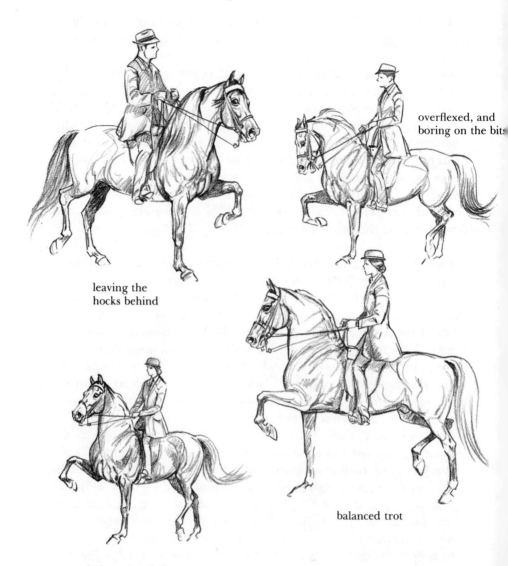

leaving the
hocks behind

overflexed, and
boring on the bit

unbalanced—all the
action is up front

balanced trot

The drawings show the one-ended horse at the trot.

- *Laboring at the Trot*

Second in appearance, as regards faults, would be the horse that is laboring at the trot: he is just working *too* hard. It is an apparent effort for him to lift his knees in the required way. He looks as though he is working in deep mud and must yank each leg out of the mire at each stride; he looks wobbly and extremely artificial. This horse is the antithesis of the oily mover. And generally he runs out of gas before the class is half over. It fills one with dismay to watch him.

There are several reasons why a horse moves this way. It may be a conformation fault: heavy, wide-chested, heavy-fronted horses often can move no other way, regardless of their training.

Overworking in elastic shackles also can lead to this fault, since a horse becomes so accustomed to the action of the elastics that he will yank up his legs at the trot even when these devices are removed. Shackles can be useful occasionally on some horses, but making a horse train in them continuously often results in an extremely artificial way-of-going. An experienced horseman can usually spot a horse that has been the shackles route.

Another cause for a horse's laboring at the trot is overweighting of the shoes. Now, shoeing show horses is a very individual thing: so many factors, often intangible, seem to enter into how a horse must be shod to perform at his best. No set rule can ever really apply to all horses since each has very different requirements. The animal standing 15.2 with a big round foot is certainly going to require a shoe far different from the one for a horse standing 14.2 and having a small foot.

Weighted shoes have caused a clatter and din in recent years in more ways than one! And some folks will never be satisfied on this point. No manner of sound argument, delivered by experienced and reputable horsemen, can prove to them that the weighted shoe is not an abomination *per se.* That the turbulence often is generated by those who do not show Park horses (or do so unsuccessfully) perhaps is the key to the vehemence with which they decry the use of weighted shoes on Morgans. However, with recent rule-changes, this whole matter is at last becoming academic. Park horses have no weight limit and a 5¾-inch length limit, which includes shoe and pad.

From watching hundreds of show horses and working with scores of them, my observations have led me to conclude that weight *sensibly used* on an individual horse not only has no ill effect on that horse but, on the contrary, can mean just the particular little difference in his way-of-going that brings him to a peak of performance, and makes him a top horse.

As in all things, though, the weighted shoe has its abusers, and I have no intention here of whitewashing them. But seldom do the users of excessive weight gain in the long haul. It is felt by most showmen that if a horse performs *freely and smoothly*, what is on his feet—within reason—should be of little concern. Of course, if a horse is laboring and/or flipping his toes or landing on his heels, something is physically wrong and should be immediately recognized and corrected. And it may not be the shoes at all.

Often, even the most natural show horse may require corrective shoeing, which sometimes might mean the addition of weight to either the heel or toe of his shoes. The really good horsemen recognize this need, and don't abuse the privilege.

- *Other Faults in the Trot*

Hitting on the heels, forging, hitching or hopping, winging and paddling are all faults in a horse's way-of-going. Some are as genetic as a tendency to mix gaits or to pace. Some are the result of poor

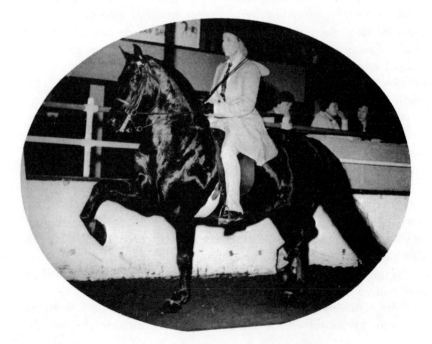

conformation, injury or sickness—a foundered horse will often hit on his heels or flip his toes even when and if he is restored to usefulness.

Hitching and hopping can be the result of poor training, or because the horse is overeager or fussy in the mouth. Forging often can be corrected by shoeing, or by keeping the horse from "going on" too fast and as a result becoming strung out and unbalanced in his trot. Winging and paddling generally have their origin in conformation faults or hereditary tendencies; corrective shoeing may help to some degree but will not eliminate these conditions if they are the result of poor conformation.

The Canter

In the show ring a Park horse must always be brought back to a walk from the trot before being asked to canter.

Ideally, the horse must take his canter smoothly on the correct lead as soon as he is asked, whatever the aid used. At the outset, being on the correct lead is elementary and imperative. He should have his head set correctly—up and flexed in, as at the trot—and he must be parallel to the rail as he goes. The canter should be smooth, slow and collected, and the horse should look alert and responsive while staying in form. When asked to return to the walk, he should come back to the slower gait smoothly without dropping his head down or boring on the bits.

FAULTS IN THE PARK CANTER: We run into interesting difficulties at the canter in Park classes. A horse's training very clearly is apparent when the ringmaster calls for this gait. Some horses scramble and leap into their canter as though someone shot them out of a cannon, and if they come back to earth on the correct lead it seems a miracle (though they often do). You may get away with this sort of start if the judge's back is turned and you get the horse back in hand before he sees you. But what do you do if the call comes to canter just as you go past him?

• *Results of a Poor Start*

Very often, too, the horse that charges into its canter never can be brought back into form, and he will exhibit poor manners and lack of discipline. It is impossible to have his head set correctly: his nose is out, consequently putting him all out of balance. This leaves him strung out and going too fast. Usually when you try to take up on him once he is cantering, he will fight you, boring on the bits. Even

The Park Canter

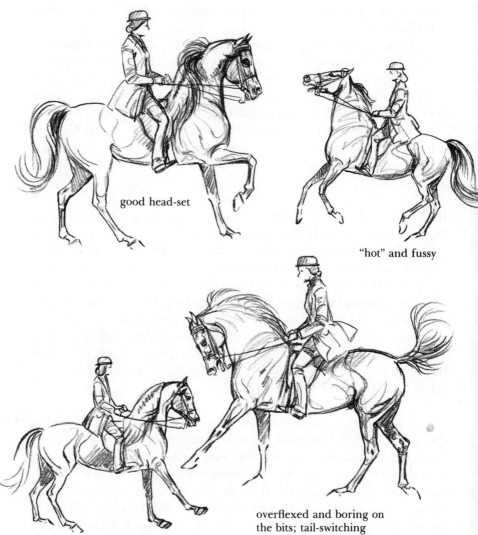

good head-set

"hot" and fussy

hitting on the heels

overflexed and boring on
the bits; tail-switching

if you succeed in getting his nose in, he often will be overflexed with his head down. Few riders have much luck getting it up again and set correctly without stopping and beginning all over—and very often there's no chance to do that anyway.

- *Cross-cantering*
Another problem we see is cross-cantering. Here the horse starts his canter on the correct lead, and then, for a variety of reasons, he switches, either in front or behind, to the other lead. It also can happen at the start: the horse will get off right in front, but be off (on the opposite lead) behind. The only solution to this is to stop immediately when you feel him going wrong, and start again. Not much use hoping he might correct himself. He might; but then again he might not, and you would have to stop and start again, anyway. A judge will often excuse a mistake if it is quickly rectified. But not if you canter halfway around the ring hoping the trouble will correct itself!

Generally, you can feel when a horse gets off wrong or switches leads. His gait becomes rocky and unco-ordinated. If you know your horse, you will instantly be able to feel when he is wrong.

- *Tail-switching*
Quite often a horse that is heavy on the bits and cranky at the canter will switch his tail excessively. This is considered a fault too, particularly if he keeps at it for the duration of the canter. A relaxed well-trained horse does not switch its tail unduly. If he does, it is a good indication that something is bothering him. Flies, perhaps? Not too likely if he is fussy in the mouth as well. Check his mouth after the class: there's a chance that the bit or curb chain was pinching him, or he bit his tongue. Or maybe the saddle wasn't properly adjusted.

A horse that constantly switches his tail at a canter (or at any gait) usually has a problem of some sort, unless he is just a sulky horse who doesn't enjoy working.

- *Wrong Cadence, Two-tracking, Flipping*
The canter should have a definite three-beat cadence. A four-beat cadence would indicate that the horse is uncollected and disunited. Experience will let you feel that the horse you are riding is moving correctly. You soon become accustomed to the rhythm and beat of each gait, and notice at once any deviation from the norm.

Even though returned to soundness, many horses that have been foundered will land on their heels in front, flipping their toes before hitting the ground. This is a definite fault which judges should, and do, penalize. Very often with this condition a horse works "out ahead of himself," causing him to always look strung out no matter how well his head may be set.

To sum up: He should have inborn presence and sparkle, exhibit the results of careful training, and perform correctly—with spontaneity, not just obedience.

THE PARK HORSE IN HARNESS

The very first consideration when choosing a Morgan to be shown in Park Harness is to decide whether that horse has ideal harness conformation. Without it, all your efforts will avail you little. For no matter how much action he might have, if he doesn't look like a harness horse he may very well be overlooked in the judging. Luckily, though, the typy Morgan is well suited to being shown in harness.

To be really suitable for Park Harness, the horse must have long, sloping shoulders with a reasonably long neck set high upon them. His crest, in the ideal, shouldn't be too heavy; nor should he be too meaty in the throttle, because this makes it difficult for him to set up properly. He should have a naturally regal bearing which allows him to appear completely unencumbered by the harness. When horsemen say of a horse that "he really can wear a harness!" they are paying him the highest compliment. The drawing shows the correct conformation and head-set for the ideal Morgan Park Harness horse. The horse has type and conformation and, as we say, "he looks the part."

Also sketched is the horse that is completely unfit for the Park Division. His neck is set on wrong, and his conformation and bearing would indicate that he will never look appropriate in a Park Harness Class no matter how high he can trot.

The horse which is properly conformed and light and airy in his gait will always prevail over the heavy-going, ill-formed animal, regardless of the latter's apparent high action.

As described in the preceding chapter, in the Park Harness Division all Morgans wear Fine Harness and are driven to a Show Buggy. Events for them include Stallions in Harness, Mares and Geldings in Harness, Junior Harness, Park Combination and Ladies' and Children's Harness classes. (Only mares and geldings are allowed in the last.)

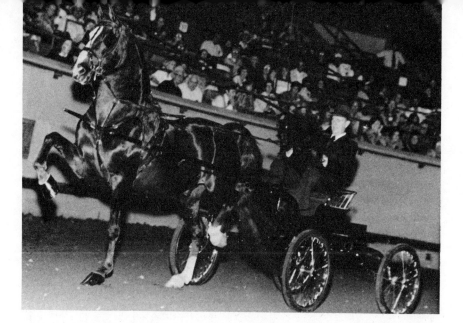

The Walk

Here the Morgan is *not* required to do a slow, flat-footed walk: rather, the gait has, in essence, almost the speed of a jog-trot, but is performed airily and regally and with great presence. The horse's gait should be elastic, animated and stylish. He should look like a show horse in every line, even at the walk. Evidence of pacing generally will disqualify him, while winging or paddling is always considered a fault.

The walk is judged when the entries are brought back to this gait prior to the judge's reversing the class. Usually the ringmaster will have the exhibitor nearest to him, at the call for the walk and reverse, cut his horse across the center of the ring. The remainder of the class follows, so that each entry passes the judge individually. It is at this stage that the walk is usually judged. Sometimes a class is asked to reverse without cutting across the ring, but this method can cause some tricky maneuvering in a large class. Whichever method is requested, your horse should be nicely in hand and displaying style and animation at this time.

The Trot

Perhaps the Morgan Park horse is at his most beautiful at the trot in harness. Here, unencumbered by a rider, with his head regally set, he seems to become more majestic than ever. There is little effort required to pull the light vehicle and its occupant, so he can expend

Suitability for Park Harness

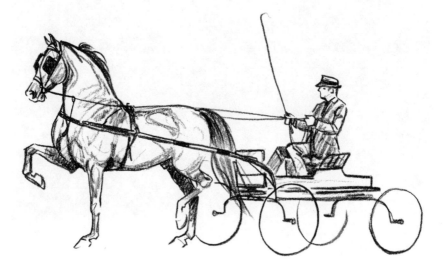

correct conformation and head-set

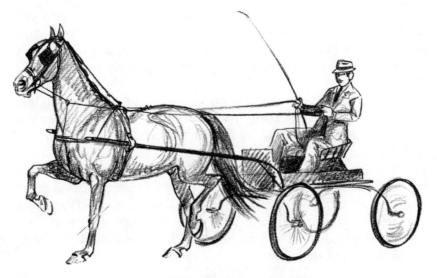

type and conformation unsuitable

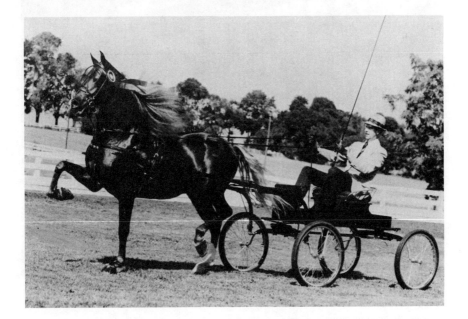

all his energy displaying his show-horse abilities to best advantage.

The Park trot here is judged on boldness and action. Your horse will be asked to "go on" a little; but, though moving slightly faster than at the Park trot under saddle, he must not extend himself to the point where he loses form. His gait should be precise and, again, "oily," with brilliance in each measured stride. His head carriage must be correct or the total effect will be destroyed. His action should be balanced, with his hocks well flexed and working in perfect harmony with his forehand. The smooth precision of the trot, and the airy brilliance which seems as though the horse were scarcely touching the ground, make the Park Harness Morgan a favorite in the show ring. When the announcer says "show your horse," it means ask a bit more from your horse than in the Park trot. This command is given, incidentally, only in Open and Amateur classes.

FAULTS IN PARK HARNESS:

- *Unsuitability*
  There is no doubt that the most serious deficiency among Park Harness horses is lack of suitability. A naturally low-headed horse will simply not make a top Park Harness competitor, for even when he is checked up (having the check-rein in place), the horse will

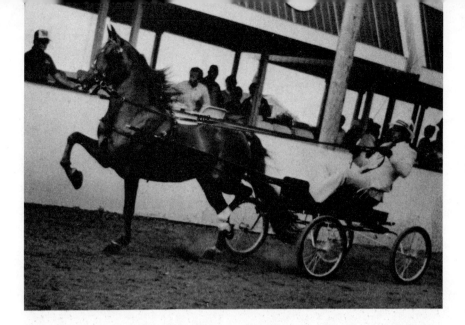

Show your horse!

not give a pleasing impression in harness, since it is almost impossible for him to carry his head correctly. Although a rather long-necked horse is liked as the harness type, a fairly short-necked horse will give a good impression if his neck is set on his shoulders at the desired angle. On the other hand, a long-necked horse with his neck set on forward of the shoulder will have little success looking the part of a Park Harness horse. These are definitely matters of conformation. But it is surprising that sometimes a horse with a fairly plain neck which looks quite unattractive when unchecked, will "wear himself" so well that his neck does not detract from his appearance when he is checked up and moving well. Learning to recognize the suitable harness horse is not difficult when the basic requirements are understood.

- *"Throwing Action Away"*
One often sees an exhibitor trot his horse on too fast in a Park Class, thus causing the horse to become strung out, often "throwing his action away" in front. His driver, thinking to achieve extra boldness and brilliance by pushing the horse on, is in reality causing the horse to go out of form instead.

A horse that is otherwise performing well but has his nose out is also impairing his chances for a high ribbon. He looks awkward and out of balance. The head should be flexed at the poll and the horse should appear responsive to the bits.

When a horse is checked too high, many times he will elevate his nose as a defense. It is then difficult for him to move consistently, because he is usually fighting the bits when he has his head in this position.

• *Hitching*

Sometimes we will see horses hitching or "hopping in front" at the trot—that is, they elevate one foreleg higher than the other at each stride, thus spoiling their timing and producing an uneven gait.

And some horses will hitch either in front or behind on the turns: they appear to be skipping as they come around, as though one end were trying to catch up with the other. For this reason many judges stand at one end of the ring to see which horses are handling themselves best on the corners. If it is a tight ring and a big class, one or two off-strides might go unpenalized, being put down to conditions. But if a horse goes along down the straightaway still hitching, he's all through!

Some Measures for a Good Performance

"HEADERS" ON THE JOB: To find your horse's best speed and how high his head should be checked for the best impression, it is almost invaluable to have a knowledgeable person watch your horse go around a few times before you enter the ring. Then any adjustments to the harness can be made; and, too, you will have some idea of how much to push your horse on in the class. If this same person will come in and "rail you"—stand on the rail during your class and advise you (with signals) on how your horse is performing—so much the better.

The header in harness classes.

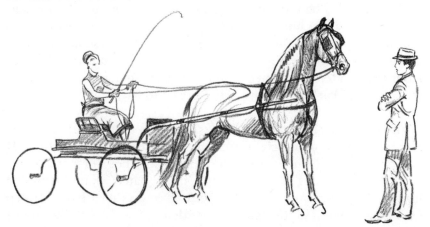

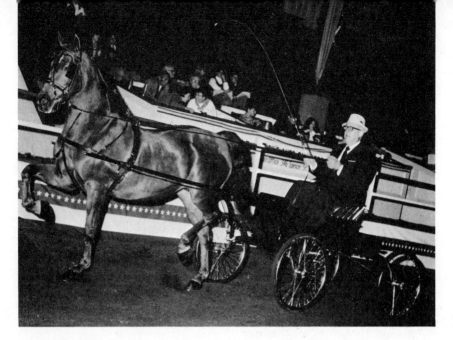

Amateur Park Harness entry.

Very few exhibitors enter a harness class—or a saddle event either, for that matter—without someone at the rail who has their interest at heart.

Generally, the same person will "head" your horse in the line-up after the class has performed on the rail. The header is simply a person, properly dressed, who enters the ring when the call "Grooms in!" is given. He stands at your horse's head in case he is needed to perform some service. He usually carries a small towel to wipe away any sweat the horse may have under the harness. In classes *other than* Ladies', Junior Exhibitor and Amateur, horses may be unchecked while waiting to be individually judged in the line-up. The header, after checking the horse up, should stand back a few paces at this time and not interfere with the horse. Ideally, the horse should stand quietly, but alertly, when being judged in the line-up. Interference from the header is frowned upon unless the horse shows signs of misbehaving. Park horses are *not* required to back.

THE WHIP'S RESPONSIBILITY: In harness classes, one must always be alert and on the defensive. Care must be taken to avoid cutting off another exhibitor on a turn or to "spook" another horse with your whip. Ring manners are important. Unfortunately, many well-filled harness classes resemble the Los Angeles freeways at rush hour. Keep your eyes open, lest you cause an accident or become the victim of

Form in Park Harness

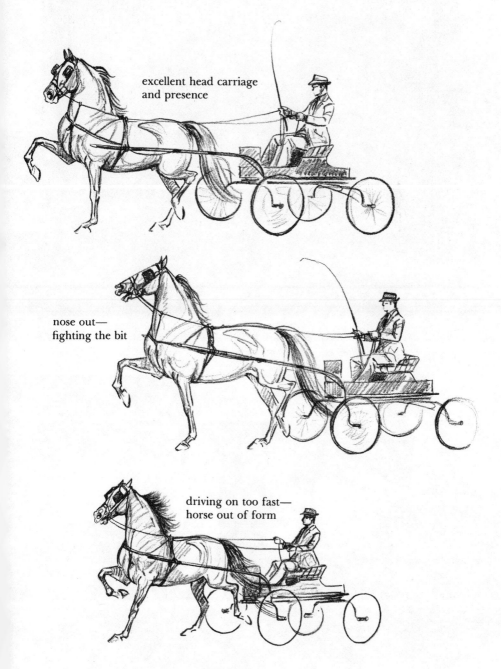

excellent head carriage
and presence

nose out—
fighting the bit

driving on too fast—
horse out of form

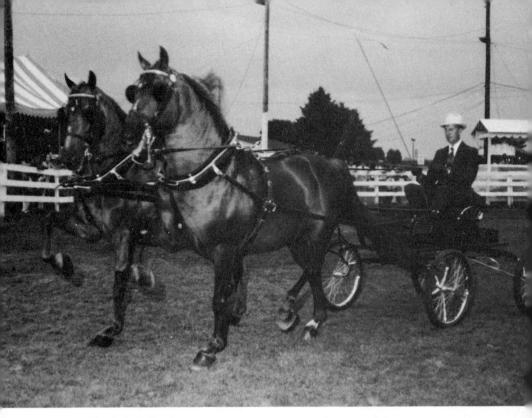

Park Harness Pairs.

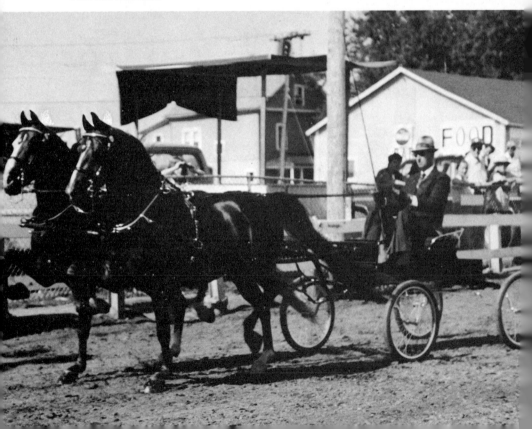

one. Many times an exhibitor will become so involved with his own horse's performance that he is oblivious to the others around him. Show your horse, but be aware that others are doing the same.

Should something unforeseen take place, always line your horse up in the center of the ring and nod to your header (who should be halfway there already!). Your horse should be unchecked and held until the crisis is over.

A runaway or other similar occurrence can cause some hair-raising moments. Keep cool. These happenings are rare, but it is best to be advised on procedure, in any case. Quick thinking on the part of exhibitors and railbirds alike can prevent a mere mishap from becoming pandemonium.

MANNERS FIRST FOR LADIES AND CHILDREN: In Ladies' or Children's Park Harness classes, manners are extremely important and are given first consideration. A horse may perform with brilliance and presence, but excessive boldness is not considered appropriate here. Save that for the Stake classes. Only mares and geldings may be shown in Ladies' or Children's classes; stallions, though perfectly mannered, are not eligible. A woman or child may drive a stallion in any other classes, however.

A Ladies' Harness horse should have quality, too: coarse, heavy-going horses just don't look the part. When choosing a Park horse for Ladies' classes always look for quality and manners as well as action.

THE PLEASURE HORSE

Observing the size of the Pleasure classes at the shows, it is easy to understand why it is here that the Morgan has his widest appeal. With his personality, disposition and a willingness that just won't quit, Morgans easily win the hearts of young and old alike. Their versatility and easy-keeping qualities make them the perfect Pleasure horse for anyone, regardless of his riding style. And Morgan horses and kids hit it off together like kittens with a ball of yarn.

Easily trained and level-headed, Morgans as youngsters' horses lend themselves to all sorts of fun projects: 4-H competition, trail rides, gymkhanas, parades and, of course, horse shows. Companions more than mere mounts, the Morgans are equal to any task, and perform with a flair that lifts them well above the ranks of simple

transporters. They perform equally well in English and Western tack—
or in little tack at all! And there just isn't a better all-around Pleasure
Driving horse than a Morgan: in temperament or performance or
endurance.

UNDER SADDLE IN THE RING

Since the show ring demands of its exhibitors impeccability in all
divisions, the Morgan Pleasure horse has just as many requirements
for excellence placed upon him as the Park horse does, for *in his own
way* he should never be inferior to the more dramatic performer. In
his action and appearance, he should display his own talents with the
same keenness and style; physically, he should exhibit equal finish
and excellent type. In other words, ideally he should in every way
be the equal of his Park counterpart, the difference being that the
Pleasure horse has a weight limit of 18 ounces and a 4¾-inch length
of toe limit, including shoe and pad.

The "only-a-Pleasure-horse" attitude has been just about elimi-
nated in recent years. Some of the Breed's most stellar performers
have been English Pleasure horses. The "new style" of the English
Pleasure horse in the show ring has evolved for a number of reasons.
In the '60s and '70s, the Pleasure horse was expected to go on a loose
rein with a relatively low head carriage; manners were considered

A typy English Pleasure Morgan.

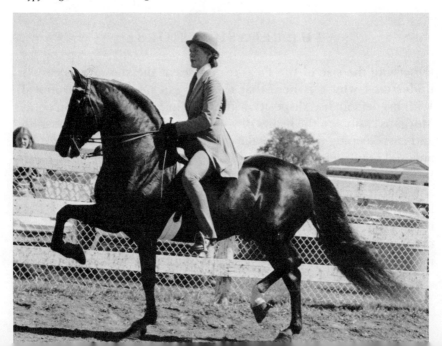

above all else; and Morgans of varied types were shown. The winners were the quietest, best-behaved animals on the loosest rein. The classes were usually *enormous!* Of course, there were always the pretty typy Morgans who "stood out in a crowd" who would take the high ribbons.

Then a few high-moving, up-headed individuals with excellent attitude and manners started to appear in classes for the English Pleasure horse. As long as their manners were impeccable, judges started giving the top ribbons to these more stylish, higher-actioned horses. With heads set like Park horses and action high and almost as brilliant as a Park horse, these new-style Pleasure horses soon had people thinking differently about Pleasure horses in general.

All this was looked upon with a baleful eye by the "old guard," who expected a Pleasure horse to be as equally at home on the trail as in the show ring. But the handwriting was on the proverbial wall, and there now appears to be no turning back, at least as far as the "A" shows are concerned. The high-headed, set-up Morgan shown with light contact on the rein is apparently here to stay. His higher action, extra presence and excellent type coupled with agreeable manners put the English Pleasure horse right up there with the Park horses for spectator appeal.

The only discordant note in regard to the metamorphosis of the English Pleasure horse are the cries from exhibitors whose horses lack both the conformation and attitude to compete with the new style show horse. And indeed a valid point could be made that many of today's top English Pleasure horses ten or fifteen years ago *would* have been considered Park horses. But take into consideration that breeders of Morgans all over the country are, or should be, striving to produce high-headed animals with natural style, presence and show horse attitude. With the improvement of type, quality and athletic ability, it was inevitable that the *show ring* would demand the type of Morgan seen in today's competition.

So what happens to the less typy, plainer, less brilliant performers? The answer: competitive trail rides, smaller shows, carriage meets and marathons, working stock horses and horses just to have fun with—the list goes on and on.

Excellent and persistent training can make *your* Morgan anything you want him to be. But the show ring always has demanded the best of the best. You must decide when you choose your first Morgan where you are going with him. Aim your sights realistically; be objective. There is a place for every good Morgan!

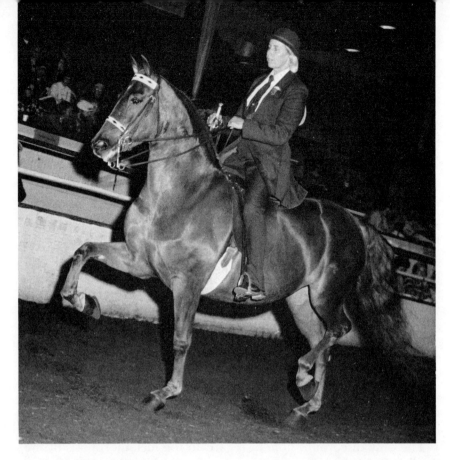

An English Pleasure mare.

PERFORMANCE OF THE ENGLISH PLEASURE HORSE

Manners in the Ring

The lack of manners sometimes seen in Pleasure classes is most usually the result of a horse's not being really ready for the show ring. His training has been incomplete or faulty, and he becomes unstrung when he is confused or frightened. Just because a horse can be ridden pleasurably does not mean that he has the poise to withstand the pressure of competition. The best-shown Pleasure horses have had days, months, even years of careful training, and as seasoned campaigners seldom are guilty of poor manners in the ring. The owners, serious about their horses' accomplishments, bring their animals to the peak of training before entering them in the top shows. Being judged Champion Pleasure horse is not often an accident or a lucky break: he has received as much attention and training as the Champion Park horse ever did.

This is by way of being a word to the wise to anyone who is planning to get his horse up out of pasture and take him to a show. Occasional wins at the local level notwithstanding, he must have his horse sharp and ready if he sets his sights on the major competitions.

I realize that this warning may seem rather tiresome to the un-initiated owner—because he keeps a Pleasure horse for *pleasure*, after all. But it is only fair to his horse, to the others in the ring—and, yes, to the Morgan breed—to have the animal well prepared in every way before asking it to compete for a *top ribbon*. And if one really likes working with horses, all the extra time and attention given one's horse can be fun too!

The Walk

On the trail there is nothing more frustrating and annoying than a horse that hangs back and must continually be urged to keep up, and therefore a good ground-covering walk is essential in a Pleasure horse.

Not only on the trail but in the show ring as well should a Morgan walk with a free-moving, flat-footed, ground-covering stride. It should

English Pleasure walk.

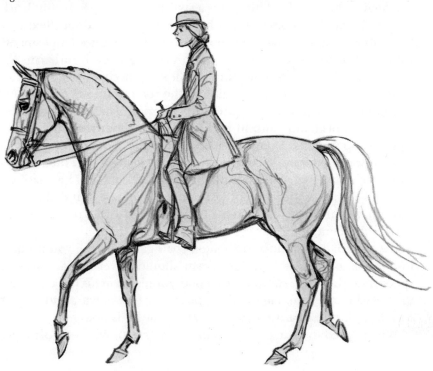

have a clear, four-beat cadence, be relatively brisk and with no tendency to jig or move sideways. He should be up in the bridle but not under undo restraint. Judges often look closely at how a Pleasure horse walks. If the horse is "mincey" or "pacey" going or looks as though he will break into a trot momentarily, he will be penalized. A horse who won't walk at all should be out of the ribbons in a Pleasure Class. So your horse's walk *is* a very important gait.

The Trot

In the English Pleasure Class, horses will generally enter the ring at the Pleasure trot. And a brisk, spanking trot it should be! The first moment the judge sees your horse should be an image of excellence. If your horse is up and showing, the impression given is one of a serious competitor, and a judge will take your horse seriously immediately. If your horse breaks, bucks, throws his head or is just not together, you must find a way on the next pass by to redeem yourself. It is far better to have your horse make that first pass at his best. In big classes you may never get another chance!

The Pleasure trot is either maintained when the class is closed or called for after the judge has brought all entries back to a walk. You must keep sharp and have your horse ready to pick up his Pleasure trot again when asked. This gait is a stylish, not too speedy, but brisk, collected trot. The horse should have his head up and set (flexing at the poll) with light contact. His motion should be balanced and smooth with knee action level, or at least approaching a level, forearm. His hocks should be well under him and flexing nicely.

When asked to extend the gait into the road trot, the horse should maintain his form while lengthening his stride. Horses that are able to move on brilliantly and in form and yet without restraint usually win the top ribbons. Excessive speed is not the criterion, however— though some exhibitors have the idea that it is and throw their horses all out of form by trying to out-trot the competition. The road trot should be neither a speed contest nor a horse race, but a chance to show that your horse can increase his ground-covering trotting speed while still maintaining his collection and form. Lapping every horse in the ring in a wild, unco-ordinated road gait will avail you nothing under a knowledgeable judge. Form should never be sacrificed to speed, and the horse should show good impulsion in his hocks, having them well under him. He should appear very free-moving and smooth with an attitude that indicates he likes what he is doing.

When asked to return to the walk, the horse should walk off easily and not jig or go sideways. As in the Park horse, the trot is the competitive gait, so excellence here is very important.

The Canter

While the Pleasure horse's trot should be brisk and ground-covering, the canter ideally should be slow, collected and exceedingly smooth— a veritable rocking chair. It should be straight on both leads—that is, the horse must move parallel to the rail—and performed on a light rein. The horse should appear relaxed and responsive to his rider from the moment he is asked to canter until he is returned to the walk.

The transition from the walk to the canter should be achieved with no apparent cue from the rider. A carefully and thoroughly trained horse will take his correct leads at once with almost imperceptible aids.

Should your horse take a wrong lead or cross-canter, stop him immediately and start again. It may cost you the class depending on the judge and the circumstances. Some judges are always looking for a horse to make a mistake, and others will excuse a small one if a horse is a superior performer. If there is a tie of sorts, that small mistake may cost you!

When I judge a class, I try to place the best horses. I will not place an inferior horse over a really good one because of a *small* mistake. If the horse canters all around the ring on the wrong lead, that's another story!

And speaking of judging, I would like to insert here a comment in regard to type. In qualifying classes, a judge must place his horses 40 percent on type and conformation and 60 percent on performance and manners. In championship classes, the percentages are 50/50. I always try to adhere to these rules, looking for the typy horse who is a good performer and giving the full percentage for type. Judges who hold cards in the Morgan Division shouldn't forget that type *is* very important and go heavily on performance only. All horses may be asked to back in the Pleasure Class.

TRAIL CLASSES—ENGLISH

In this division, the less typy Morgan can become a star. He is judged heavily on his performances over obstacles. He may be a bit lower headed or not as classic, but with careful training and a willing disposition, he can really rack up the ribbons for his owner. He will be

The English Pleasure Trot

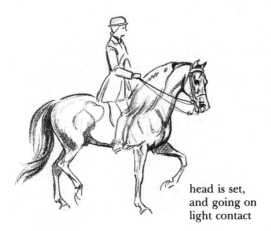

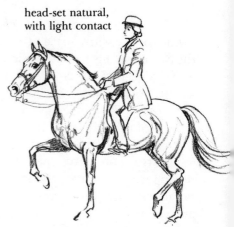

head-set natural,
with light contact

head is set,
and going on
light contact

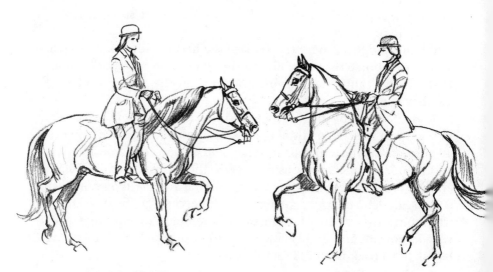

horse had been
"thrown away"—all out of
balance in carriage
and action

too "heads-up"
and "hot" for a good
Pleasure horse

The Road Trot

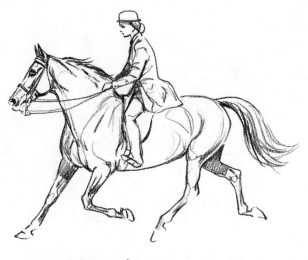

extended trot under
light contact

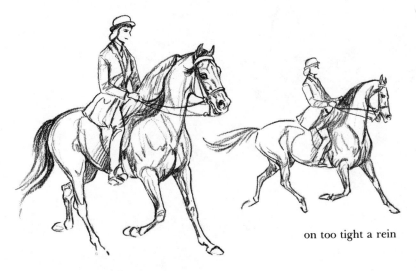

on a loose rein,
but maintaining form

on too tight a rein

The English Pleasure Canter

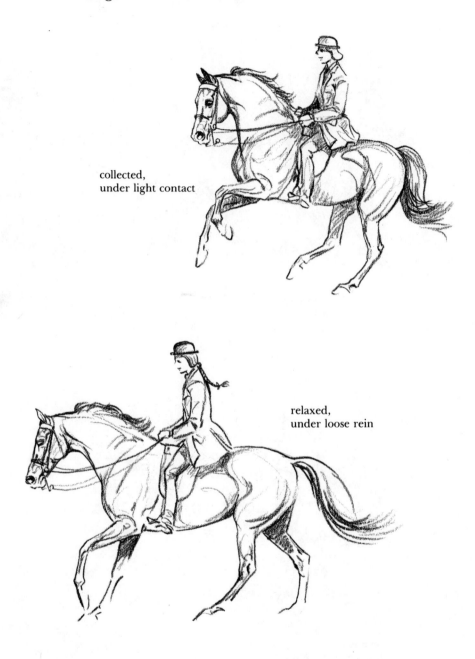

collected,
under light contact

relaxed,
under loose rein

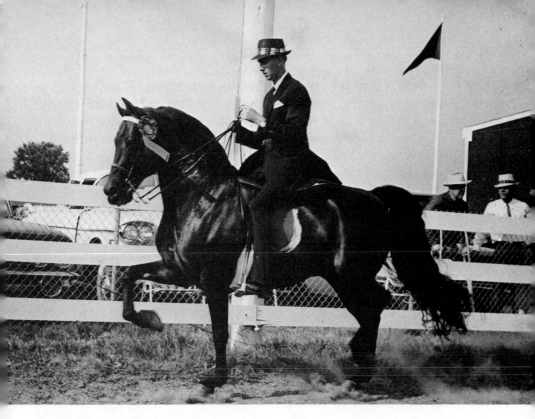

English Pleasure stallion.

asked to do a course over obstacles consisting of jumps, cavalletti, backing through rails or barrels, water, trees—anything which realistically might be encountered on the trail. This Morgan is actually as at home on a long distance ride as in a Trail Class at a show. Because he isn't expected to have the flash and style of his counterparts in the Open English Pleasure Class, he is easy-going and coolheaded. Trail horses have really changed very little over the years. They are still *fun horses* for all ages!

Some trail classes may have a quite involved and difficult obstacle course that is designed to test the horses' nerve and ability thoroughly. Others perhaps have only four or five simple obstacles to determine the horses' general willingness to negotiate them. To many a judge's chagrin, there are often horses which, though beautiful performers at the three gaits on the rail, are less than perfect (or even act downright silly) when tested over obstacles.

It has been found that either a horse is good over a course or he is *not*. Schooling at home may help him, but the naturally suspicious horse is never really trustworthy when faced with obstacles in the show ring, no matter how well he may cope with the familiar objects at home. Confronted with something he hasn't seen before, his antics can be exasperating—and his rider's efforts are usually futile. Such refusals can be a huge disappointment, especially when he has out-done himself on the rail. Surprisingly, this same horse may hardly give a second look to a log or a branch when confronted by it on the trail. Exhibitors have all run into this problem in the ring at one time or another, though. But usually if a horse is a calm, methodical performer over a variety of obstacles at one show, he will be equally sensible at most of them. By the same token, the silly horse will be quite likely to blow his chances a good deal of the time.

ENGLISH PLEASURE MORGANS ON THE TRAIL

Showing horses—especially on a season-long campaign—requires stamina not only on the part of the horse but also the same dynamic energy and competitive spirit from his owner. Still, if you simply haven't the heart for it all, for the long hours and hectic preparations

Taking no chances—English Trail Class.

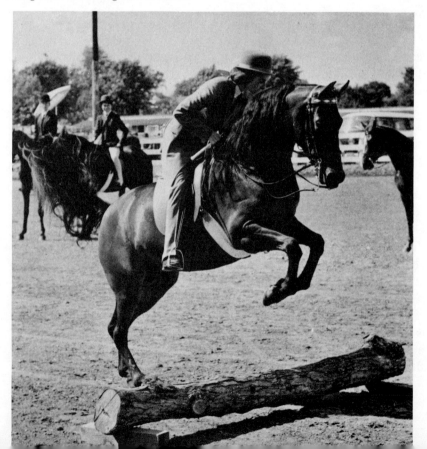

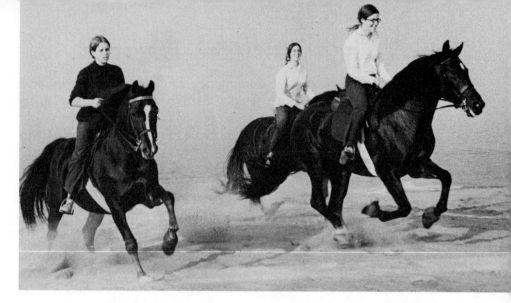

On the beach.

that precede the inevitable disappointments as well as the heady triumphs, you still will always enjoy your Morgan along the wooded trails and the open road. Here, far from crowds and blaring PA systems, you can share a companionship with your horse that is difficult to describe: a sense of oneness with the beautiful and intelligent creature with whom you experience each sight and sound.

It is on the trail that you have the leisure really to learn to know your horse and appreciate his smooth gaits and his pleasant disposition. As the miles clatter away under his feet you establish a rapport with him composed of admiration, affection and esteem. Your feelings for this alert, friendly animal seem to grow almost with each excursion. That he too always seems to enjoy your hours spent together makes your relationship with him something quite special. A Morgan Pleasure horse, quite possibly because of his intelligence and personality, seems to be well out of the simple "beast-of-burden"

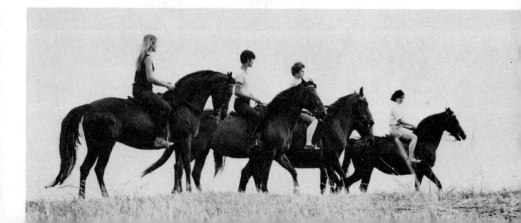

category. He really does share experiences with you. With his alert ears and interested manner, he almost converses with you as you go along. There is communication as surely as though there were words spoken between you. All of us who have had our Morgans on the trails have enjoyed these "conversations"—especially when, riding alone along some scenic ridge or open field, you tell him it is a lovely view and he informs you that there may be a deer down there in the woods!

This is companionship of the best sort with a horse, and it is certainly highly recommended to anyone who hasn't tried it. Many a Pleasure Morgan is considered no less than a member of the family.

English Trail Tack

When riding the trails or bridle paths, use tack that is comfortable and well fitting for both you *and* your horse. An improperly fitted saddle can turn your ride into a nightmare of rubs and aches for you and chafes or bruises for your horse, so choose your saddle carefully. If your Morgan has a high-set neck or prominent withers, a cut-back or modified cut-back saddle is ideal. But actually any type of saddle you like and which fits your horse without pinching or rubbing is fine on the trail. A light string or mohair girth will not chafe him the way leather girths sometimes do, since the air circulates through it as the horse moves. You may also want to use a saddle pad. The white quilted type is practical because it can be laundered easily when it becomes excessively soiled with mud and sweat.

Bridles are an individual thing. Some horses go well on the trail in a snaffle bit; others require a bit more restraint, and perhaps a

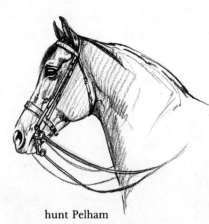

hunt Pelham   hunt snaffle

Pelham would be more practical. The full show bridle, while certainly the best-looking bridle on a Morgan, is not necessarily required on the trail, though it can be used if appearance is important. The light snaffle with double reins and running martingale, mentioned in Chapter 7, makes a practical bridle for English trail-riding too. Here the horse's mouth is comfortable with an easy bit, yet, should the need arise, leverage can be applied from the curb rein running through the martingale. However, there are no rules for tack on the trail, so use what you like and the one in which your horse goes best.

If you are in hunt country, you will probably ride your horse with hunter equipment, especially if you plan to ride him over fences. If you do, a jumping saddle is both appropriate and comfortable. A snaffle or Pelham hunt bridle (no colored browband here!) would then be used. And it is essential that you outfit yourself with a hard hat if you are planning to do any jumping.

Manners

Some of the basic requirements of the English Pleasure horse on the trail are that he be good with other horses, be a brisk walker without jigging or breaking gait frequently, and be relaxed and yet alert, going on a loose rein.

A horse that flattens his ears every time another horse looks his way and, with switching tail, indicates that he would kick without too much provocation, is a maddening animal in company. With this horse you must keep your distance in a group and thereby miss out on much of the good fellowship.

You miss out, too, when you ride a slow walker. You must constantly urge him along if he hangs back, and you are worn out after a few miles of the seemingly endless need to nag at him with your heels. Morgans usually do not suffer this fault, however; you are much more likely to find yourself reining him back till the others catch up to you!

On the other hand, a horse who continually breaks gait or jigs when he should be walking is also a trying and tiring mount on the trail. He makes it hard on both himself and his rider, and a few miles seem like many.

The ideal Pleasure horse on the trail is generally sensible and good-natured, and agreeable with other horses. He goes along in an easy, relaxed manner on a light rein, and with his ears up and with an alert appearance. He returns to a walk without fuss even after a brisk trot or canter with a group of riders across a field or down the road.

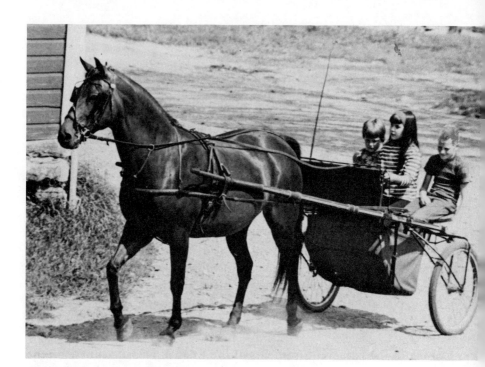

A Pleasure horse for the children.

He is cool-headed about obstacles or hazards in his path, crossing them carefully and deliberately. And he doesn't spook at shadows. He will stand quietly when tied (of course you never tie a horse with the reins: you will bring a halter and shank if you may be tying your horse out).

A Morgan is the sort of animal that makes your hours on the trail pleasantly memorable.

PLEASURE MORGANS IN HARNESS

Most young Morgans are broken to harness as a basic part of their early training, regardless of whether they are Park or Pleasure prospects. Most of them accept this schooling willingly and well. Indeed, Morgans in general seem to enjoy harness work naturally.

Since their conformation and gait create a pleasing appearance in harness, Morgans make better Pleasure Driving horses than any other breed.

A person of any age can derive great enjoyment from his Pleasure

Driving Morgan because this horse, properly broken to harness, is tractable and sensible to handle and drive, and children and older folks can harness him, and drive him with equal aplomb. For the youngster he provides something unique; for the older person a bit of nostalgia, perhaps, is mixed with the fun—the remembrance of a frosty day with bells jingling and jets of steam from a horse's nostrils and a sleigh skimming down a hard-packed road through snow-laden pines. . . . Or the kids may have other thoughts: piling as a group into a rattling, yet sound, old surrey or express wagon and driving to the lake for a swim and a picnic.

How well the Morgan fits scenes like these! Whether in the past or in the future, he *belongs*.

Tack for Pleasure Driving

When you plan to show your Morgan in Pleasure Driving classes, there are a few points to be aware of before you head for the ring.

First, of course, is equipment. Fond as you are of your handiwork, that old, refinished, four-wheeled buggy you spent so many hours lovingly repairing and repainting is just out of place in today's Pleasure Driving classes. Since these classes have grown so large, and quick maneuvering is so essential, this is just as well, for it is almost a matter of necessity to use a smaller vehicle for showing your horse. Although one used to see the Show Buggy used in these classes, jog carts are the recommended vehicles now. Trim little vehicles, with a leather "boot" for your feet, the jog carts are versatile and can be used on the road as well as in the show ring.

A neat, trim harness with a martingale is correct for Pleasure Driving classes, and the bridle with it should always have a cavesson included. Bits can be an over-check and snaffle. Some exhibitors will use a snaffle with the side-check bridle.

A buggy whip, whether you use it or not, should be carried; and a driving apron, while not a requirement, is certainly appropriate.

Showing

In the show ring the Morgan Pleasure Driving horse must have a relaxed, flat-footed walk when called for. Unlike the Park horse, which need not be brought back to a distinct walk, the Pleasure horse must really *walk*. Jigging or breaking gait will go against him. He should be characteristically high-headed; but—though stylish in appearance—he should be relaxed on the bit and have the look of a horse that would be a pleasure to drive on the road. At the

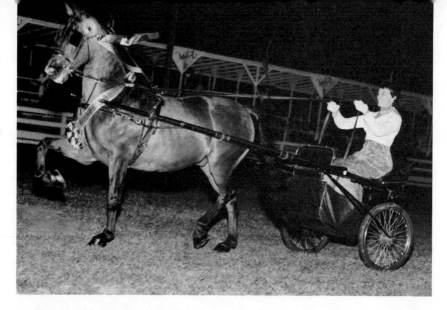

A champion Pleasure Driving horse.

walk he should move freely with an elastic, ground-covering stride.

The trot in a Pleasure Class should be the same brisk, ground-covering gait as seen in the English Pleasure Saddle classes, and have a two-beat cadence; hitching or going off-gait is penalized. When asked to extend, the horse should show proper impulsion and speed. He should be apparently easy to maneuver among horses, and, when called back to a walk, return to that gait at once and without undue resistance.

In the line-up, when entries are judged individually standing, a groom, or header, is permitted. If your horse is truly dependable while standing in a line-up, you may not require such an attendant. However, in classes for junior horses (four years old and under) a header is almost imperative, due to the unpredictable nature of young horses in unfamiliar surroundings. The header, should he attend you in the class, will help stand the horse squarely on his feet, and then step back from the horse as it is being judged. When asked, the Pleasure Driving horse should back readily and in a straight line.

Manners

With the tremendous increase in competition in the show ring in recent years, the Pleasure Driving horse should be outstandingly well mannered and stylish at all times. It is frequently the mistaken notion that, just because a horse is shown in Pleasure Driving classes, he can be low-headed and doggy-moving. Particularly in classes for Morgans only, a great amount of presence and style are required of a horse.

Pleasure Driving

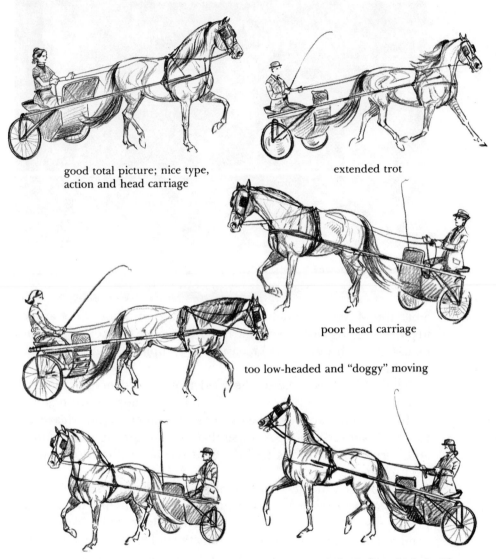

good total picture; nice type, action and head carriage

extended trot

poor head carriage

too low-headed and "doggy" moving

excellent type, and good head-set

no type, and checked too high for Pleasure

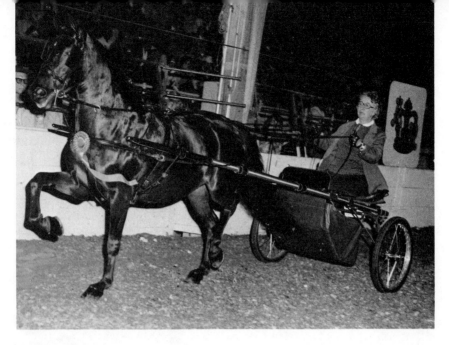

A Pleasure Driving mare.

Since the Morgan is a naturally stylish breed, he should not appear in public jogging along like some harried nag. He must exhibit perfect manners—with just a small measure of completely controlled gusto in his attitude.

Speed, while required at the road trot, should not be confused with the speed required of the Roadster. Your horse must maintain his form and not appear to be racing everything in sight!—leave that for the Roadster classes. A horse that appears strong in the mouth and boring on the bit is faulted, as is the horse that is choppy or laboring in his trot.

As evidenced by the huge size of Morgan Pleasure Driving classes at the shows, many people thoroughly enjoy exhibiting their horses in harness. Often it is necessary to divide classes three ways to accommodate all the entries and simplify the judge's task. In these large classes you need your wits about you every minute. One horse out of control can cause a chain reaction comparable to a Roman chariot-race pile-up. So not only be sure that you have your own horse under control, but "watch out for the other guy"! It is really a very grave injustice to your fellow exhibitors to enter a horse in any harness class unless he is properly trained and ready for the show ring. Of course accidents can happen to horses of any age, regardless of training: equipment breakage, flat tires, poor driving practices, etc. But if you feel deep down that your horse isn't really ready to show, be fair to him and to the other exhibitors. Hold off awhile until you feel your horse can take the noise and excitement of competition in a large class. Some pretty hair-raising scenes can occur in these large classes, and a badly frightened horse can be difficult to rehabilitate after an accident in the ring—to say nothing of the splintered jog carts and tattered harness (or worse) left in his wake.

THE WESTERN PLEASURE MORGAN

Many of us, though we neither live on a ranch nor possess the stock for working cattle, really enjoy Western riding. And even if you've always "ridden English" you owe it to yourself to try your Morgan under Western tack, for he is a natural in this sphere. He looks the part, and his smooth, easy gaits are made to order for the stock-horse scene. It has always been my feeling that if a horse is well-trained he will perform equally in English or Western tack. If he is supple and responsive, teaching him to neck-rein is achieved with little difficulty. And he soon learns to enjoy the slow, easy performance required of him.

Since good Morgan type and stock-horse type are so similar— short-coupled bodies, well-muscled quarters, straight sound legs, and

A young stock horse on a Montana ranch.

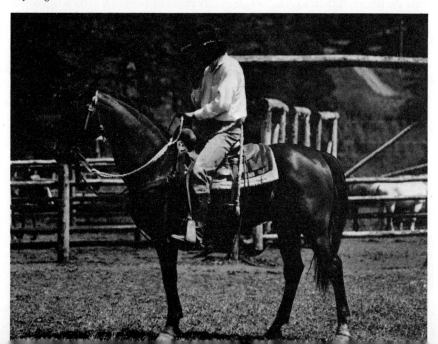

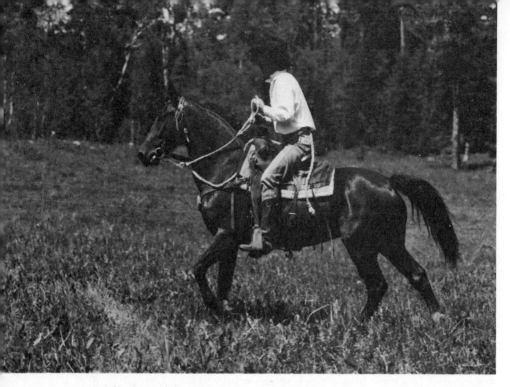

A stock horse in training.

clear-headed intelligence—Morgans have excelled in the many phases of Western riding.

Depending upon the training they have received, they have become superior stock horses and cutting horses, as well as superlative Western Pleasure mounts. Although often carrying their heads somewhat higher than other breeds do, thanks to the unique Morgan type, their savvy and agility are overshadowed by none. As working horses they have always been popular on the ranches in the West. Many Morgans were brought to the Western territories during the Gold Rush days and after. Their blood was mixed with the range stock to upgrade the quality of the native horses. Morgan stallions headed many a roving herd, imparting strength, substance and good looks to their offspring.

As working horses today, Morgans continue to be popular on the ranches. Leading unsung and unglamorous lives, they may never see a show ring, but in their own way they contribute much to the lives of their owners.

Now, with the interest in Western riding increasing tremendously throughout the country and the Western Pleasure classes at the shows filled to overflowing with entries, the Morgan has begun to gain some long overdue recognition in this field. No one can fail to see the unsurpassed smooth gaits of the Morgan or can overlook his beauty; and his abilities can be developed with expert training to satisfy the most astute stockman.

UNDER SADDLE IN THE RING

Having chosen your stock saddle carefully, you are ready to spend many enjoyable hours in the show ring and on the trail. It must be re-emphasized here that ill-fitting saddles on poorly gaited horses have soured many a new-to-Western rider. And, conversely, a great many English-style riders have become addicted to Western riding by the acquisition of a really comfortable stock saddle and a smooth-gaited Morgan!

Most Morgans that have worked in a full bridle will accept a Western curb readily, and will quickly learn the fundamentals of neck-reining. For the young horse starting his Western training, there are many excellent training bits, as well as the hackamore widely used on colts and green animals.

Since the training of working stock horses is a whole field in itself, we will deal only with the Western Pleasure horse here. It should be stressed at the outset that, before you enter a Western class, you have all your essential appointments. The American Horse Shows Association has definite requirements for horses shown in this division: a well-fitting stock saddle, Western hat, cowboy boots, chaps, a rope or reata.

Your saddle may be elegant and fancy with buckstitching and silver, or plain—but it should be clean and workmanlike. Beat-up, scruffy-looking saddles are not appropriate in the show ring any more. Even if your saddle has gone a good many miles, it will still look presentable when cleaned and polished. Perhaps you might treat yourself to some bright new silver conchas for it, plus a colorful, just-for-showing saddle blanket to enhance its appearance.

Many exhibitors use a braided leather reata in lieu of a bulky (but required) rope. A reata is a neatly coiled rope of sorts which fits on the pommel of the stock saddle. If you use split reins on your bridle (they are open-ended), technically your horse should "ground-tie" (stand quietly when the reins are dropped—seldom asked of an exhibitor these days). If romal reins are used, you must carry hobbles on your saddle as part of your appointments. Use of a slicker or

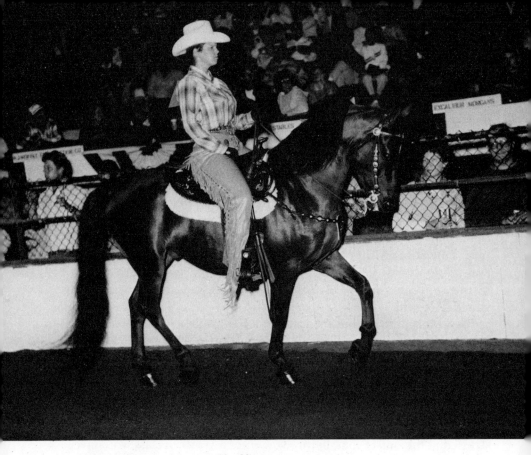

A Western Pleasure three-year-old gelding.

raincoat is not required in a Western Pleasure Class at most shows unless perhaps in a Trail Class. Always check with your show steward before a class if you have some question about appointments.

The Walk

The Western Pleasure Morgan should have an extremely smooth ground-covering walk. His head carriage may be somewhat lower than the English horse, but he should flex at the poll and be light on the bit. He should go on a relatively loose rein with light contact desirable to maintain his head-set even at the walk. The Western horse should have a catlike gait that enables him, when reined, to turn or move quickly and easily and be backed readily if asked.

A horse is penalized for being fussy in the mouth or breaking gait when being asked to walk. Head-tossing and fighting the bit are definite faults at any gait as well as when asked to back.

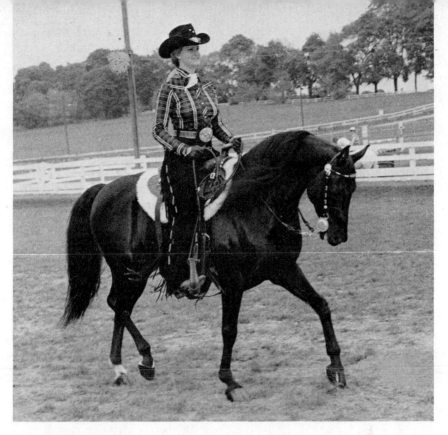

A Western Pleasure stallion.

The Western Jog

The jog is a slow, smooth, easy trot, performed as though the horse could maintain the gait for hours on end without discomfort to himself or his rider. The good rider on a horse jogging properly, scarcely seems to move in the saddle, for horse and rider are one unit in appearance. A good jog is all-important in the Western horse.

Some of the short-pasterned bone-crushers we see in the ring and on the trail leave much to be desired, and one wonders why a stock saddle was ever placed on their backs. Padded seats on the saddles notwithstanding, the heavy-going, choppy, hard-gaited joggers really are out of place in Western tack. One has only to go out cross-country on a rough mover to see (and feel!) why this is true. If you plan to ride Western be sure your Morgan is gaited for it. Most are.

As previously stated, the Morgan Western Pleasure horse must carry his head up, flexed in at the poll and showing proper response to the bit. His mouth should be quiet: no tongue-lolling or heavy bit-chomping. At the jog, the rider's position and ease in the saddle show

The Western Jog

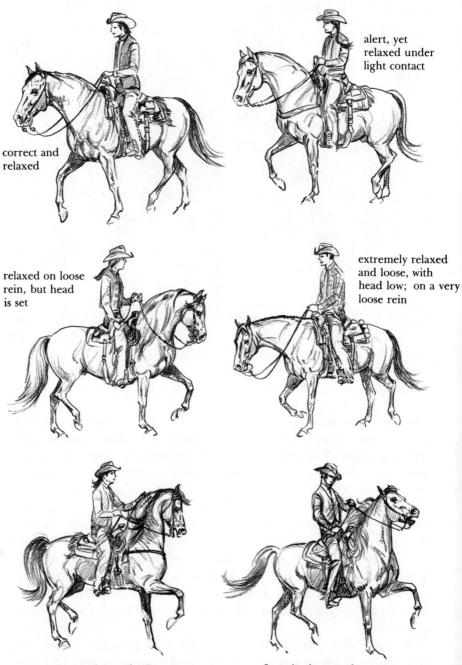

correct and relaxed

alert, yet relaxed under light contact

relaxed on loose rein, but head is set

extremely relaxed and loose, with head low; on a very loose rein

much too "hot" and high-headed

fussy in the mouth, with head tossing

a judge just how comfortable the gait is. Naturally, a superb rider can make a not-so-smooth jogger appear *quite* comfortable.

The jog itself should have a clear trotting cadence with *no* tendency to mix gaits. It should be slow but not so slow that the horse looks as though he will break back into a walk at any moment. A sloppy jog does nothing for a horse and—hind feet just barely clearing the ground and sending up dust clouds at every stride—gives the animal a bored, lazy appearance. Conversely, a horse that jogs with too much animation can be just as undesirable. If he is hot and fussy as well, you are in for a rough go. It is just about impossible to "fake it" with a horse who is too keen.

A fine-tuned performance, the result of very careful training and natural ability, is what makes the Western Pleasure horse a winner!

It might also be mentioned here that this same Western paragon will be equally satisfying on the trail as well. Smooth gaits, alert yet relaxed countenance and quiet but energetic action are all pluses.

In a class or on the trail, it is almost as unnerving to have to keep after a horse with your legs to keep him going as it is to constantly have to rein him back in his eagerness to go on. So, keep your horse moving at a jog with a catlike agility: slow and relaxed but alert and free-moving.

Often judges will ask for an extended jog in a Western Pleasure Class. This is accomplished by urging your horse to move on at a speed that is noticeably different than the jog but not quite as fast as the English Pleasure trot. The transition should be smooth. Evidence that the faster gait is comfortable to sit to should be apparent. The horse's head-set and rein should remain the same.

The Lope

Seeing a top Western horse perform the lope, one is indeed reminded of the proverbial rocking chair. It is the *pièce de résistance* of the Western horse. A slow, extremely comfortable, easy canter, the lope is a gait a horse can maintain over long periods without fatigue to himself or his rider.

Ideally, he should be relaxed and light on the bit with his head carried just slightly lower than that of the English Pleasure horse at the canter. There should be a definite three-beat cadence to this gait, and by its smoothness it should give the impression of a total unity of horse and rider. Horses must move without restraint and should

The Western Lope

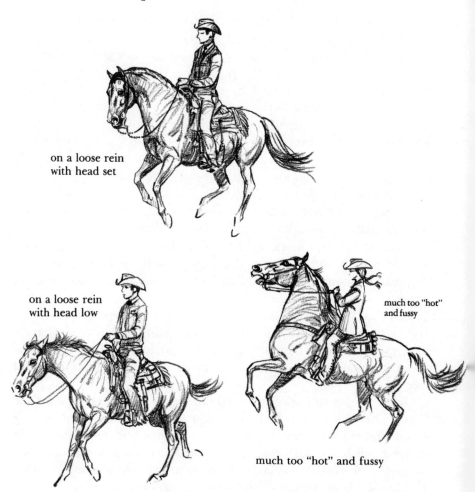

on a loose rein
with head set

on a loose rein
with head low

much too "hot"
and fussy

much too "hot" and fussy

be quiet in the mouth. Going with the mouth open, or with head-tossing or any evidence of tenseness in the horse, is faulted at the lope. The horse should be responsive and supple in his movements, giving the impression that any quick turns or maneuvers could be achieved without his becoming out of balance.

Horses which appear to be bunched-up and tight-going, or moving on too fast under a snug hold are not fulfilling requirements. Cross-cantering, side-passing, or being strung out are all faults to be penalized.

ON THE TRAIL

Requirements for the Western Pleasure horse on the trail are quite similar to those for the English horse: an amiable disposition, easy gaits, a responsive mouth, cleverness over obstacles, and stamina. In addition, some Western Pleasure horses are also taught to ground-tie or to wear hobbles. In Trail classes at the shows, you are often required to show that your horse will ground-tie or stand quietly in hobbles. He should also stand quietly when you mount or dismount.

Perhaps the greatest bar to becoming a good Western Pleasure horse on the trail or in the ring would be a tendency to be too hot (nervous and overly keen). A horse with this trait often has a fussy mouth as well, and it is impossible for him to be completely relaxed. He jigs when he should be walking; he tosses his head whenever you rein him; or he is snorty and spooky about objects in his path. This disposition is not ever going to allow a horse to be a reliable and pleasurable Western ride. His gaits, being erratic, are tiring to him (though this type seldom runs out of gas) and extremely uncomfortable and frustrating to his rider. It seems impossible for him to lower his head and relax, being always on the defensive, rebelling against the bit, the weight on his back, and his surroundings.

We see this type in English tack and pity the rider, but in Western tack he is totally *impossible*!

The lazy, doggy horse is at the other end of the spectrum and,

Relaxed and sensible: dealing with obstacles in a Western Trail Class.

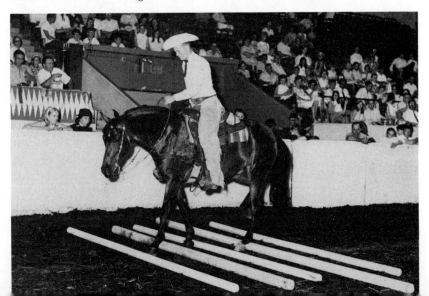

though somewhat of an improvement over the hot horse, will not give you a really pleasurable ride: you simply must work too hard to keep him going. In company he will lag behind; alone he will go like an auto with the brakes on. Except when you turn him toward home—and then there is an immediate and remarkable transformation. It is amazing how these old fakers can appear so tired and worn out until the change of direction comes! Wearing spurs on the lazybones may help, but constantly prodding a horse becomes tedious.

To sum up: When choosing a Morgan that will be really suitable for Western Pleasure riding—either in the show ring or on the trail—you will look for a horse that has appropriate conformation, smooth, ground-covering gaits, and a good mouth. He should neck-rein readily and have no objection to working over, around and through any obstacle either on the trail or in the ring.

Size is rather a matter of preference, depending on your height and weight, but in general a horse between 14.2 and 15.0 hands gives the best appearance in Western tack because he usually fits the stock-

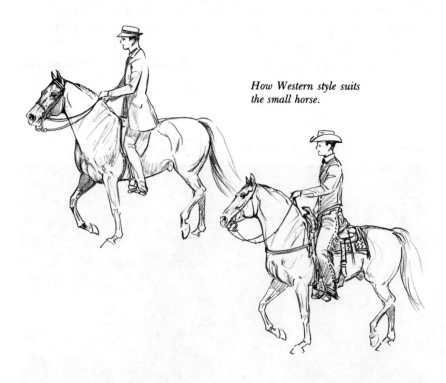

How Western style suits the small horse.

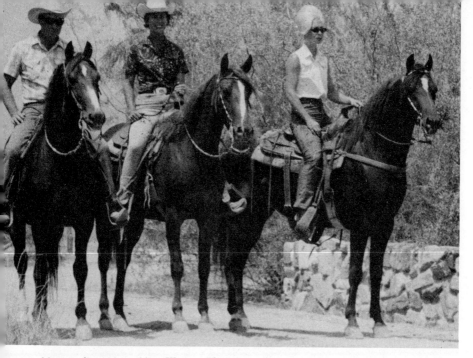

Morgan disposition adds to Western Pleasure on the trail: a mare flanked by two stallions, in Arizona.

horse type and thus looks the part. And an interesting note, in reference to size: a tall or heavy rider will look more appropriate riding a fairly small horse with Western tack than he will when riding that same horse in English tack.

Large, rangy horses tend to lack Morgan, as well as stock-horse, type, and very often are not gaited well for Western riding. A reachy, jouncy trot or a rollicking, lumbering canter are quite uncomfortable in a stock saddle.

9

The Morgan Roadster, Road Hack and Hunter/Jumper

THE ROADSTER

An exhibition of speed always generates interest no matter where it is performed, for there is invariably a great measure of excitement when horses are in competition at speed. Since the chariot-racing days of ancient history, the compelling fascination of the speed contest has been inspiration and challenge to people everywhere. However, the Morgan Roadster Class is not technically a race *per se*, although entries vie with each other to show speed, form and brilliance.

Any versatile Morgan possessed of a brisk natural trot may seem to the novice to be a terrific Roadster prospect. Caught up in the apparent glamor and excitement of this division, such an owner may think that he is fulfilling requirements merely by donning silks and bringing his horse clockwise into the ring. But the Morgan Roadster showing with top contenders must possess much more than a brisk trot: he must show the speed and style which, in competition, will bring the spectators to their feet.

Cheers and whoops of delight signal the "Drive on!" call of the announcer as the horses skim around the ring at a speed quite breathtaking considering the area in which they are required to perform. Your horse must be able to extend himself to the limit, yet maintain his gait and style even under the pressure of crowding by other horses, tumultuous noise from the stands, and the constant demand that he give everything he can to his performance.

Special and intensive training goes into making a top-ranked Roadster. As with Hunters and Jumpers, natural ability plus serious,

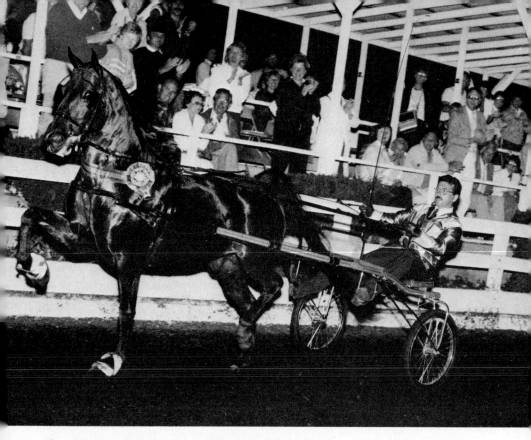

The style and elegance wanted in a Morgan Roadster.

qualified training produce the best performers. Anyone can put his horse in the ring with the correct appointments and a trot a bit better than average, but if you really want to excel, you will find that the Roadsters that are consistent winners are those which are shown exclusively in this division and trained with it in mind. Certainly the very nature of the versatile Morgan will allow him to do a creditable job in a Roadster event, but if you have your sights on blues and championships, keep him *just* a Roadster that season.

Several top Morgans that were previously shown in the Park Division have later turned out to be outstanding Roadsters—with additional training in this direction. They have the natural style to begin with, and it is quite amazing how they seem to enjoy the opportunity to extend their trot, once they understand that they are actually being allowed to go on!

Working a horse on a track or a dirt road, especially in the company of another horse or horses for competition, is a good beginning for Roadster training.

IN HARNESS

Hitched to a "bike" (sulky) with drivers in stable colors, horses enter the show ring in a clockwise direction at a jog, which in this class is a brisk road trot. It should be noted that only in Roadster classes do horses show clockwise first; all other classes require entries to perform first in the counterclockwise direction.

From the jog, the horses are next asked for the fast road gait. This is a very speedy trot but still not top speed, which is saved for the reverse direction.

After the judge has looked them over sufficiently, the horses are asked to reverse direction and continue jogging. When all entries are traveling counterclockwise, they are then asked again for a road gait. This is a *very* fast trot. Brilliance of form and presence as well as speed are required of the Morgan Roadster here. He should be well balanced, folding up his knees while his hocks are working well under him in perfect co-ordination. He should have his head set correctly and be responsive in the mouth, enabling the driver to take him back on the turns if necessary, and to regulate his speed easily at all times. He should stay on the rail except when passing.

When the announcer calls "Drive on!" horses are asked for their top trotting speed, maintaining form while showing what they can do. Even at extreme speed, the trot should be balanced and correctly

An old-fashioned vehicle on a modern road horse.

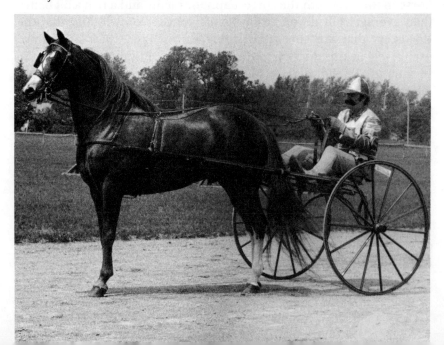

cadenced. Hitching the turns or pacing and mixing gaits are penalized as is *any* breaking of gait. It is important to know what to expect of your horse—how much to push him before he becomes dangerously close to going off his feet, and how much to take him back on the turns. Unlike a horse race, where getting under the wire first at the correct gait is all that is required, the Roadster Class demands that a horse be a show horse too. Not only must he be able to show speed at the trot, but he also must add brilliance and presence to his talents.

A horse with a short, choppy trot—no matter how speedy he may seem—will not make a first-rate Roadster, for in reality the impression of speed may be the result of the quickness of his gait rather than the ground-covering stride demanded. So, although style is required, the horse must possess a lengthy stride as well. The choppy-gaited horse will use more energy and cover less ground, and he seldom can fulfill the requirements for the Roadster in the ring.

The Morgan to be shown in Roadster classes is allowed a bit longer leg and length of body than may possibly be found in the ideal in hand type, but nevertheless he certainly should possess good basic Morgan characteristics.

Performance faults include speed without style, unco-ordinated action with hocks trailing, spraddling action behind, forging, breaking gait or mixing.

After the horses have been judged at three speeds of the trot, they are asked to line up in the center of the ring. Since no attendant or header is allowed in this class, the horse should be prepared to stand quietly in the line. The driver remains seated in the bike unless there is need for some adjustment to be made to tack. The horses are judged individually for quality and manners, having already been judged for manners on the rail. If a workout is called for, two or more horses are asked to work again on the rail. The exhibitors lined up in the center may uncheck their horses if they wish and hold them by the head for the duration of the workout.

Requirements for attire in Roadster classes are racing silks in stable colors with cap and jacket to match. Kentucky jodhpurs, or pants with tie-down straps, and boots complete the outfit. Gloves are almost always worn.

The Morgan is permitted to wear quarter boots in Roadster classes, both in harness and under saddle, to protect him should he overreach when going at speed.

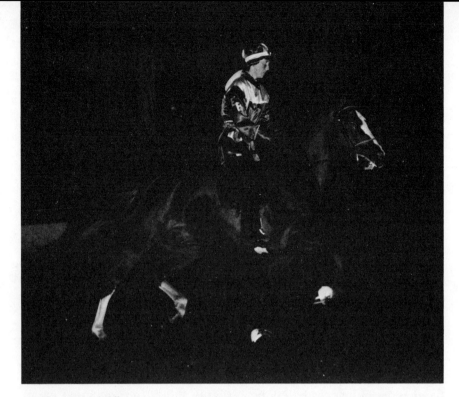

Roadster under saddle.

UNDER SADDLE

Long before New England roads were suitable for vehicles driven at speed at the trot, riders most assuredly raced their horses under saddle at this gait whenever a stretch of terrain seemed to lend itself to the sport. Albeit without the cheering crowds and flashing silks, it was heady fare, nonetheless, to speed down the narrow lanes with dust flying and the staccato beat of trotting hooves starting birds from their nests and field mice scurrying for cover in the grass.

This same excitement is generated in our classes for modern Roadsters under saddle. Where the colonial farmer raced perhaps for a beaker of rum at the local tavern, today Morgans display their speed and form with equal zest as (side bets notwithstanding!) they vie for blue ribbons in the show ring.

Requirements for the Roadster under saddle are the same as regards to performance and appointments in harness. Class procedure is also the same, with horses entering the ring in the clockwise direction.

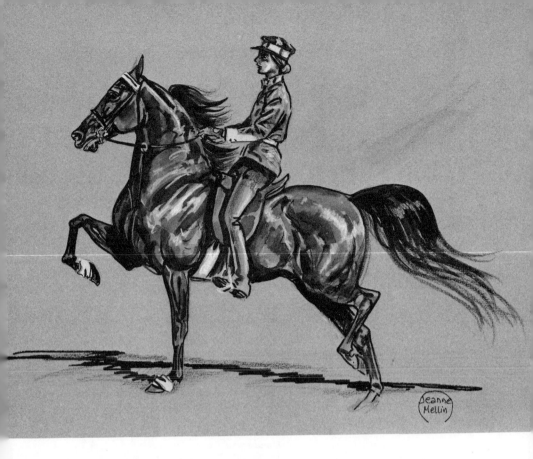

Roadster under saddle showing the action and style that are required along with speed.

The rider again wears stable colors. The horse is shown in a snaffle bridle with a running martingale, generally without the neckstrap. A flat saddle, usually a cut-back show saddle, is used, and the horse may wear quarter boots or bell boots at the rider's discretion.

THE ROAD HACK

Almost any Morgan that performs well in English Pleasure events, displaying manners, a strong trot and a good mouth, will also make a topnotch Road Hack entry. It takes a speedy trot, a brisk, lively walk, and an abundance of manners to qualify, and since Morgans excel at these gaits and are practically born with manners, they make formidable competitors—not only against each other, but against other breeds in open classes as well.

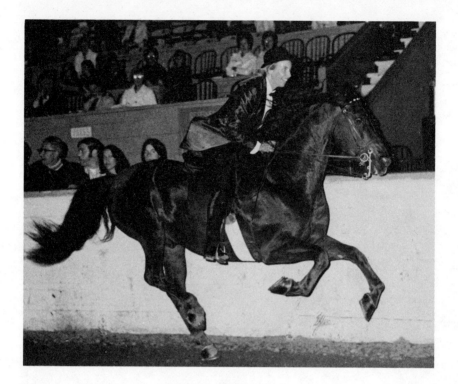

Hand gallop.

APPOINTMENTS

Requirements for tack and dress are generally the same as for the English Pleasure classes. You may of course show in hunt attire and tack, but bear in mind that if the class consists of a majority of Saddle Seat riders, you may look somewhat out of place in a Morgan Road Hack Class in a hunt outfit. Still, in an open class, where you will be competing with other kinds of horses and styles of riding, your Hunt Seat clothes would be perfectly permissible. Conversely, if you are showing your Morgan in hunt country in a Road Hack or Bridle Path Hack Class and everyone is attired in keeping with local usage, your saddle suit would be equally conspicuous!

The saddle suit and its variations, both formal and informal, are described in Chapter 12, and any truly knowledgeable outfitters or seasoned Hunt Seat exhibitors can advise you on the fine points of hunt apparel for the ring. Then, use your own good judgment in regard to clothing compatible with your tack—which in turn can be dictated by the circumstances.

And remember that it is the horse's performance and manners, not the rider's clothes, that are the really important factors.

PERFORMANCE

While the Road Hack should always work on a relatively loose rein, it is inadvisable to "throw your reins away" regardless of how reliable and relaxed your horse might be. This is especially true in large classes, where extremely loose reins make it much more difficult for you to cope with the unexpected, such as another horse cutting you off and obliging you to pull up suddenly to avoid a collision. Drooping reins can really present an immediate and often embarrassing problem here as you suddenly find your horse's head in your lap and seemingly miles of flopping reins to gather up in frantic haste in order to avoid a mishap.

The trot and road trot are performed much as they are in the English Pleasure class. They should be brisk and well balanced, with the horse moving in under himself in the hocks to produce the propulsion and speed required. When asked to walk, a horse must return immediately to that gait, and stride off in a resolute manner and on a light rein.

The canter should be slow and collected, with the horse appearing relaxed and responsive : If the class is small, the ringmaster will call for the entries to hand gallop. (If a class is large, it is lined up, and only eight entries are asked to hand gallop at a time. This does away, somewhat, with the cavalry charges and attendant chaos that a large group of horses can cause in the ring when asked for speed.)

The hand gallop in essence is an extended canter. From the slow canter, the horse moves on, lengthening his stride and increasing his speed while remaining in hand and in form. Mad, headlong galloping is usually penalized and, though the temptation is often strong, obviously racing another exhibitor before the judge is not recommended!

From the hand gallop, the horse must pull back to a walk again as soon as the call is given, and walk off quietly. Often a judge will order "Halt!" Horses should immediately stop and stand quietly— no moving about. This is part of what is meant by "manners."

In the line-up the horses must stand quietly without fidgeting. They will be asked by the ringmaster to back individually, or a few at a time. They should do so with their noses down, responding to the bit and stepping back a few steps in a straight line. Horses which fail to back are of course penalized for the disobedience.

A horse that seems unable to extend his trot or refuses due to laziness is not a good candidate for Road Hack competition. Hard mouths and jiggy walks result in wasted entry fees too. Morgan type and outstandingly good conformation may not be a strong requirement in the Road Hack Class, but a horse's performance must be exemplary to make up the deficit. You should bear in mind, however, that an attractive, well-conformed Morgan *will* have a slight edge if he is an equally good performer. Also, a well-turned-out, correctly appointed horse and rider will get the judge's attention over a carelessly groomed pair every time.

In any case, it is always well to do your utmost to have your horse as well as yourself properly and neatly attired for the show ring. Sloppy clothes and dirty tack and unkempt horses really add nothing to enjoyment of a show on the part of spectators or exhibitors.

THE HUNTER/JUMPER

Much has been said and written about the Morgan's qualifications in the hunt field and over fences in the ring. Various conclusions have been drawn in this regard, with the proponents staunchly defending the Morgan in the field in every respect, while the opponents, needing to be convinced, regard the breed as not "looking the part," as too small and often as inconsistent.

Concerning conformation, you will have seen from the illustrations that the *ideal* Morgan type possesses a high-set neck which he is not wont to carry down. A horse of this type very often would find it difficult to use his neck and head over fences, as the requirements for a good Jumper demand. This does not necessarily indicate that a horse of this type will not have a talent for jumping: it indicates only that, due to his conformation, his form over fences might leave something to be desired in the eyes of a "hunter man."

TALENT AND TRAINING FOR THE RING

Talent in jumping, as in any other phase of horse activity, depends on the natural ability of the individual horse and his training in this field of endeavor. Some Morgans are natural Jumpers, with many performing very well over fences; others are not. Breed seems to

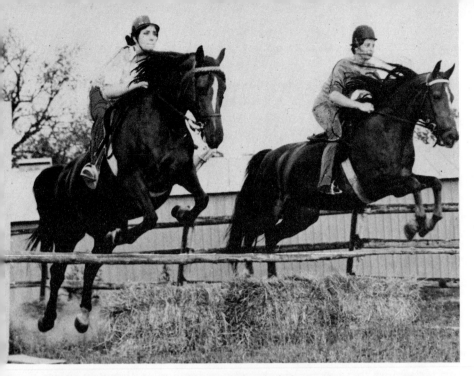

Training good Pleasure mares with a natural aptitude for jumping.

have little to do with it. Not all Thoroughbreds make good Jumpers, and, by the same token, some Pintos and grade horses are tops. A horse must have the will to excel at jumping. Without it, he will never be a consistent performer, whether he is a Morgan, an Arabian or a grade—or a Thoroughbred, for that matter!

His initial training also is of the utmost importance. It must be conducted by a knowledgeable person under appropriate conditions. Popping a horse over an occasional obstacle on the trail or in the ring does not constitute Hunter/Jumper training!

If your forte is the hunt field and you are determined to prove your Morgan can excel there and make a name for himself, carry out his training from basics to advanced requirements in a conscientious and methodical way: cavalletti in the ring, jumping on the longe-line, experience in the field. If your horse is genuinely inclined in this direction, as the top Park horses appear to be in theirs, he will consistently improve with this regime.

However, if he performs well over fences one day and for no apparent reason is cranky and sticky in the ring the next, you have reason to doubt his dependability in classes over fences. And, realistically, what is to be gained by putting into the show ring a Morgan— or any horse for that matter—with which you stand a 50/50 chance of being made a fool of? The odds would seem to be pretty dismal, yet fairly often one sees people do this with untalented or under-trained Morgans. Would it not be better to keep such a horse on the flat where he can do himself *and* his breed credit, rather than to insist that he jump in the show ring?

SHINING IN THE HUNT FIELD

Morgans in the field are another matter. Many horses—and partic-ularly Morgans, perhaps because of their intelligence—are happy and enthusiastic Jumpers cross-country, even though they are less than sold on jumping in the ring.

With natural fences and the apparent freedom of the open coun-try, they respond by performing second to none. Many Morgan horses take part successfully with recognized hunts, staying up front and proving that they are capable, and often outstanding, Hunters in any company. They are quick, enduring and sensible. Smaller size will not be against them except in the case of having a tall, heavy rider; certainly it will not affect their jumping ability. And maintaining a good Hunter pace between fences has never been a problem, for

Morgan Hunter performing capably in Hunter Over Fences Class.

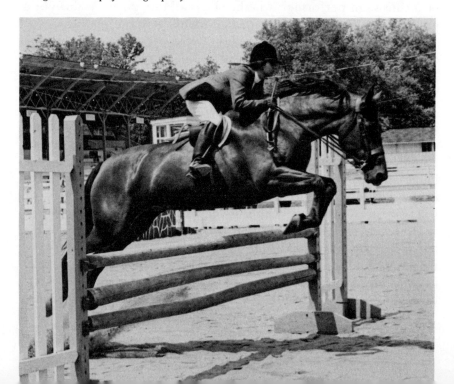

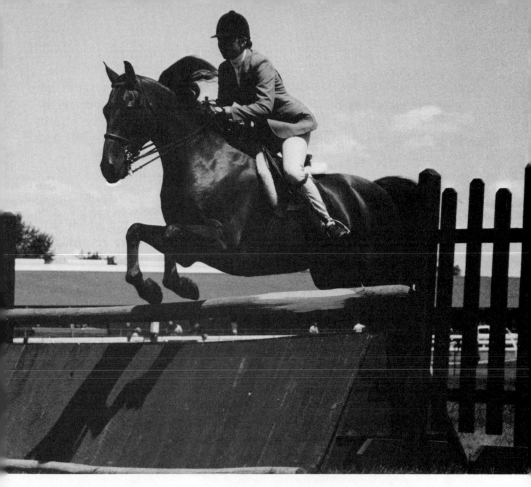

Another Morgan on the course.

they can move out with the best of them and love every minute of it! Especially in rough country, the clever, sure-footed Morgans can outdo their larger, heavier companions with satisfying regularity.

There is no reason why a Morgan, raised and well-trained in the hunt-country environment and with a qualified and enthusiastic rider/ trainer, can't sell the Morgan breed to newcomers to the sport of hunting—and perhaps even gain some guarded approval from hitherto resolute partisans of another breed.

APPOINTMENTS

If your Morgan is really well qualified to be shown as a Hunter, it goes without saying that you owe it to yourself and him to turn him out properly. He will make a better impression on the judge (who quite frankly may be prejudiced against Morgans) if he is correctly braided—mane and tail—and wearing appropriate tack, i.e., hunt bridle and jumping saddle. Naturally, you also will be properly appointed.

These things may seem "picky," but they do really make a difference in the ring or in the field if you want to be taken seriously by either the judges or your peers. After all, keeping abreast of current trends and requirements is necessary for any division in which you plan to exhibit. Subtle changes in tack and clothes are continually taking place, and, whether we like it or not, we must know what they are; then, if their acceptance seems universal, we should adopt them too. Failure to keep in step with approved trends in the show ring can place an exhibitor at a psychological disadvantage. Be alert, aware and always respect tradition.

Morgan Jumper showing form over fences.

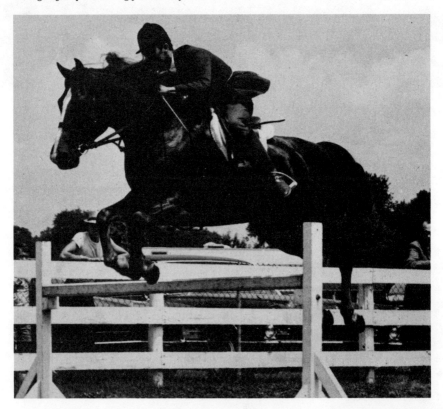

CLASS REGULATIONS

There are many technical and general rules with which you should familiarize yourself if you plan to show in the Hunter/Jumper divisions. A current American Horse Shows Association Rulebook can be acquired by joining the ASHA; a membership blank can be found in the prize list for any recognized show. The rulebook will give the requirements, procedures and changes for that year, and answer any queries you may have. Briefly, the rules are as follows.

In Jumper classes *only* performance counts. If your horse has a clean, correct round over the course and no other horse does, you take the high ribbon. If two or more entries go clean, the fences are raised and you go again until the tie is broken. This may amount to several jump-offs if competition is keen. Style is unimportant so long as your horse negotiates the fences without fault. More and more we are seeing events that are timed—in which case the time factor will affect the results. Lesser ribbons are awarded on the basis of the number of faults against a horse in the final jump-off.

It is a bit more complicated in Hunter classes, however. Not only must a horse put in a clean round over the course (rubs and ticks may not count unless they are the result of poor jumping), but he also must move at the correct Hunter pace between jumps and show good form over his fences. He is judged on his apparent suitability as a mount that would carry his rider safely and pleasantly cross-country to hounds.

Upon completion of the last entry's round over the course, the highest-scoring horses are led back into the ring or judging area to be jogged for soundness. Here they trot by the judge one by one, and then are lined up in the order of their final placing after the judge has looked over all of them individually.

Although your Morgan has performed well over the course, he must still look the part here as he stands for judging. In top competition he should be, as mentioned earlier, braided both mane and tail. Since, in order to be braided correctly, a Hunter's mane is pulled to facilitate making smaller plaits, the exhibitor does run into a problem if he plans to show his Morgan both in Hunter and Morgan classes, because a long, natural mane is a Morgan trademark if not technically a requirement. Being familiar with the demands of the Hunter/Jumper Division is very important, for nowhere else does tradition so emphatically call the turns!

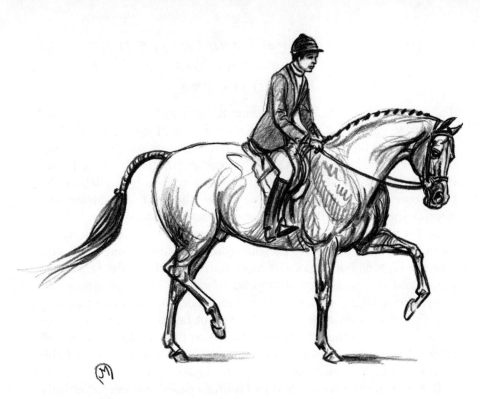

Morgan on the flat.

Hunters under saddle and Bridle Path Hacks, Hunter Type and Hunter Hacks—all are classes for the Hunter on the flat at a walk, trot, canter and hand gallop. Hunter Hacks are also required to jump two fences in the ring. However, in classes specifically for young or green horses, the entrants are not required to gallop.

Morgans shown in any of the classes mentioned above will, if they are well qualified and are outstanding performers, contribute greatly to the breed's reputation for versatility. But a sincere word of caution: be sure, before you enter and exhibit in these classes, that your Morgan is really a consistent performer who will be a credit, not a detriment, to his breed, for if his performances in this area sometimes seem a fiasco with refused fences, running-out, and going off-course, you hurt more than just yourself.

In short, be sure that he is properly schooled at all times, that you and he are both correctly turned out, and, above all, be thoroughly acquainted with all the rules of the division.

10

Fitting and
Showmanship in Hand

A HORSE SHOW is many things to many people. For some it is simply a sporting event, with all the recreational benefits attending any sport; for others it presents an opportunity for brief personal glory and a chance to enjoy fleetingly the hero worship accorded the winners; for still others it offers a possibility of being rewarded for the efforts expended in perfecting a horse's abilities. But to most of us who respect and love the Morgan, it is a showcase for our breed. It is at a horse show that we have the opportunity to display the Morgan's varied talents in the most distinctive fashion. The promotional ramifications are endless, a fact well-known by exhibitors and breeders everywhere.

Because a show indeed places its performers under the cold, critical scrutiny of the horse-conscious public, every effort should be made by exhibitors to foster admiration for, and bring honor to, the breed. The responsibility is ours. Anything less is an injustice not only to ourselves and our horses but—and this cannot be overemphasized—to the Morgan as a breed.

We have already discussed the various show divisions for the Morgan and their individual requirements, so this chapter is devoted to the technicalities of preparing the horse physically for the show ring, with some hints on showmanship for good measure.

FITTING

Any horse that is to be shown—either in hand or in performance classes—should first be in good physical condition and, as the ASHA

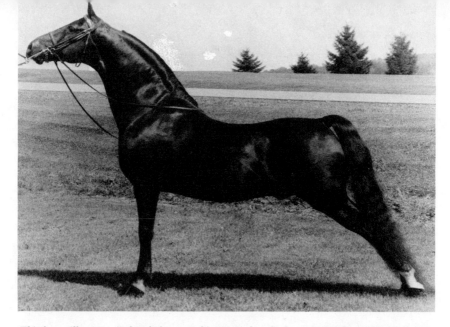

This horse illustrates in-hand showmanship. Note that the horse is standing with his forelegs perpendicular to the ground. He is overstretched somewhat, but his weight is correctly over his forelegs. This horse is well-fitted: his coat is clean and glossy, his hoofs blackened, his tail picked out and his bridle clean.

Rulebook states, "serviceably sound." He should be fat enough to look his best, but not hog-fat and soft. The horse is an athlete, and thus should be in top athletic condition for the performance expected of him. His muscles should be firm and in good tone; his coat should be glossy and sleek. And he should be clipped and trimmed where necessary to give him a "bandbox" finish.

To prepare a horse for a season on the circuit, or even only one or two shows, you should give him the benefit of regular sessions with the grooming kit and clippers before each outing.

Trimming off Hair

To facilitate keeping him looking his best you should have a pair of electric small-animal clippers, with two sizes of blades: No. 40 for ears and No. 10 for general clipping and trimming. It is all-important to have your horse's head neatly trimmed of excess hair just prior to leaving for the show. If you do it a week before, the hair will grow back and you will have to go over him again.

The ears, especially, look unkempt if not clipped inside and on the edges just before the show. Since most horses which are being shown are kept stabled, flies are no great problem to the show horse with clipped ears (although horses kept in pasture much of the time *will* need the long hair in their ears for protection from flies). The "before and after" photographs show the great difference trimmed ears make in their appearance.

If you have never clipped your horse's ears before, it is advisable to have someone assist you. Some horses allow their ears to be trimmed with electric clippers without any fuss at all. Others resent it with a vengeance—sometimes violently! (When you purchase a horse, be sure to ask his former owner how the horse reacts to clippers, so you will know what to expect of him.) If he has never been clipped, proceed cautiously.

Should the horse not stand quietly to have his ears done, and should he seem quite touchy when you attempt to handle them, don't fight him; and don't have him in the cross-ties. Instead, if he is just too rebellious about the operation, put a twitch on him, having someone hold it while you operate the clippers. Nothing is gained by losing patience and whacking him. It is far easier on his—and your—nerves to employ the twitch. It doesn't hurt him, but, being uncomfortable, it merely takes his mind off his other troubles. Since using a twitch usually puts an end to his foolishness, it is far better than beating on him and taking a chance of subsequently making him head-shy.

When you have finished the ears, trim the mane behind them for

Heads: trimmed and not trimmed.

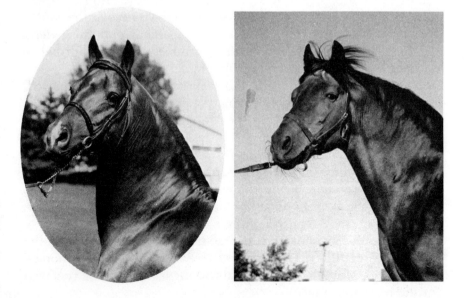

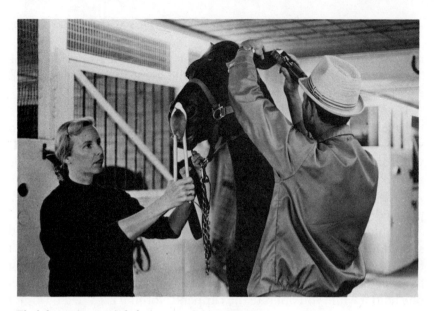
The helper using a twitch during an ear-trimming session.

approximately four or six inches, depending on the length and shape of your horse's neck. The illustrations show you some variations. It is a matter of preference how far back you go, but don't overdo it: you don't want him to look bald. Some owners take off just a bridle path behind the ears to accommodate the crownpiece of the bridle. If one is showing in Hunter classes this is customary; but the general standard for Morgans is to have them trimmed back a bit further to enhance the line of neck and throttle.

The long hairs on the muzzle and over the eyes should be removed, and the hair on the lower jaw trimmed smoothly. This trimming gives the horse's head the clean-cut, sleek appearance that is well worth the effort. It facilitates the work if you use a grooming halter for the entire procedure. And it is wise *not* to have the horse on the cross-ties for the clipping session; have someone hold him with a shank during the operation of the clippers if he is at all snorty about it. Once a horse gets the notion to fly back in the ties and break a halter, he is often on the verge of making a habit of it.

Most professional horsemen like to trim the long hair around the coronary band of the foot as well as the fetlocks of their show horses. Indeed, with Morgans any long hair on the legs should be removed for the best appearance.

Trimming the Mane

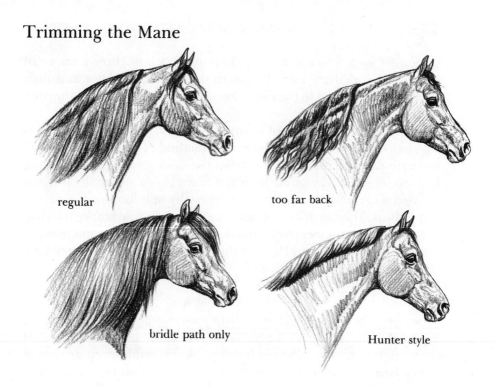

regular

too far back

bridle path only

Hunter style

Shampooing

The washing of manes and tails should also take place just prior to leaving for a show; or it may be done at the show if facilities and time allow. The mane should be washed with warm water and either a good shampoo for human hair or one prepared especially for horses. Using plain bar soap will take the natural luster and gloss out of the hair. Work the shampoo well into the mane, being sure to get the underside clean right to the roots; rinse thoroughly with warm water until there are no traces of shampoo left. When the mane is dry, brush it carefully with a not-too-firm hairbrush such as you'd use on your own hair, and pick out any snarls with your fingers. If a horse has a particularly heavy mane with a tendency to tangle easily, use a creme rinse after shampooing to facilitate later brushing. Always rinse all products out thoroughly after each application.

Before washing your horse's tail, you should carefully pick it out with your fingers to remove traces of bedding and other debris. Then it should be shampooed and rinsed till it squeaks. Pick it out again and brush it gently with the hairbrush.

You may want to braid it up to keep it clean till he is due to show. Tear some strips of old bed-sheets about an inch wide and about three feet long. Place a strip of cloth over each of three sections of hair and braid them into the tail to the end. Tie a knot and then loop the tail back up to the dock, using the dangling ends of sheeting to tie it up.

There are several ways of doing the braiding, and here again it is a matter of your own preference. The method of making many small separate plaits that hang down from the dock sometimes makes the hair extremely kinky or bushy when taken down, especially if it was braided when damp. Overly kinky or bushy tails look very artificial. Either braid the tail dry or remove the braids a while before the class so some of the kinkiness will fall out. Tails should be silky and blowing free to give a pleasing effect: if they are stiff and bushy, they look like a mat rather than a banner.

Currying and Polishing

When your horse is at a show, a bath with complete over-all sudsing is probably unnecessary—unless he has really made a mess of himself in the stall due to insufficient bedding. A thorough, deep grooming puts a better shine on his coat anyway, because water tends to make the hair stand up and appear dry and harsh, especially in coarse-coated horses.

Start by currying him with a rubber currycomb to lift loose scales of dander and all surface dust. Then go all over him with a stiff dandy brush (rice-root or plastic-bristle), removing as much as you can of the dirt loosened by the currycomb; keep the currycomb in your free hand and clean your brush with it frequently during the process. Don't spare the elbow grease: they still haven't invented a commercial product that can beat it!

Brush the insides of his legs and the underside of his barrel—we tend to miss these places sometimes.

Use a soft brush on his head, stroking with the direction of the hair. Go carefully around his eyes. Horses don't like to have their heads brushed, and if you are rough about it they really resent it.

Next, go over his body with a soft white-fiber brush or body brush. You'll find that most of the dirt you brought to the surface with the currycomb and dandy brush will disappear when the soft brush is used. Finish with a thorough wiping from head to tail with a soft terrycloth towel or linen stable rubber.

Wait until you have a class coming up soon to put the finishing touches on your horse. His feet may be blacked with a self-shining liquid hoof polish, or rely on your favorite hoof dressing. There are also a number of patented coat-conditioners and dressings available for show horses. In spray containers, they are successful in putting a nice gloss on a horse just before his class—but they do tend to collect dust, so apply them sparingly and only at the last minute. Of course one never uses a spray container of any sort around a horse's head.

To make his head look sharp and clean, apply baby oil to your fingers or on one corner of a towel and smooth it around his nostrils,

Last-minute details for that "bandbox look" in the show ring: applying corn starch to white socks.

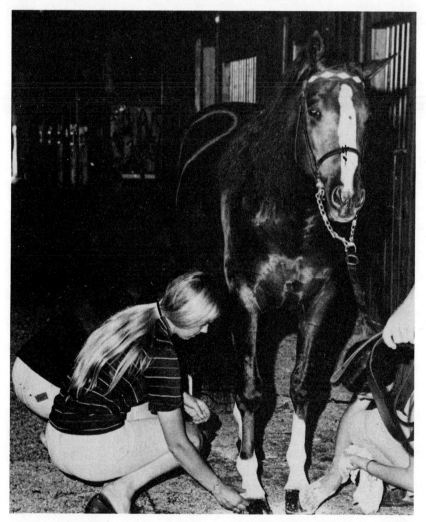

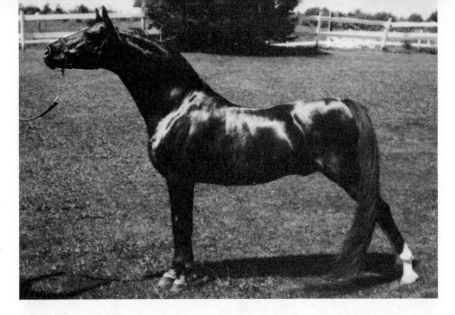

After a thorough bath.

muzzle and eyes. The insides of his clipped ears should also be done. This eliminates any dusty look on the surfaces.

SHOWING IN HAND

Now that your horse is gleaming from all the time you have invested in preparing him for his class in hand, the next item to consider is tack.

Tack

If he is a suckling or weanling, you will show him in a halter. The halter should fit quite snugly (but not so tight that it will pinch), because weanlings tend to slip out of them if they become excited in a class, and a suckling is especially likely to do so if his mother is calling anxiously for him outside the ring. These young horses are always unpredictable at best, so be constantly on the alert.

Yearlings, too, may be shown in halters. Most popular are the narrow, round-leather cheek type with a narrow, colored browband. These are usually equipped with a matching chain lead-shank.

Two-year-olds may be shown in a halter or a neat bridle with a small snaffle bit. It is not at all advisable to use a curb bit on a two-year-old unless he is thoroughly accustomed to it. A young horse who isn't well acquainted with a curb can get himself into some really

In-Hand Tack

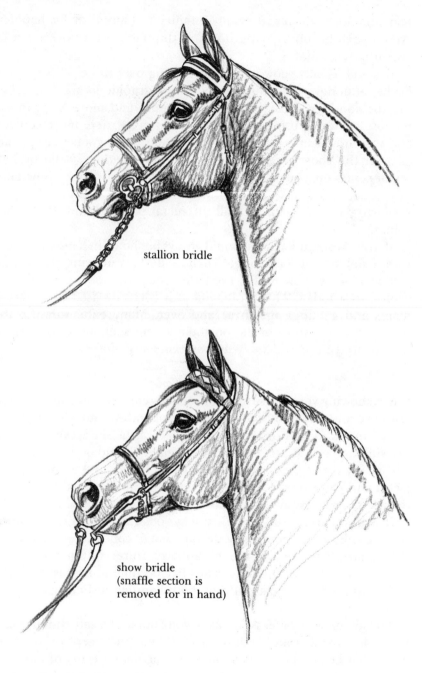

stallion bridle

show bridle
(snaffle section is
removed for in hand)

bad situations which can result in injury to himself or his handler. And a curb bit on a young horse in the hands of a novice can be absolute dynamite!

You will usually show a mare or gelding over three years old in a bridle, although, depending on your geographic location, a halter may be considered correct. However, more and more Morgan exhibitors prefer to use a bridle, because it gives them more control, and somehow seems more appropriate and making a better appearance in the show ring. Still, your choice of either bridle or halter depends on your point of view, the location of the show and, of course, on the age of your horse. Whatever you use, be sure it fits neatly and is clean, with all the metal polished and the leather shining.

Mature Morgan stallions should always be shown in hand in a bridle with a stallion bit, or a single curb made by removing the snaffle section from a show bridle, the latter being the most generally accepted style today. This arrangement is correctly used on stallions, mares and geldings age three and over. Many exhibitors use the stallion bit in a show bridle on their young stallions as well as on mature studs; *it should not be used on mares or geldings.*

Duties of the "Tailer"

When showing your horse in hand you may carry a whip, but it should not have any sort of attention-getting appendages attached to it.

You may also have a helper—or "tailer," as he/she is called—when showing in hand. Both you and your helper should be appropriately and neatly dressed either in a saddle suit (ladies and girls) or sport jacket and pants or saddle suit (for gentlemen). Many exhibitors and their helpers dress alike as an added bit of showmanship.

It is also correct to wear Kentucky jods (and boots), a white or colored shirt and tie and a vest or waistcoat of contrasting color. Both ladies and gentlemen can use this apparel. In recent years, however, the "dress code" in in hand classes has become more casual. But *I* feel a co-ordinated, neat outfit on both handler and tailer is important.

The job of your tailer is to follow your horse at a safe distance and keep the animal from hanging back or "going to sleep" on the line. There has been much discussion on the actual necessity of having a tailer in in hand classes. But from personal experience I can state with firm conviction that a good tailer can make a tremendous difference in a horse's performance. The top teamwork of header and

Pointers for Showing in Hand

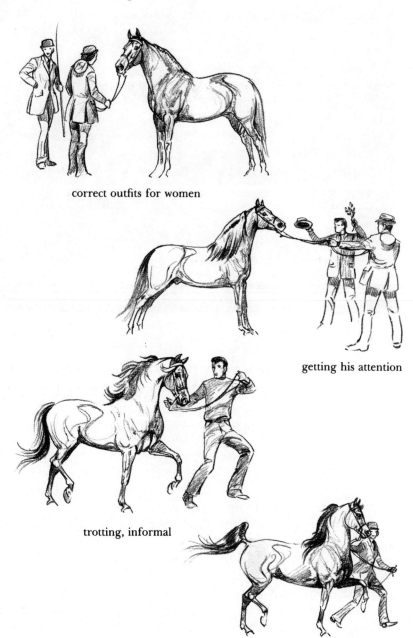

correct outfits for women

getting his attention

trotting, informal

trotting, in a show

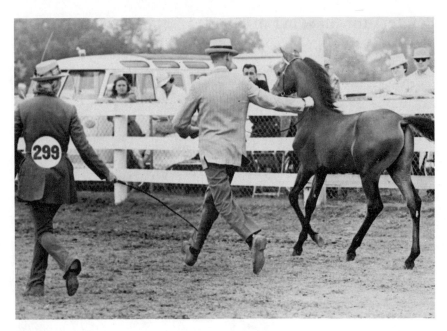

The job of a tailer.

tailer can be a great asset to a horse, because between them they keep him looking sharp. The tailer may carry a towel and possibly a mane brush into a class.

Handling in the Ring

Never forget that your horse is on display from the moment he enters the ring. Depending on how he acquits himself, he will be a credit to your training, or the butt of criticism. And most of the time his performance is entirely up to you.

As in other events in the show ring, any in hand class requires showmanship and a conscientious effort on your part. Never let down until the judge hands in his card. Show your horse well every minute. If the class is a huge one, where the judge is occupied at the far end of the ring, you may let your horse relax a bit; but bear in mind that once the judge has seen your horse, he just might look back your way again to make a decision. You won't want to have him find you and your horse asleep at the switch. After observing a few in hand classes at the shows, you will see that the exhibitors who seem to be consistent winners really work at it.

Again depending on the locality in which you are showing, you will enter the ring with your horse at a trot, make one pass down the rail or through the center, and then line your horse up with the others. In some areas, particularly where Morgans are shown primarily in halters by exhibitors in Western attire, entries will come in at a walk and quietly line up to await individual judging.

The manner in which you show your horse often can have a distinct bearing on how he places in the ribbons. Regardless of whether you are showing quietly in a halter or you have the horse up on the bit and displaying presence and action, he should always be alert. The illustrations show the tremendous difference it makes to have your horse shown correctly.

HOW HE STANDS: While the judge is examining him, you should have the horse standing squarely with his forelegs perpendicular to the ground. His hind legs should be placed together and straight, or slightly, back.

It is advisable to place a horse's hind legs correctly first, and then to bring him up straight in front: handled thus, he will stand with his weight distributed evenly *over* his front legs. If he seems to pull his weight back and overstretches his legs in front, back him up and set him up again.

Nothing spoils a horse's appearance more than letting him overstretch in front and throw his weight behind his shoulders, for then his back will appear low and he will look high in the croup: a glaring fault. (One sees this situation when horses are allowed to keep "creeping up" in front—a habit acquired often by overschooling—until they are way overstretched and awkward-looking.) Sometimes it will help to keep a horse standing straight on his forelegs if you have a bit of apple or carrot or grass in your hand and hold it out to him. In the process of reaching for the tidbit, he will lean forward, bringing his weight up front. It is very important to have your horse standing correctly and looking bright and alert at this time. The judge is forming his opinion, and it is up to you to see that he will remember the animal favorably and keep him in contention.

So keep working every minute—and stay sharp yourself!

GETTING THOSE EARS UP: Keeping a horse's ears up can be somewhat of a problem, especially in large classes where he becomes bored with the waiting. Horses' individual temperaments enter the picture here too. Some are naturally alert and interested in the goings-on no matter how long the class, while others easily become blasé or even downright sulky after only a few minutes in the ring. And when they

For the Line-up in Hand

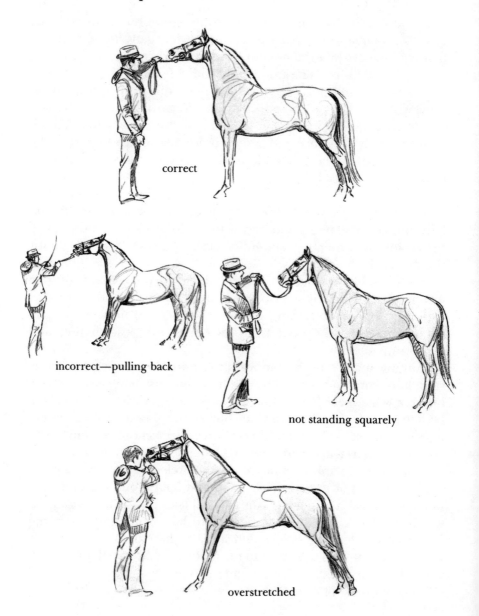

correct

incorrect—pulling back

not standing squarely

overstretched

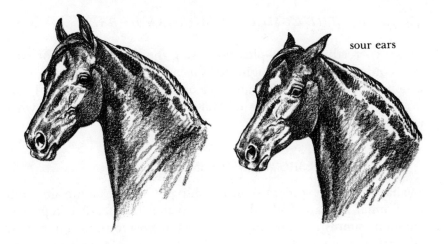

sour ears

put their ears back, they can look unattractive no matter what their other attributes are. It is best to try to learn the secret of keeping your horse bright and with his ears up for in hand classes. But remember, all horses are individuals, and the little trick that works for one will not necessarily work for another. Experiment!

Meanwhile, the tidbit that lures him to put his weight well forward may also get him to use his ears with interest, thereby imparting the ideal expression that all Morgan exhibitors strive for. There was a time when you could have ribbons or streamers or a small plastic bag on the end of your whip to get his attention and cause him to use his ears. But no more: too many exhibitors were guilty of spooking other horses with these innovations, and such novelties have been banned for understandable reasons.

The True Criteria

Every judge has his own method for judging his classes. Many will ask each entry individually to move down the rail at a walk, turn and trot back to him. Standing by the rail, the judge can then see how the horse handles himself both going away and from the front. Winging, paddling, going wide or close behind will all be noted if the condition is present. Hitching, pacing or any variation from the correct cadence of the walk and trot are considered faults and are penalized accordingly.

There has been criticism heard that judges have a tendency to pick high-going horses, thus giving such animals an advantage in the ring. To remove any ground for misunderstanding, a rule has been made which states: "height of action will not take precedence over a correct way-of-going." If a horse has much natural action and presence *and* moves correctly as well—plus possessing the requirements for type and conformation—he might get the nod over a horse with little action or bloom even if the latter is a basically good individual. However, a judge must be able to evaluate what is obvious and what is not.

SHOWMANSHIP IN PRACTICE

We have all seen excellent showmanship put a horse on top although the animal perhaps had a fault or two that the handler kept well "hidden" simply by knowing his horse and how to show him to best advantage. Conversely, a very good horse will suffer when he is inefficiently handled. Observe as many classes as you can. You will soon become acutely aware of the various methods of *ethical and courteous showmanship* which seem to bring a horse to the peak of his performance in the ring.

Unfortunately, quite often we do see deplorable behavior in the show ring, both on the part of exhibitors and their horses. The animals that leap and plunge and just won't seem to stay on their feet, and the handlers who have acquired the reputation of being "whip artists" seem to combine forces to render suspect the entire procedure of the in hand class. While most of the exhibitors are mindful of the rules and show their horses correctly and well, a few rascals, without regard for their fellow exhibitors, keep their horses spooked every minute, regardless of the effect on others. And of course a whip is valuable and essential if you wish your horse to be brilliant and bright-looking, but overuse of it leads to so much criticism that those who do use a whip judiciously suffer opprobrium along with the guilty. It is important to keep your horse alert and looking his best, but he should not be so agitated that his manners suffer as a result. Certainly one should not prevent another exhibitor's properly showing *his* horse.

Showing a horse in hand, whether it be a weanling or a mature animal, requires that ample time be spent preparing the horse for the ring just as you would prepare for any other class. Working a horse in hand at home until he becomes accustomed to the procedure will do much to improve his manners when actually in the ring.

Foals or weanlings are naturally unpredictable no matter how much time you give them, but if you are planning to show a suckling foal in hand, let him become used to being taken away from his mother. Work with him at home. Don't wait until his class comes up and then without warning, suddenly, separate him from his dam! He will usu-

Showing in a Halter

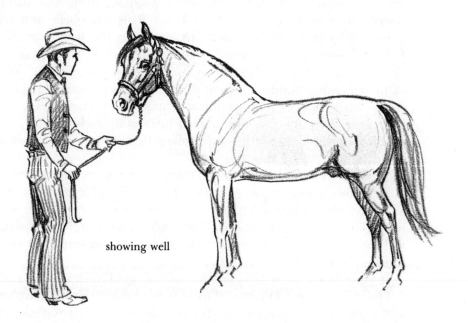

showing well

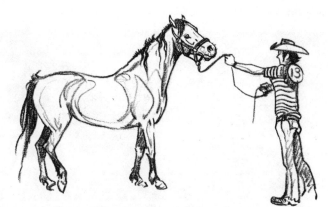

not the way to do it!

ally react with violence, his truculence asserting itself with flailing
hoofs and screaming indignation. Many foals have been seriously
injured as a result of fear and anxiety about the whereabouts of
Mother, especially when in strange surroundings. Weanlings and
yearlings can be unpredictable too, so always be watchful for signs
of their coming "undone" Should a young horse rear in panic or
temper, never, *never* pull on him to bring him down: instead, slack
off immediately and give him rein. If he goes up and over, he could
injure himself permanently—especially if he hits his head or the back
of his neck in a vital spot.

Mature horses which are up on the bit and snorty will sometimes,
out of sheer good spirits, give a couple of playful leaps when they
enter the ring. These shenanigans can be excused if they are done
in fun and are not prolonged. But don't confuse high-spiritedness
with bad manners: the former is spontaneous and brief; the other
can reflect a sustained state of agitation.

If your horse (and stallions, mares and geldings can be equally
guilty) is overly keyed up over the excitement of the show atmosphere
and seems about to come out of his hide, let him get some of the
kinks out of his system by moving him *before* the class begins. Trot

A present-day descendant of Justin displays inherited type and spirit.

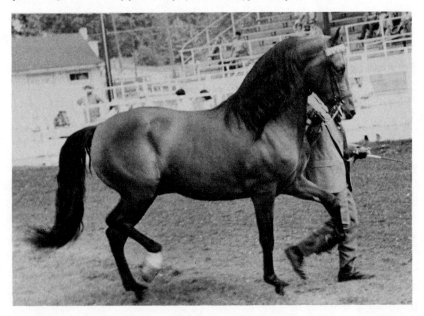

him out a few times on the line. Or better yet, put him on a longe-line a few minutes before taking him over to the ring. Either procedure might prevent him from giving you a merry time of it once he gets in the ring.

On the other hand, if your horse appears lacking in enthusiasm and apparently bored before he starts, it certainly does not harm him to wake up a bit with a couple of pops of the whip behind him or with clatter from a few pebbles in a tin can. If he has any spirit at all, he'll soon be bright-eyed and bushy-tailed as he heads for the ring. Be considerate, though, and *don't upset other people's horses* in the process.

To sum up: The basic requirements for showing a Morgan in hand are as follows:

- Your horse should be well-groomed and well turned out.
- You and your assistant should be appropriately and neatly dressed (sport clothes or saddle suits for men; saddle suits or Kentucky jods or neat trousers with a shirt, tie and vest for ladies; or in some areas neat Western attire for both).
- The horse should be wearing a good show bridle or a neat, well-fitting show halter.
- You should have your horse as well-trained for this class as any other. He should move correctly on the line at the walk and a trot and stand alertly with legs properly placed while being judged. Excessive use of the whip is definitely frowned upon, so keep your horse bright but don't overdo it. Keep your horse always looking his best in class; don't "fall asleep": if you stay sharp yourself, so will your horse. Letting him rest one hind foot or hang his head, for example, makes you both appear uninterested.
- Remember that you and your horse are, in fact, "on stage"—so don't forget your cues!

11

Pleasure Horse–Fun Horse

JUST EXACTLY what is a fun Pleasure horse? How is it difficult from, say, a field Hunter or a working stock horse or a polo pony? The difference is specialization. The Hunter is required to excel at a specific task: to follow and keep up with hounds. The stock horse's job is working cattle, and the polo pony is trained specifically to twist and turn at speed and keep his eye on the ball. Many people who are fond of horses indulge in these special fields and prefer to limit their horse activities to their own sphere of interest. People who have show horses of various breeds, and prefer the excitement and glamor of the show ring to the sound of the hounds and the crack of a polo mallet confine their interest to the call of the show circuits.

But the vast majority of horse owners keep horses for pleasure riding. They find, in the easy companionship of a good horse on the trail, more downright enjoyment in just following a path in the woods than they would in sailing over walls at a mad gallop or trying to outrace a competitor for a white wooden ball.

The Pleasure horse has become increasingly popular, with a growing number of people becoming interested in horses and riding. More and more adults are finding that the relaxation and healthful exercise which go along with owning a horse have benefited them greatly in the frantic rush of the times. A good horse is a companion that does not make unreasonable demands; nor does he back-talk you when all you wish for is peace and quiet, and he will greet you with a friendly nicker when you come to the stable. Even the tending of him, if you truly like horses, becomes a ritual rather than a chore. There is a certain satisfaction in carefully grooming your horse and

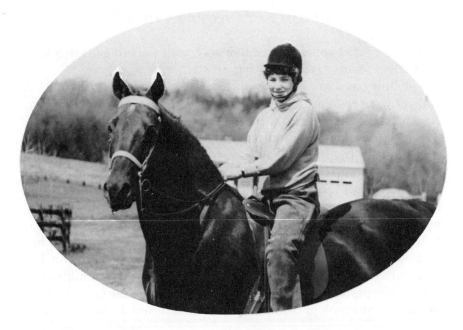

Young girl and her "friend."

seeing the reward of your efforts in his gleaming coat; or in putting down a fresh, crisp bed of straw in his stall and watching him roll luxuriously in its clean, crackling softness. If you like horses, your own stable, no matter how modest, is your pride and your retreat from the hustle and bustle of everyday living. To saddle up and head for the hills is the best prescription ever written for jangled nerves and frayed tempers. A good Pleasure horse can make you forget you had words with the boss or that tomorrow a big conference is waiting with its attendant headaches. All the worries and frustrations seem to fall away with the gentle clop, clop of your horse's hoofs on the soft ground. Many are the people who never thought to own a horse who have found and are finding horse ownership a most rewarding experience.

The Morgan has proved himself in countless ways to be the ideal Pleasure horse for young and old. His natural docility, coupled with a personality that almost defies adequate description, makes him the favorite of owners everywhere. His hardiness and easy-keeping qualities, his endurance and versatility make the Morgan in demand the country over.

Regardless of whether you prefer Western tack and style of riding or English, the Morgan is equally at home. And indeed many owners ride them both ways depending on whatever whim seizes them. Morgans give a good appearance either way, with smooth gaits that lend themselves to any task.

The little bay mare who was my first horse stood only a slight 14.2, and yet her versatility and temperament amazed all who knew her. At the age of three years she had negotiated every jumpable stone wall within a radius of twenty miles of her stable. She hauled us all over the back roads in a heavy cart for hours at a time and whether she was tacked up in a stock saddle or a forward-seat jumping saddle or ridden bareback, it made little difference in her outlook. Long hours on the trail with frequent all-out gallops, racing against friends' hunters, or a myriad of walls and logs to jump en route never seemed to wear her out. She would always come home with a spring in her walk and ears cocked eagerly for the familiar road. She won her share of ribbons at the shows and taught innumerable children to ride. She experienced parades and picnics and even the Grand March in a rodeo. She took us swimming in the sound, and in a work harness

Your Morgan "at home."

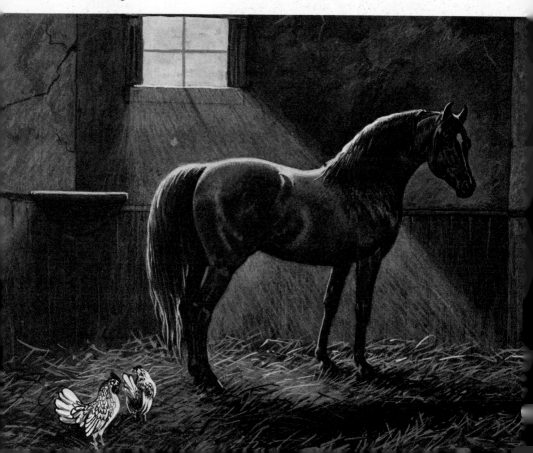

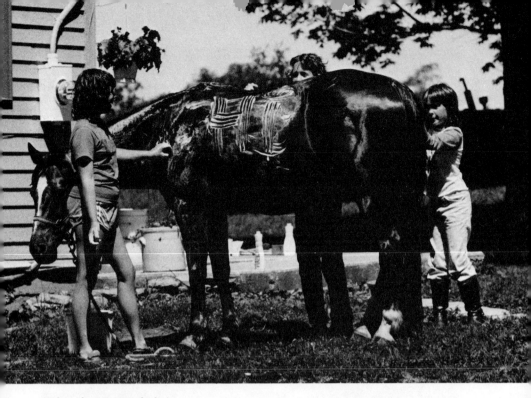

Kids and a Morgan: bath time.

raked hay with a creaking old horse rake swaying behind her. At the age of *nineteen* she won blues at the shows, amazing people by her youthful appearance and action. Her legs were free of any blemishes all her life and never was she lame despite her varied tasks. This little mare was a Pleasure horse in every sense of the word. She was companion and friend and confidante. She was a member of the family, a pet who would eat ice cream and apple pie; was a means of transportation when the car was gone; and was the heroine of the neighborhood kids. This is the way Morgan Pleasure horses should be: equal to any task and willing and eager to go along with their riders' whims. No assignment should be too difficult for a Morgan at least to try.

THE COMPETITIVE RIDE

As an example of the competitive trail ride available to the Morgan owner, it might be interesting here to give some information about the famous 100-Mile Trail Ride which is held annually in the "Morgan country" around Woodstock, Vermont.

A successor to the old 300-Mile Endurance Rides held in Vermont by the cavalry (Vermont was chosen because it offered the best riding country and afforded the most variety in terrain), the 100-Mile Trail Ride was first held in 1936. It was sponsored by The Green Mountain Horse Association and is the oldest competitive trail ride of its type in the United States.

Although only eleven entries turned out for the first ride, each year the event attracted more and more horsemen to the Woodstock area in the late summer. From all parts of the country they came

A veteran trail rider and his Morgan—winner of 1985 Sweepstakes—on The Green Mountain Horse Association 100-Mile Trail Ride.

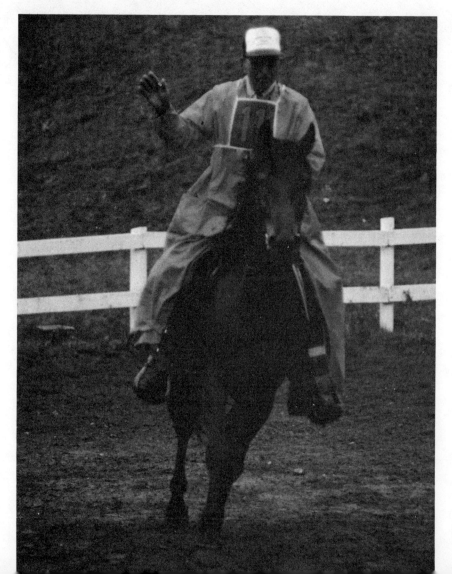

with a mixed variety of horses in tow. The increasing interest brought so many entries that soon a limit had to be placed on the number allowed to compete in the ride. A 50-Mile Pleasure Ride was inaugurated to give more people a chance for group trail-riding in the Vermont countryside. Non-competitive, this ride offers a less grueling, equally enjoyable experience on the lovely Vermont trails.

In the 100-mile ride, 40 miles must be covered each of the first two days. Seven hours are allowed for the 40-mile distance, with penalties given for extra time used. On the third day the riders are allowed three hours to complete 20 miles. And all these miles are over rough, tortuous trails that test to the fullest a horse's condition and endurance. Needless to say, the riders must be made of the same stuff as their horses, for the long hours in the saddle can take their toll with the improperly prepared human or equine. Yet it is interesting to note that despite the arduous experience the 100-mile ride affords, the waiting list of those who wish to enter the ride grows each year.

Judges and official veterinarians follow the riders each day and no one escapes their careful scrutiny. Each horse is checked for condition throughout the ride and the judges make their scorings. A rider must time himself carefully during the periods on the trail because no extra time is allowed for unscheduled stops.

The official timer checks every horse as it returns to the stable and records the exact time on each entry. For every three minutes over the time limit, a penalty is imposed. No boots, pads or bandages are allowed on the horses, and equally taboo are liniments or other medications. A horse *must* be in top condition: any sign of soreness leads to disqualification.

You may ask what purpose the 100-Mile Trail Ride serves. The answers are many and varied, but the most important reasons are that it increases interest in trail-riding and provides a model for other rides, it is a stimulus for developing the endurance of horse and rider, it proves the rewarding knowledge that selection, conditioning and proper care of horses pay off in added enjoyment, and it puts sportsmanship and horsemanship above the glory of winning honors. Riders participate for various reasons, too—for the zest of competition, the camaraderie of kindred spirits and a pure love of horses and riding.

Morgans have always done well in the 100-mile ride since its inception. Over large fields with their representative breeds of light horses, they have won much acclaim and racked up phenomenal records.

A WORD ABOUT DRESSAGE

Although "dressage," as a term, simply means "training," there is much more involved than merely teaching a horse to carry a rider and perform whatever gaits are required. Dressage, in essence, is a harmony of horse and rider performing simple or extremely intricate movements together. They are a unit: the horse an extension of the rider—supple, keen, under perfect control.

There are several stages of training in dressage, each leading to the next level. In the U.S.A., tests include the following: Preliminary, First, Second, Third and Fourth levels. The highest standards are seen in the F.E.I.(Fédération Équestre Internationale): Prix St. Georges, Intermédiaire and Grand Prix.

Dressage training at any level will do much to improve a horse's abilities. Collection, impulsion, cadence and lightness in the rider's hands are all accomplished by dressage training. Since Morgans have the temperament and natural style required of dressage performance, it is only a matter of correct training to develop the tremendous potential already there.

Much could be written here concerning dressage training, but the subject is material for a book in itself and space here allows for only a mention of the Morgan's aptitude to become tops in this field. It takes *time*, knowledge, *patience* and perseverance to achieve the highest levels. If you and your horse have these qualities—*go for it!*

CARRIAGE DRIVING

With the fast growing interest in antique vehicles in this country comes another enjoyable equine sport that you might say was virtually designed with Morgans in mind—Carriage Driving.

Basically, the Morgan used in Carriage Driving is often the same animal used for Pleasure Driving, except somewhat more is demanded of him.

In regard to the vehicle and harness used, the vehicle must have wooden spoked wheels, and your harness should fit well, be heavier and sturdier than the show harness. Both carriage and harness should

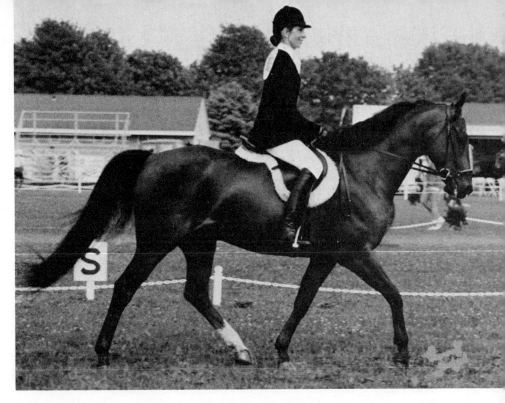

Dressage: First Level, working trot, using jumping saddle and pad.

Dressage: First Level, extended trot.

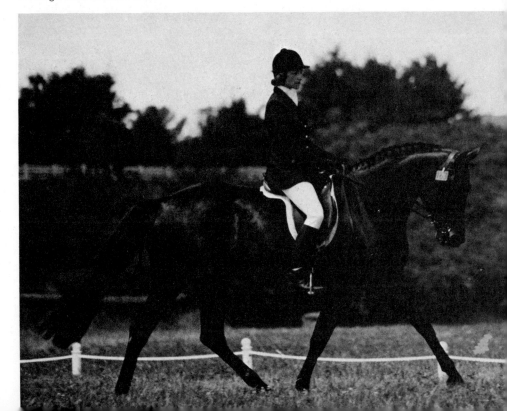

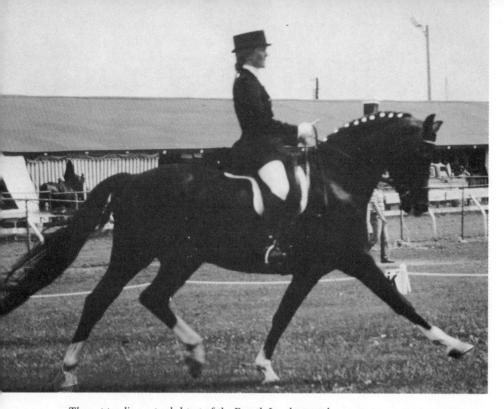

The outstanding extended trot of the Fourth Level contender.

A champion through the Fourth Level, this Morgan performs a canter pirouette to the right.

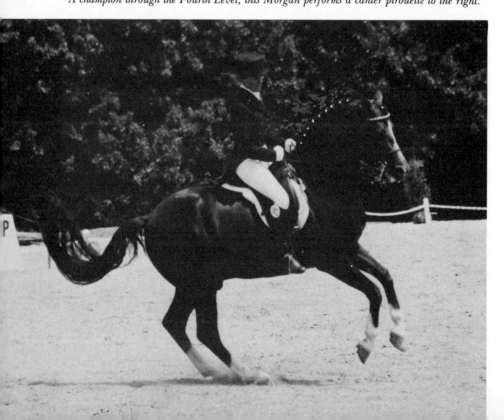

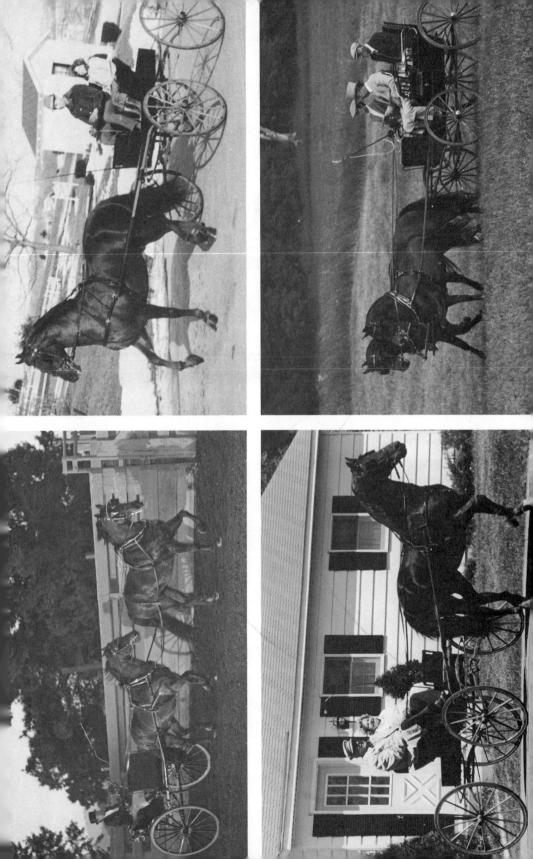

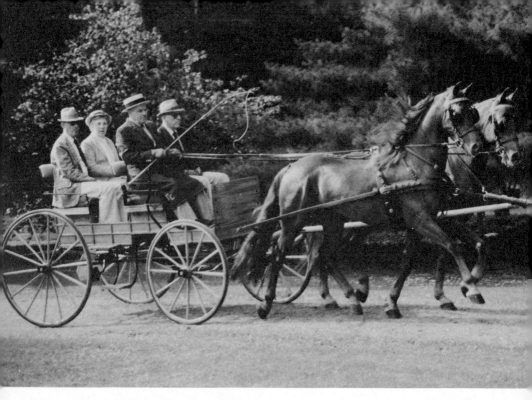

Carriage Driving.

Marathon Driving.

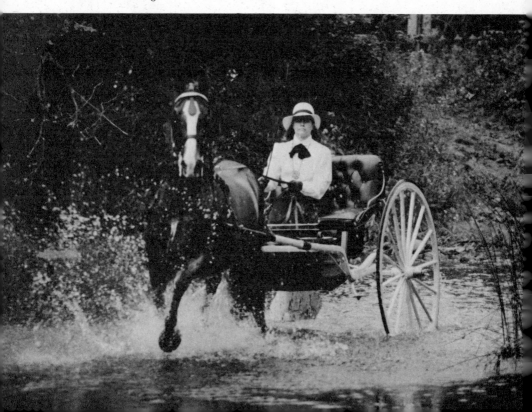

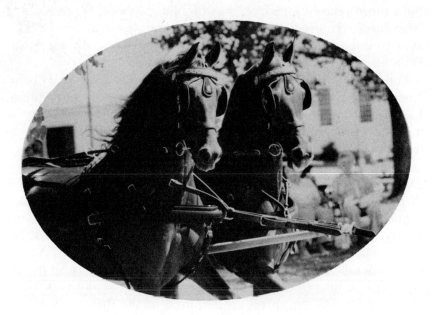

be in excellent condition—clean and appropriate for the competition or class entered.

In Pleasure classes, you will be asked to perform a walk, a collected trot, working trot and to trot-on. Style is not foremost, though certainly appreciated, in carriage classes, but manners, handiness and a good elastic, ground-covering way-of-going are. Your horse must stand quietly and back readily when asked.

At the walk, your horse should move freely, with no hint of breaking gait. This point is taken more seriously here than in judging Pleasure Driving classes at the shows. Both the collected trot and working trot must show a horse that is supple in his way-of-going and alert. When asked to trot-on, he should lengthen his stride noticeably so that he is performing three distinct speeds at the trot.

Since Carriage Driving is a traditional sport, etiquette, correct appointments and procedure as well as over-all elegance should be much in evidence.

Training for Carriage Driving consists of the same general methods as for the Pleasure Driving horse, except that the horse is asked for a more relaxed and freer way-of-going without any tension or "showiness" required. Working a well-started horse in small circles as in dressage training teaches the horse to bend to the rein smoothly. He is often judged on how well he performs these patterns.

For a really finished carriage horse, some competitions offer combined driving events. This, in essence, is a three-day competition. Each day is devoted to one phase: dressage driving, cross-country or marathon and a cone obstacle course. You are judged on your three-day over-all performance.

Another competition for only Morgan carriage horses is the Morgan Heritage Class at some of the All Morgan shows. Drivers and their passengers are dressed in authentic period costume that is appropriate to their style of vehicle. It is judged by the same standards as any carriage class, entries being asked for a walk, collected trot and working trot; they will also be expected to back readily. A trot-on is generally not required in this class. The driver must sit on the right side of his vehicle and must carry his whip at all times. Hats, gloves and a driving apron are required of the drivers. Not only performance, but condition of vehicle, costumes, harness and appointments are all judged.

Carriage Driving is a sport that can appeal to people who are not

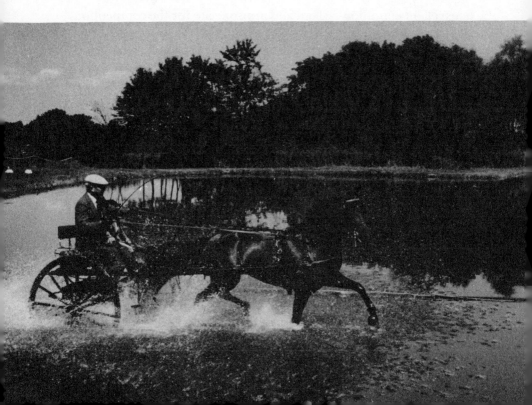

interested in the show ring, particularly. They may want to have some fun with their Morgans yet like something competitive that, while challenging, is more natural. It is noted here that inquiries to the American Driving Society or the Carriage Association will probably bring a deluge of further information about the sport of Carriage Driving.

12

Further Points on Dress and Equipment

REGARDLESS of whether it is English or Western style of riding you have chosen to enjoy with your Morgan, there are certain basic items of tack and equipment that you will need. There are also a number of other things which, while not actually "musts," will make caring for—and showing—your horse easier, and so will add to your fun.

In preceding chapters we have considered the specific types of tack required or regarded as suitable for the various show classes, with brief comment in passing on the garb considered appropriate for the exhibitor. Therefore, this chapter is designed merely to amplify some points and to fill some gaps with handy information. It could almost be called "Guidelines on Dress and a Few Helpful Hints on Tack and Equipment for Home and the Show Circuit." Let's look at clothing first.

WHEN TO WEAR WHAT

If you aim for success at the "A" shows where the competition is keenest and the numbers greatest, you must present yourself, as well as your horse, in the best possible manner. This means clothing that is appropriate, with neatness a prime consideration. It is truly inexcusable to appear in the show ring in sloppy attire, for it strikes a discordant note among exhibitors who have taken pains with their personal appearance—and isn't it also an injustice to a good horse? After all, you are asking him to make a winning impression: you can show your pride in him by not being unkempt yourself!

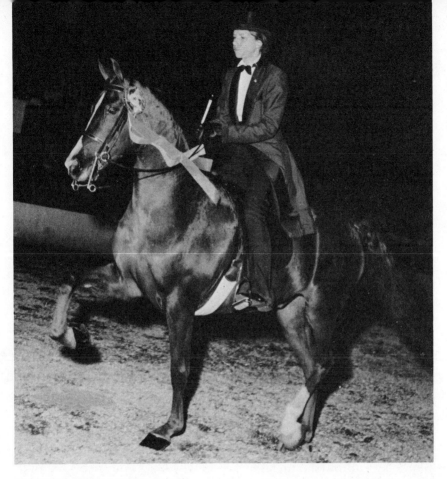

Rider in formal attire for evening.

The following are simple guidelines for what is worn in the various classes. As can be seen from the photographs appearing throughout this book—and as will be stressed again here—correlation of one's clothing with the type of tack, good taste and practicality are the governing principles.

The attire for showing in hand has been discussed in Chapter 10. Following are details of dress for saddle and harness classes—much of it already shown, but without comment, in photographs up until now.

Park and English Pleasure Saddle Classes

In Morgan Park and English Pleasure classes the saddle suit is the accepted attire for both ladies and gentlemen. Originally designed for the American saddle horse people, it has won favor with exhibitors of all breeds on which the cut-back show saddle and the Weymouth show bridle are used in the ring. The Saddle Seat and saddle suit certainly emphasize the Morgan's modern image.

THE INFORMAL SADDLE SUIT, ACCESSORIES AND VARIATIONS

The saddle suit is composed of a jacket cut with rather long skirts having inverted pleats at the sides, and of matching jodhpurs in "Kentucky style"—that is, with a flare at the ankle and no extra fullness above the knee. In morning and afternoon Park and English Pleasure classes, the suit is informal either as to color—such as the grays, blue-grays, brown tones, etc.—or as to accessories, for the more formal darker hues may be "dressed down" with informal accessories for daytime wear.

These accessories include matching or black derbies for ladies; gentlemen may wear a street hat or derby, with most preferring for morning and afternoon a neat, narrow-brimmed street hat of straw or other lightweight material and often with a colored band. Shirts are white or conservative light colors that blend unobtrusively with the jacket. Neckwear for all daytime exhibitors is the four-in-hand—plain-colored, striped or discreetly patterned. Gloves are always worn. Well-buffed or patent-leather jodhpur boots complete the outfit.

A variation on the informal saddle suit that has become really popular in recent years is the combination of contrasting jacket and Kentucky jodhpurs. The latter are usually black; the jacket, cut like its saddle-suit counterpart and having self-collar and lapels, is a solid and *non-garish* blue, red, green or yellow, white or it occasionally is a subdued plaid. Accessories would then be black.

Juniors wear informal saddle suits or the variation just mentioned; the accessories are as noted. The little folk in Lead-Line classes wear any trim jacket with jodhpurs or trousers, jodhpur boots or dark oxfords, and an appropriate hat if desired. In most Lead-Line classes today, the youngsters are small duplicates of their older counterparts.

FORMAL SADDLE SUITS, ACCESSORIES AND VARIATIONS

Technically, 5 P.M. is the point that divides afternoon from evening classes, and informal from formal show-ring attire. But as every follower of horse shows can testify, a number of factors can throw the best schedule awry, so observance of the demarcation hour for dress is not rigid by any means. Furthermore, there are lesser degrees of formality that are quite acceptable in Morgan evening classes, and this leeway is a boon to exhibitors who do not want the expense of a wide variety of outfits for themselves.

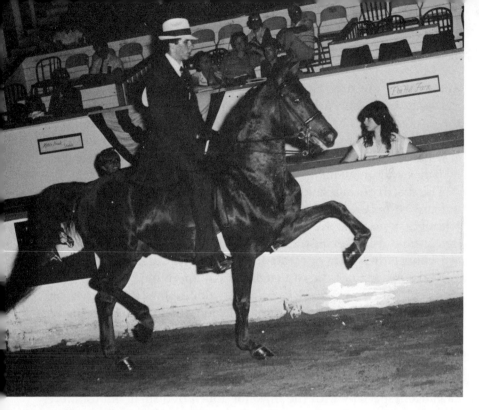

Men's informal attire.

Ladies' informal attire.

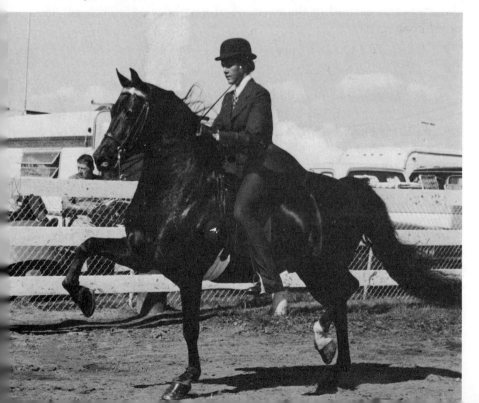

Yet, while not making classically formal dress obligatory, evening classes in both the Park and English Pleasure divisions do suggest the darker tones in saddle suits, or "dressing up" a lighter suit with appropriately dark derby or street hat, four-in-hand and gloves. Several photographs show the attractive touch of a boutonnière worn by ladies and gentlemen.

The strictly formal saddle suit resembles men's formal dinner suits in many respects. It is black, with the gentlemen also opting for navy/midnight blue. The Kentucky jodhpurs have a silk or satin stripe down the outside seam; the shawl collar is again silk or satin. Shirts are white, either plain or pleated, and are worn with a cummerbund.

Neckwear is a bow tie to match the cummerbund. The top hat is worn only with the bow tie. Gentlemen seldom show in a top hat, but it is being seen more and more on the ladies. One will also see some well-turned-out men in a dark street hat of the sort that would be worn at night with a formal dinner suit.

Black gloves and black boots—with patent-leather boots an innovation now accepted in the show ring—round out the picture of elegance, especially with the finishing touch of a small boutonnière.

Other variations on strictly formal attire are solid-color jackets, cut like a dinner coat with long skirts, and having a silk or satin shawl collar. Overly bright or gaudy jackets tend to be distracting, to say the least, and carried to the extreme of garishness, are certainly in questionable taste.

Road Hack and Hunter/Jumper Classes

ROAD HACK ATTIRE

The dress worn in English Pleasure classes is also appropriate for Morgan Road Hack events. This generally means a saddle suit, since the cut-back saddle and full, or double, bridle are by far and away the most popular tack for Pleasure competitions in Morgan shows. Although hunt tack and attire are not a breach of etiquette in Morgan Pleasure classes, riders who wear hunt outfits *do* look out of place when surrounded by the great majority of exhibitors in saddle suits. If the usage in your area leans toward the Hunt Seat for Morgans in hacking classes, however, you will feel less conspicuous in hunt clothes for evening, and wearing less formal versions in the morning or afternoon (high boots or conventional jodhpurs or even gaiters, a hacking jacket, four-in-hand tie and a soft hat).

The basic rule to go by is *never mix your outfits in the show ring*. Go

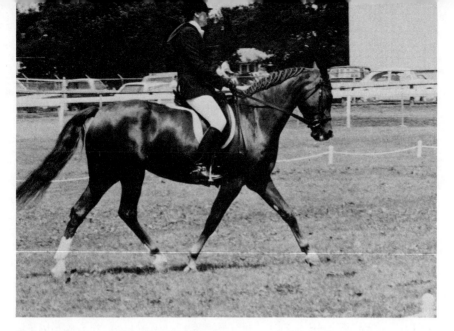

Hunter attire; horse with a French braid.

totally Hunt Seat or totally Saddle Seat, and then dress accordingly. It looks amateurish to ride in one style and dress in another.

And of course one would never wear hunt clothes in a Morgan Park class.

HUNTER/JUMPER DRESS

Attire for Hunter/Jumper events is much easier to decide upon: when your Morgan is showing in classes that are being judged specifically for this type of horse, you will use a hunt bridle and jumping saddle and you will wear high boots, hunt jacket and a hard hunt cap. Juniors may also wear conventional jodhpurs. Consult a reliable outfitter concerning the variations in formality in hunt clothes, then strike a happy, practical medium.

Western Pleasure Classes

Although fashions come and go in Western show riding, certain requirements of dress are mandatory. You must always wear cowboy boots, a Western hat, belt and chaps; also a long sleeved shirt and tie or bolo. Vests or jackets are optional. Jump suits were popular, but shirts and Western pants always seem in style. A carved belt with a silver buckle and silver initials or conchas on the belt of your chaps dresses up your outfit. Chaps should fit properly and can be either of smooth or sueded leather. They can be trimmed with buckstitching

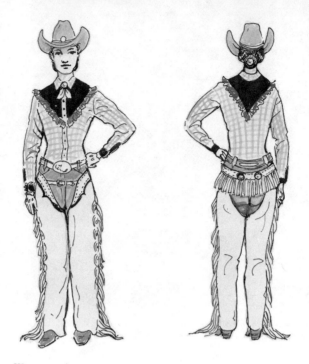

Western attire.

or silver and usually have fringes that come down over the heels of your boots. Too short chaps are a definite no-no! Colors are optional but, as in everything else, be tasteful in your selections. Wearing gloves completes the outfit.

Your choices can be made according to current styles for the basics and for additional appointments, but colors should be consistent and not scream at each other; nor should you sport parade touches in a straightforward Pleasure class. But whatever your personal preferences for styles and colors, it is important that you be neat and well-turned-out for your Western classes. A sloppy or excessively gaudy outfit doesn't do you justice. With such wide selections in this clothing available now all over the country, there is just no excuse for entering the show ring looking like a refugee from either a three-month trail drive or from a psychedelic dream of the Golden West!

Harness Classes

In all harness classes, gentlemen usually wear a business suit and street hat—and here again the conservative choice of color and pattern is considered best, for loud colors and *avant garde* styles have no place in the show ring. Saddle suits are also correct in harness classes, but worn with a soft hat for evening as well as for daytime events.

Ladies showing their horses in Ladies' Park Harness or Pleasure Driving classes will wear neat, attractive dresses, and always be gloved. A hat is appropriate if it is small and secure on the head (but great floppy confections are distracting and out of place).

In an Open Class, or if an impossibly tight schedule precludes changing into a dress, a saddle suit is always correct too. If possible, though, wear a dress: it simply looks attractive—particularly in the classes specifically for ladies.

EQUIPMENT

Every trainer, whether he is amateur or professional, has his own methods and equipment with which he achieves good results on the horses in his care. These include time-honored tricks of the trade and special pieces of tack he has possibly developed and used successfully—and about which he is undoubtedly not just a little secretive. If you are lucky enough to be able to pry one or two hints from a respected individual, they could greatly facilitate your own horse-training activities. Much can be learned from conversations with these trainers and by observing the methods they put to use.

Tack for the Home Stable

A clear knowledge of quality tack and its functions is of prime importance when you are about to launch yourself seriously into the rewarding world of horse ownership. There are many basic items you will need, as well as a number of others which, though not necessarily required, will serve a useful purpose and make owning your horse easier, and thereby more fun.

Perusal of any saddlery catalogue will often confuse and bewilder the novice horse-owner. What equipment is needed to fulfill requirements? How can one keep from overstocking on some items, and at the same time lack equipment that is important and necessary.

No matter which style of riding you have chosen, the basic items will be about the same. Depending on your individual situation and resources, you can invest various sums on these things. We have already covered saddles, bridles and harness in an earlier section. Stable supplies and training equipment will be mentioned here.

Fred Herrick's Longe-Line

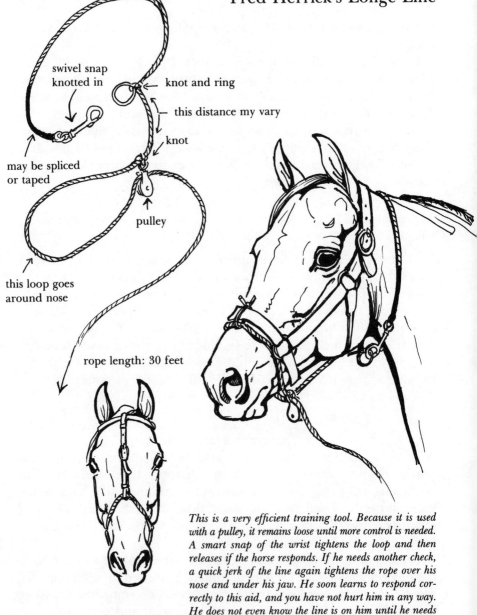

swivel snap
knotted in

knot and ring

this distance my vary

may be spliced
or taped

knot

pulley

this loop goes
around nose

rope length: 30 feet

This is a very efficient training tool. Because it is used with a pulley, it remains loose until more control is needed. A smart snap of the wrist tightens the loop and then releases if the horse responds. If he needs another check, a quick jerk of the line again tightens the rope over his nose and under his jaw. He soon learns to respond correctly to this aid, and you have not hurt him in any way. He does not even know the line is on him until he needs to be restrained. You have great control without any injury to the horse. It teaches him manners very quickly, and it is super for putting a "whoa!" on him.

When used in conjunction with a halter, tie the loop at the top of the noseband with a piece of rawhide, shoestring or even baling twine. This will keep the loop from slipping down over the horse's nostrils. If used with a bridle, we use a Western curb strap hanging from the browband, as shown. Or it can be tied to the top of the cavesson. Note: be sure the rope you buy for this longe-line will go freely through the pulley.

HALTERS AND LEAD-SHANKS

You will need a good everyday halter. This can be one of the several varieties of woven nylon halters available. They come in a number of colors and are very strong and durable. You may later want to invest in a show halter of doubled and stitched leather, possibly with your horse's name engraved on a brass plate on the cheekpiece. A halter with a snap at the throat is convenient and heartily recommended.

Lead-shanks are also essential. They can be of rope, nylon or leather, and with or without a chain. So long as a shank is sound, it will fulfill its purpose, but remember that rope and nylon are tough on your hands should a horse resist the lead. Nylon can also be rather slippery and difficult to hold, especially with a fractious colt or a snorty stallion. Leather lead-shanks, while more expensive, are still your best investment. They have a chain and snap attached to one end and will give you more control of your horse than any other type.

It is recommended that the chain be used as shown in the illustration when leading a stallion—or any high-spirited horse, for that matter. With the snap merely on the bottom ring of a halter, you have very little control should your horse leap forward or shy away from you. It is just good insurance to put the chain over his nose (or under his jaw) and snap it into the other side. There is no need for letting a horse drag you all over the yard when a chain over his nose will quickly curb any such impulse on his part as you lead.

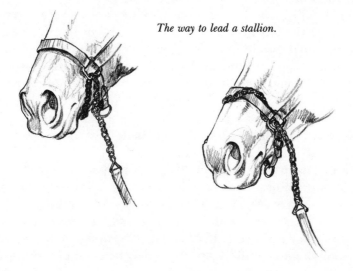

The way to lead a stallion.

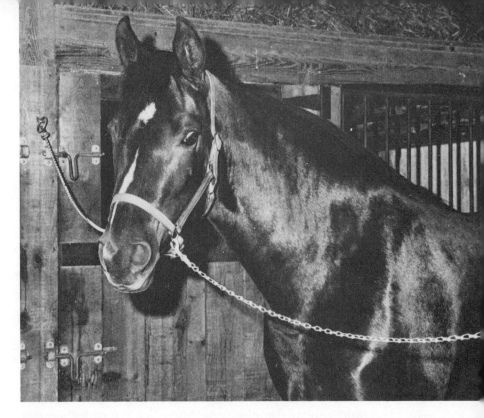

On the cross-ties.

THE GROOMING AREA

It is of the utmost importance that your barn or stable be equipped with a grooming area where you can keep handy all the paraphernalia needed to keep your horse looking his best.

You should have enough area to allow you to rig up cross-ties, which have the advantage over the single tie in that they keep the horse confined in one place so he won't keep moving around while you are working on him. Be sure the ties are neither too snug *nor too long*. Set them so the horse's head will be in a natural and comfortable position when he is standing in them. When they are too tight he may panic and fly back, breaking a halter and thereby implementing bad habits about standing tied; have them too loose, and he will be moving backward and forward as you work on him—and this can be a very exasperating habit on his part, to say the least.

You should build shelves or bins to contain all your grooming gear close to your cross-tie area. This way the items will be handy as you need them: It is also recommended that you have several hooks near by to hang tack up as you finish with it. A cleaning hook is also handy, with sponge and saddle soap on a shelf or counter close by. With these things conveniently placed, you will find the care of your horse and his equipment no chore at all. Have a systematic set-up and you won't always be wondering what happened to the currycomb or trying to remember the whereabouts of the saddle soap.

THE TACK AREA

If possible, you should have a clean, dry place in which to keep your saddles, bridles, harness, etc. It is helpful if this too is near the grooming area, but certainly it should be dry, because dampness raises havoc with leather equipment. If you must use a feed room for your tack, always cover saddles and harnesses to protect them from the dust and chaff.

Saddle racks can be homemade from scrap lumber or purchased from the saddlery shop ready to hang. The same applies to bridle and harness racks. Tack is expensive and should be cared for properly both in use and in storage. Don't just throw it down in a heap.

GROOMING AIDS

For grooming you will need the following: a rubber currycomb; a stiff rice-root brush; a soft white-fiber dandy brush or a body brush; a hoof-pick, a sweat-scraper, and a medium-firm human's hairbrush.

Also handy are a shedding blade, a waterbrush for the mane, and a good group of old terrycloth towels for rub rags.

A mane comb is a controversial matter, because so much mane is pulled out with it that it is not recommended for general use in a Morgan stable. Manes and tails should be carefully picked out with the fingers and then brushed gently with the hairbrush so as not to pull out any more hair than necessary. I shudder to think of how much Morgan mane and tail has ended up on the floor of the grooming area when someone has raked carelessly through it with a stiff brush or mane comb! Luxurious, long manes and tails are a Morgan trademark and should be preserved.

You should have electric clippers, whether you plan on showing or not. There are two types: small-animal ones for fine work (with two heads) and large ones for all-over clipping. If you can avail yourself of only one type, probably the large ones would do more jobs for you, although they will not accommodate the ears. If you plan to do much showing, however, you almost have to invest in a pair of small-animal clippers too; if you are not planning to show, you will not need them.

You will need a twitch. These come in a variety of styles and all are useful and effective. Certainly they are a necessity around any stable—not only for trimming but for "doctoring" and occasionally for shoeing or whenever it is necessary for the horse to stand quietly.

You also should rig up a medicine cabinet in your grooming area. It should be stocked with such items as horse liniment, hoof dressing, Victor's gall remedy, wound ointment, cotton, colic medicine, a dose syringe and a veterinary thermometer, body wash (such as Bigeloil or Vetrolin), and cough medicine. And don't forget a first-aid kit for the human element!

A cooler and scrim sheet, a stable sheet and a heavy blanket are also necessities, and it is handy to have blanket racks attached to one wall on which to hang them when they're not in use. Many Morgan

A tail such as this can be achieved only by care and heredity. It must be washed and picked out frequently—and kept braided and tied up when not being shown. The hereditary factor is a strong point, however; some horses just seem to have a tendency to grow long, thick tails, and some do not!

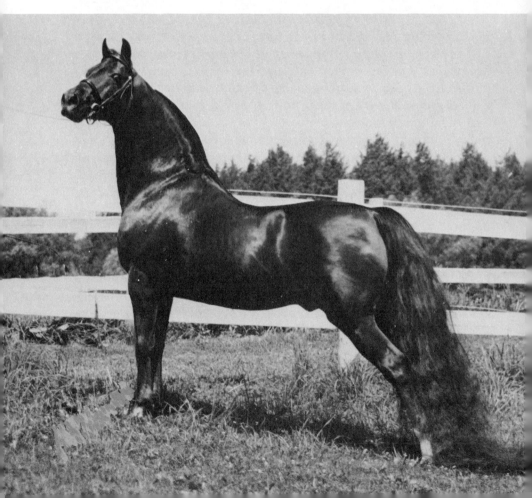

owners who want to keep their horses from getting overly heavy in the throttle area will use a jowl-wrap on them (illustrated in Chapter 6). They aren't a necessity, but they do help to keep the throatline neat and trim for the show ring.

THE STALL

Your horse's stall should be equipped with a feed bucket or corner manger, and a water bucket. It is best if the water bucket is put up with a screw-eye and snap, so it can easily be removed when putting a horse back in his stall after work. Even horses which seem to be cool can break out in a sweat again when returned to their stall, and it is best if they do not have access to water until they are thoroughly cooled down inside and out.

A removable water bucket also makes cleaning chores easier because it can be taken out, scrubbed, and hosed down when necessary.

Some stables have built-in hay racks, but they are not absolutely necessary: as a matter of fact, many horsemen prefer to have their horses eat hay from the floor of their stalls to reduce the amount of dust and chaff that can get in their nostrils.

For stall cleaning, you will need a manure basket or wheelbarrow, a fork and a shovel. A watering can with a disinfectant (such as pine oil) is recommended to use when the stall is cleaned thoroughly and before adding fresh bedding.

On the Show Circuit

A large trunk to store assorted items of tack and accessories is also handy and can do double duty by carting all the pieces of equipment you will need when you go to a show. The tack trunk can be painted in your stable colors further to identify you and your horse at the shows. If you have a farm name or trademark, this can also be painted on the tack trunk for added identification. But regardless of its decor, its tray at the top is good for keeping all sorts of small items—such as double-ended snaps, curb chains, saddle soap and sponges, extra lead-shanks, a leather punch, a white web show girth, saddle whips, etc.—so you can have everything you need for your horse when away from home. Some horsemen keep duplicates of all necessities in the tack trunk so as not to be caught with something vital missing just before a class. If you have ever discovered that you had a jodhpur strap missing or broken just as your class was called, you know how important it is to have a tack trunk well stocked for running repairs to your personal gear as well!

You should always bring a cooler and scrim sheet to a show for walking your horse out after his classes. Usually a light stable sheet will do in the stall during warm weather after the horse is cool. It will help keep him clean and prevent flies from annoying him. In the late season, it is recommended that you bring a heavy blanket with you, as often the nights become quite chilly and show stalls can be drafty.

Your tack trunk might also include a pair of rubber bell boots and, if your horse is a Park contestant, a pair of "rattlers" and/or action chains (used in training *only*); if you will be showing a Roadster, you will probably want a pair of quarter boots. Always include an extra pair of cross-ties to take to the shows too.

Other items useful anywhere are a web stall-guard and an electric water heater to be immersed in a bucket or tub, for heating water quite rapidly. Another item that's very handy is an extra cleaning hook to take along to facilitate doing up your tack after a class. A lightweight portable saddle rack is useful, and so is a similar rack for bridles and halters.

As you go along, you will think of many odds and ends to include in your tack trunk both for use at home and at a show.

And having things in order when you are at a show makes exhibiting far less nerve-racking for everyone concerned. How many times have we seen people flying around looking for a vital bit of tack in a welter of equipment all scattered about?

THE SHOW TACKROOM

Many of the larger stables set up elaborate tackrooms at shows in an adjoining stall to handle all their saddlery and give the exhibitors a pleasant place to rest before a class or to entertain friends. These tackrooms consist of curtains of a heavy material, which are attached by staples or grommets to the sides of the stall. There is usually a ceiling included, and this is stapled tightly across the top of the stall. The dimensions of the tackroom drapes are usually seven by ten feet and the ceiling twelve by twelve.

Appointments for a show tackroom include saddle racks, bridle racks, whip rack, girth rack, mirror, chairs, table, lamp and other accessories; the fixtures are all in stable colors, brass or chrome. Once it is set up, the tackroom is a cozy, attractive haven, eminently practical and as elegant as you please. A banner proclaiming the farm name is hung over the door, while often pictures of the show string are hung on the draped walls on each side. The banner makes a fine

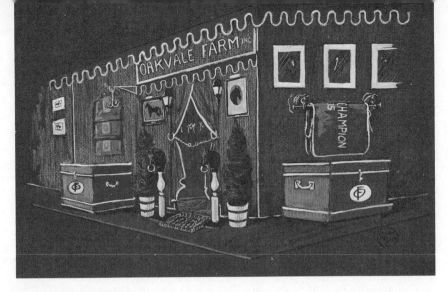

Horse show tackroom.

place to hang any ribbons won, and, needless to say, there is a great deal of satisfaction derived from looking up at a row of blues pinned to your banner at show's end.

If you will be shipping your horse anywhere in a trailer or van, you should have a set of bandages and cotton to wrap his legs. Called track bandages, they come in sets of four in various colors, and you may use sheet cotton (available at tack shops) or quilted leg-wraps under them. Also available are shipping boots lined with foam rubber which attach with zippers or Velcro tape. Whichever you use, it is good to know that your horse's legs are protected during transit. Some horses, uneasy about traveling, will step all over themselves en route, doing themselves damage if not protected.

Harness should be carried in a heavy twill bag designed for the purpose and with a drawstring top. Also available are canvas saddle-carriers to protect your saddle while on the road. Bridles may be packed in the tack trunk. Place them carefully in the trunk and don't lay anything heavy on top of them lest they be damaged.

Training Equipment

SPECIAL BRIDLES

A bitting harness is a useful and necessary piece of training equipment, but you should be familiar with its use before putting your horse in one. A few instructions from a reputable trainer should set you on the right track.

It is handy to have a snaffle bridle and a running martingale hanging in your tackroom. The training bridle as described in an earlier chapter is very effective on young horses, as well as simply being useful for general riding. You may not need a great assortment of bits, but a good Pelham, a couple of snaffles (one for riding and one for driving), a Western curb bit in an "everyday" bridle are all useful on occasion when you own a Morgan Pleasure horse.

THE LONGE-LINE

A longe-line is also a necessary piece of equipment. And it is very practical if you have a day when you lack the time to ride and yet want to give your horse some light exercise. The longe-line you will use is made of a tough webbing, and should be about thirty feet long with a snap at one end. If your horse is broken to harness, you may want to longe him on long lines (two lines attached to the bit) and used in conjunction with the bitting harness.

It doesn't take an intelligent horse long to learn to work on the longe-line if you are careful and patient with him. A helpful hint in this regard: stand about opposite your horse's hip so he is a little ahead of you, for if you get too much ahead of *him*, he will keep trying to turn in to you. By being a little behind him, you can "drive" him forward in the circle.

Always use a longe whip with a lash to keep him working and staying out to the end of the longe-line. Make him respect you and you will soon have no trouble with his manners. Work him at the walk and trot, and if he wants to dog it, pop the whip behind him a time or two to remind him that this is serious business and he'd better stay sharp!

You may canter your horse on the longe-line, but be sure he remains calm and relaxed. Many horses that are unused to cantering on the line will scramble at the start and bunch up, cutting the circle smaller with every lap. It is very important that a horse be relaxed at the canter on the line and stay out as far as the line will allow.

Always work a horse in both directions on the longe. If you have only half an hour to spend, vary his exercise and work him fifteen minutes in one direction, then turn him and go fifteen minutes in the other. This way he will be using all his muscles equally, as well as keeping from getting bored by going for long periods in one direction.

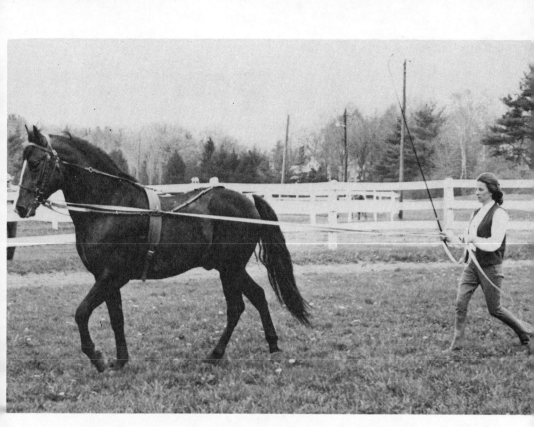

A bitting harness used in training, above, here with long lines, which are fastened to the bit and run through rings on the side of the back-pad; the bridle has a side-check and side-reins. Below, exercise on the longe.

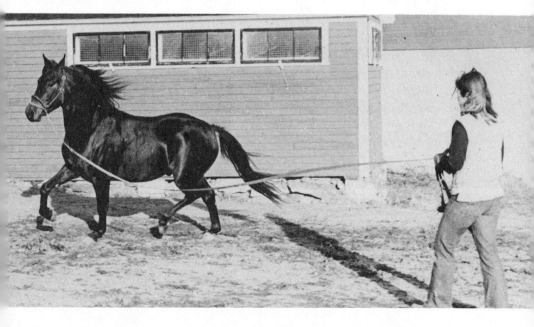

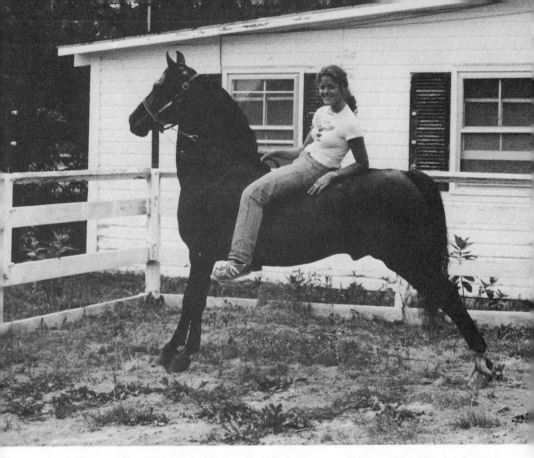

What the Morgan is all about.

As time goes by and your experience and horizons broaden, you will continue to add pieces of equipment and stable supplies to your collection. And if you follow the route of many a new Morgan owner, you'll soon be adding on stalls to your barn, as well. One Morgan almost always leads to more.

You may have to search a while to find that very special Morgan, since your standards should be high, but be assured you will find him.

A FINAL WORD

Now that you have read this book from cover to cover and have a clear understanding of what the Morgan horse is all about, I hope you will want to join the burgeoning ranks of Morgan owners.

There is indeed something special about Morgans: not only their beauty and versatility but the amazing personality of so many individuals. Morgans share your experiences. They almost seem, with their body language, to communicate with you in a way all their own. Their intelligence is really quite phenomenal on so many occasions. Times when most horses might come "unglued," Morgans take a crisis in stride. They love attention from people—not just handouts, but just being with people and being admired and praised. All this can't help but lend truth to the old statement, "The Morgan horse is one thing, every other kind of horse is something else!"

Horsemen's Terms:
A Glossary

Italicized words in definitions indicate those words are defined elsewhere in the glossary.

BALANCE. Carriage in *way-of-going* that permits a horse to get the utmost from all gaits and from the horseman's aids.

In connection with *conformation*, means symmetry of body.

BALANCED TROT. Equal high action of knees and hocks—not having "all the action up front."

BEHIND THE BIT(S). A horse's refusal to exert any pressure at all on the bit(s). The neck is *overflexed* to the point where the rider cannot seem to achieve the contact needed to steady the animal when it is moving, and then all communication between the horse and the rider's hands is lost.

BITTING HARNESS. A training harness used to teach a horse the correct carriage of head and neck; can be used in the stall or when working on the longe-line or in long reins.

BORING (ON THE BITS). Bearing down strongly and with excessive heaviness on the bits when taken in hand by the rider.

CHECKED/CHECKED UP. When the check-rein (which runs from the bit—or through an arrangement on the crownpiece—to the harness pad) is in place and fastened to the hook on the back-pad, to ensure correct carriage of the harness horse's head.

COLLECTED. When the horse *flexes* his neck, lightly responds to the action of the bits and works responsively in accord with his rider at all gaits, moving in balance.

The horse is "uncollected" when he is sloppy in his carriage and out of balance in his action.

CONFORMATION. Over-all physical symmetry. A horse may be well conformed and still lack *type*.

CROSS-CANTERING. Cantering on one lead in front and on the opposite lead behind.

DISHING, see *paddling*.

DOGGY. A lazy, uninterested and plodding *way-of-going*; the horse is slow, disunited, and needing constant prodding.

EXTENDED TROT. A brisk, relatively fast trot where the horse extends himself to cover more ground in each stride—a reachy, smooth, well-coordinated and cadenced gait.

FIGHTING THE BITS. *Fussy in the mouth*. It can be caused by poor bitting, tooth problems, overbitting a young horse, or the rider's poor (i.e., heavy, jerky) hands on the reins.

FINE HARNESS. A special light and elegant harness designed for show-ring use, which can be used in both *Pleasure* and *Park* classes. An over-check or combination bridle may be correctly used.

FLEXED. The horse's head properly set at a pleasing angle, with nose dropped in response to the rider's light pressure on the bit or bits. See also *overflexed*.

FLIPPING (THE TOES). Elevation of the toe before the hoof hits the ground. A horse with this problem will also generally *hit on his heels*.

FORGING. Striking the front shoe with the toe of the (opposite) hind shoe when trotting.

FUSSY IN THE MOUTH. Excessive champing the bits, lolling the tongue, or tossing the head. See also *fighting the bits*.

"GO ON." Horseman's term for asking the horse to work harder, or to increase speed.

GOING ON TOO MUCH. Said of a *Park* horse when he extends his trot beyond the point where he can be maintained correctly *collected*.

GROUND-TIED. Dropping the Western split reins and letting them hang freely to the ground, thus obliging the well-trained horse to stand quietly even when his rider moves away from him.

HAND GALLOP. In essence, a speedy—but *collected*—gallop where the horse is completely under the rider's control, i.e., well in hand.

HEADER. The groom allowed in the ring to stand at the horse's head during the line-up in harness classes; he may wipe off or uncheck the horse temporarily. See also *checked*.

HEAD-SET. Correct carriage of the horse's head for the job he is to perform.

HITCHING. Unequal action in elevation of knees or hocks; going higher on one leg than on the other, and with a resulting break in the correct (two-beat) cadence of the trot.

HITTING ON THE HEELS. The horse's forefoot hits the ground with heel first, instead of with heel and toe simultaneously. This fault can occur with a horse that has been foundered. See also *flipping*.

HOPPING (IN FRONT OR BEHIND). Lifting one leg higher than the other in an unco-ordinated fashion at the trot.

HOT. Said of a horse that is over-anxious and agitated.

INBREEDING. Mating of closely related individuals (father-daughter, etc.). See also *line-breeding*.

JIG. A slow, fretful and nervously executed trot when the gait called for is a quiet, flat-footed (relaxed) walk.

JOG (TROT). The slow, relaxed, easy trot in Western riding.

LABORING (AT THE TROT). Lifting the feet in a heavy, inelastic manner.

LINE-BREEDING. Mating horses of the same bloodlines though not closely related. See also *inbreeding*.

LONGEING. Working a horse in a circle with a long rein or rope attached to the halter. Can also be done with a horse in the bitting harness and a bridle, using the longe-line or long reins (the long reins may be attached to the snaffle bit and run through rings on the harness back-pad).

LOPE. In Western riding, a slow, relaxed, easy canter.

MANNERS. Term denoting a horse's deportment in hand, under saddle and in harness.

NECK-REINING. In Western riding: the horse moving away from the pressure of the reins laid against the side of his neck; i.e., he moves to the left when the right rein is pressed against the right side of his neck, etc.

"ONE-ENDED" GAIT. Usually at the trot, when action in front greatly exceeds action behind. See also *balanced trot*.

ON THE RAIL. Term used to indicate the horses are to stay close to the rail rather than travel a smaller circle by cutting to the inside.

"OUT AHEAD OF HIMSELF." When a horse appears to extend his forelegs out beyond the limit of collection; also said to "throw his action away."

OVERFLEXED. When the horse appears to tuck in his chin excessively when *flexed*. He may be either heavy on the bits or, conversely, *behind the bits*.

OVERWEIGHTING. Placing an excessively heavy shoe on a horse; usually will cause an awkward, artificial *way-of-going*.

PACING. Gait (opposed to the trot, which employs diagonal action) where the legs on the same side strike the ground simultaneously. An hereditary tendency in many horses, but judged a fault in Morgans.

PADDLING. Seen from the front, the horse swings his forelegs sideways as he goes, and appears wobbly in his *way-of-going*. Also called "dishing."

PARK HORSE. A horse with high, natural action whose forte is as high-stepping performer in the show ring.

PLEASURE HORSE. Good-using individual often having diversified talents.

PRESENCE. Deportment characterized by animation, enthusiasm, and sparkle.

ROAD GAIT. Very fast trot called for in Roadster classes.

ROAD TROT. Increased speed at the trot called for in English Pleasure classes.

ROADSTER. A horse with natural trotting speed—enhanced by specialized training—both in harness and under saddle.

SET UP. To carry head and neck correctly—either sometimes naturally due to excellence of *conformation*, or generally as the result of good training. A well-set-up horse also is said to "wear himself" correctly.

SHACKLES. Elastic training device sometimes used on a horse's forelegs to encourage him to elevate his knees in a stylish manner at the *Park* trot.

SHOW BUGGY. Light, four-wheeled vehicles used primarily in the show ring; more usual in Park Harness than in Pleasure Driving classes.

SOUR EARS. Carrying ears back in a disagreeable manner—the horse appears bored and lacking in enthusiasm.

STRUNG OUT. Unco-ordinated at the trot or canter, with hind legs lacking correct impulsion and flexing of the hocks; the horse generally is completely unbalanced.

TAIL-SET. A point of *conformation* where placement of the tail is too high, too low, or correct (see illustrations in Chapter 6).

TIE-DOWN. Strap or device used to keep a horse's head down when working. Used most generally on the Western horse; may not be used in the show ring.

TWO-TRACKING. A forward movement whereby a horse gains ground in front and to one side simultaneously without turning his neck or body. Actually, he is making two tracks instead of one as he swings his hindquarters to the inside, rather than keeping his body parallel to the rail.

TYPE. Evidence in an individual animal of the maximum number of breed characteristics. A term not interchangeable with *conformation*. See ideal stallion, mare and gelding illustrations in Chapter 6.

UP ON THE BIT(S). Accepting the bit or bits willingly and working with eagerness.

"USING HIS EARS." A bright, alert attentive attitude. The horse works his ears or keeps them alertly forward.

WAY-OF-GOING (OR-MOVING). How a horse moves—whether correctly or incorrectly.

WINGING. Twisting of cannon and foot to the outside, as opposed to moving straight.

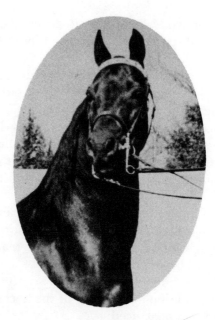

How the Author
"Judged" Them

STALLIONS (page 193)

First—E: Excellent over-all symmetry, outstanding neck-set and head.

Second—C: Nice type and topline, good over-all symmetry, neck-set not as high as E.

Third—B: Equal in type and refinement as C but not as good in the back.

Fourth—F: Nice length of neck and excellent topline, but not as distinctive in type as E.

Fifth—A: Good over-all symmetry and depth, but a bit heavier and with less refinement.

Sixth—D: Slightly straight shoulder, high in the croup; low neck-set, good head.

MARES (page 203)

First—F: Excellent neck-set, refinement; good topline and type.

Second—C: Very good neck-set and topline, but not as good in shoulder as F.

Third—E: Excellent over-all type, placed lower only on neck-set.

Fourth—B: Over-all good individual, but not as good in topline as E.

Fifth—A: Nice refinement and type, good topline and symmetry.

Sixth—D: Very typy mare with good refinement, but very short in neck and long-bodied; good topline, however.

GELDINGS (page 207)

First—E: A young animal with excellent neck-set, shoulder and topline.

Second—C: Very good over-all symmetry and type, but neck-set could be higher.

Third—B: Good neck-set, but quite sloping croup and typy head.

Fourth—F: Good refinement, topline and over-all symmetry.

Fifth—D: Good shoulder and depth of hip, but not as good in topline as F.

Sixth—A: Over-all a nice individual with a good shoulder and head, but slightly coarse in the throttle.

All the above horses could be placed differently by different judges. Preference is an individual thing, as each person sees something in a horse he might like over another point: i.e., some judges prefer a very high neck-set and would excuse, say, a bit of a slope of the croup if the horse carried himself with style. Another might look for absolutely correct legs and feet, etc. It is always well to remember, though, that you are judging a *type* breed—and perfect conformation does not insure that a horse is a good *Morgan*. Learn to recognize type and judge the best of the typiest!

Illustration and Photo Credits

Page

i, Author's collection/Photo by Judy Buck
ii, Author's collection
vii, Author's collection/Photo by Judy Buck
2, D. C. Linsley
5, 6, *Het Friese Paard: Vroeger en heden [The Frisian Horse: Then and Now]*, by Wouter Slob (Algemeen Publiciteitskantoor, Leeuwarden, 1963), with 6 by Volmer Photo.
9, Author's collection/Photo by Fred Sass
10, 12, 14, Author's collection
17, Courtesy C. D. Parks
21, Author's collection
24, Courtesy Vermont Historical Society
27, 28, 30, 31, Author's collection
34, Courtesy Vermont Historical Society
37, Author's collection
38, Courtesy E. Paquette
40, Author's collection
42, Courtesy Vermont Historical Society
44, 45, *The American Morgan Horse Register*
47, Author's collection
48, D. C. Linsley
51, *The American Morgan Horse Register*
52, 57, The Harry T. Peters Collection, Museum of the City of New York
60, *The American Morgan Horse Register*
63, 65, Author's collection
67, D. C. Linsley
69, 72, Courtesy Vermont Historical Society
74, Author's collection
75, Author's collection/Photo by Judy Buck
77, Author's collection
79, *The Morgan Horse Magazine*
82, 85, Author's collection
86, 90–92, *The American Morgan Horse Register*
93, Courtesy Vermont Historical Society

Page

95, The Harry T. Peters Collection, Museum of the City of New York
97, 99–101, Author's collection
103, *The American Morgan Horse Register*
104, 106, 108 top, Author's collection
108 bottom, Ted Freudy
109 top, Randy Myers
109 bottom, 111, 114, 115, 118, Author's collection
120, Stephen P. Davis, University of Vermont
122, Courtesy Polly Quinn
123, Author's collection
124, 126, Stephen P. Davis, University of Vermont
127, Author's collection
129, *The American Morgan Horse Register*
130, 132, Author's collection
134, W. A. Cowan, University of Connecticut
135, H. R. Hoover
136, Author's collection
137, Author's collection/Photo by Judy Buck
139, Author's collection
141, Courtesy Mary DeWitt/Photo by Judy Buck
142, Author's collection/Photo by Judy Buck
143, Author's collection
145 top left, Author's collection/Photo by Fred Sass
145 top right, Author's collection
145 bottom left, Barbara Hipsley
145 bottom right, Author's collection/Photo by Judy Buck
148–169, Author's collection
173, H. R. Hoover
175, 177, Author's collection
179, Courtesy Tara Farm
181, 182, 184, 186, 188–191, Author's collection
192, Author's collection/Photo by Judy Buck
193A, Author's collection
193B and C, Author's collection/Photos by Judy Buck

Index

Abdallah, 61
Allah F-1, 96, 107
American Cultivator, 50
American Driving Society, 335
American Ethan, 54, 91
American Heritage Class, 218, 219
American Horse Shows Association
   (ASHA), 279
   rulebook, 301, 303–304
American Morgan Horse Association, 117
American Morgan Horse Register, 2, 5,
   52, 64, 66, 100, 144, 170
   rules for admission, 138–40
The American Morgan Horse Register,
   Inc., 114, 116–117
American Saddle Horse Register, 97,
   105
American Saddlebred horses, 47, 66, 109
   Cabell's Lexington, 97–98
   Coleman's Eureka, 99–100, 102
   Denmark, 96–97
   history of, 96
   Indian Chief, 102–103, 105
   Justin Morgan's influence on, 105–107
   Peavine, 105
   Upwey Ben Don, 106
American Trotter, 7, 94, 96
   See also Standardbred horses

American Trotting Register, 55
Anacacho Denmark, 105
Anacacho Shamrock, 105
Annie C., 103
Arabian horses, 3, 4, 61
Aristos, 92
Artemisia, 126
ASHA. *See* American Horse Shows Asso-
   ciation

Babbitt horse, 67
Balch, Donald, 134, 136
Barbs, 3, 4, 22
Barnard Morgan, 89
Battell, Joseph, 110–13, 114, 118, 121
Beautiful Bay. *See* True Briton
Ben Franklin, 92
Bennington 5693, 124–25
Beppo, 66
Billy Barr, 54
Billy Direct, 47
Billy Root, 143
   owners, 49
   picture of, 48
   qualities and background, 48–49
Black Hawk Maid, 53
Black Hawk 20, 20, 25, 75, 88, 143
   influence on other breeds, 47

Black Hawk 20 (*cont.*)
offspring, 46–47, 49–59
owners, 41, 43, 45, 46
picture of, 42
qualities and background, 40–46
record at stud, 46
trotting contests, 46
Blood's Black Hawk 20, 47, 102
Bourbon Chief, 98
Bourbon King, 47, 103, 105
Bradford's Telegraph, 107
Bread Loaf Stock Farm, 64, 121
Breast-collars, 228
Breeders' guidelines
applying the guidelines, 172–74
choosing mates, 144, 146–47
guidelines for novice breeders, 171–72
obligations to the breed, 174
percentage of Justin Morgan's blood,
143–47
points on breeding, 170–71
rules for admission to the Morgan
Register, 138–43
size, 138–41
standard of perfection of the Morgan
horse, 147–49
type, 141–43
Bridles, 222–25, 226, 228, 231, 270–71,
310, 311, 312, 351–52
The British Morgan Horse Society, 118
Buggies, 228, 229, 230, 273
Bulrush, 5, 20, 89
compared to Sherman and Woodbury,
35–37
descendants, 81–87
owners, 32, 33, 35
picture of, 31
qualities and background, 30–33
speed and endurance, 33
standing in New England, 33–35
"Burbank horse." *See* Woodbury
Bureau of Animal Industry, 131
Butler's Eureka, 99

Cabell's Lexington, 97–98
Cameo Kirby, 105
Canadian pacers, 98
Canfield, 128
Carriage Association, 335
Carriage driving, 328, 332–35
Cassandra, 129
Championship classes, 218–21
Clark Chief, 92, 94, 124, 125
Cobden, 92
Coleman's Eureka, 97, 99–100, 102
Comet. *See* Billy Root
Copperbottom, 98
Cox's Eureka, 100
Cream Hill Stock Farm, 62

Daisy 2nd, 105
Daniel Lambert, 54, 91–92
background, 61
offspring, 60–61, 64, 66, 91–92
owners, 61, 62, 64
qualities, 62–64
record at stud, 62, 64
and standardbred horses, 91–92
Danville Boy, 87, 89
DeLong's Ethan Allen, 54, 91
Denmark, 88, 96, 97
Denning Allen, 54, 91, 121
Dexter, 55–59
Diamond, 4
Diamond Denmark, 96
Diomed, 61
Dorsey's Eden Stock Farm, 89
Draco, 87, 89
Dress. *See* Tack and dress requirements
Dressage, 328, 329–30
Duroc, 61
Dutch horses. *See* Frisian (Dutch) horses

Edna May's King, 47, 105
English pleasure
canter, 263, 266
equipment for, 25, 270–71, 337–40

manners, 260–61, 271–72

"new style," 258–59

stallion, 267

on the trail, 268–70

trot, 262–63, 264

walk, 261–62

English trail classes, 263, 267–268

Equipment. *See* Tack and dress requirements

Ethan Allen (50), 20, 46, 88, 143

and Dexter, race with, 55–59

monument in Kansas, 59

offspring, 54, 60–66, 91–92

owners, 51, 53, 54, 59

qualities and background, 49–50, 51–54

racing record, 50, 54, 55–59

and Standardbred horses, 90–92

Ethan Allen 3rd, 126, 143

Famous Saddle Horses, 102, 106

Fanny Allen, 54

Fanny Cook, 61

Fanny Scott, 122

Fearnaught, 85, 86, 87, 89

Fédération Équestre Internationale (F.E.I.), 328

Fenton horse, 5, 20, 39

50-Mile Pleasure Ride, 325

Figure. *See* Justin Morgan (Figure)

Fitting show horses, 303–304

currying and polishing, 308–10

shampooing, 307–308

trimming off hair, 304–307

Friendly, 129

Frisian (Dutch) horses

description, 7

and Morgan horses, 4–7

and Norfolk trotting horse, 8

regulations, 7

The Frisian Horse Studbook, 7

Gaines Denmark, 96

Geldings, Morgan, 204–205, 206, 208

confirmation, 205

judging them, 207, 361–62

General Gates, 54, 91, 121–24

General Hibbard, 67

George Wilkes, 47

Gifford Morgan, 66, 89, 143

offspring, 70, 71–77

owners, 68, 70

qualities and background, 67–70

record at stud, 70, 71

Gist's Black Hawk, 97

Golddust, 89–90, 91

Green Meads Princess, 106

Green Mountain Black Hawk, 97

The Green Mountain Horse Association, 326

Greyhound, 94

Grooming aids, 347–49

Hale, Silas, 71, 75

Hale's Green Mountain Morgan, 49, 70, 80, 100, 143

offspring, 76

owners, 71, 73, 75

picture of, 72

qualities and background, 71

as show horse, 71, 75, 76, 215

at stud, 71, 73, 76

Halters, 310, 319, 345

Hambletonian, 54, 81, 87, 88

Hamburg Belle, 94

Handling a show horse, 314–15, 316

getting ears up, 315, 317

how a horse stands, 315

Harmony Brook, 106

Harnesses, 228, 229, 230, 273

Harrison Chief, 94, 98, 124, 125

Hawkins horse, 5, 20, 39

Hero. *See* True Briton

Hippomenes. *See* Daniel Lambert

Hoke mare, 89

Holabird's Ethan Allen, 54, 91
Honest Allen, 54, 91
Hotspur, 54
Huijing, L.E., 7
Hunter/jumper horses, 296
  appointments, 299–300
  class regulations, 301–302
  shining in the hunt field, 298–99
  talent and training for the ring,
    296–98

Indian Chief, 47, 66, 101, 102–103, 105

The Jennison colt, 83–84
Jog carts, 229
Jubilee de Jarnette, 66, 103
Jubilee Lambert, 66, 92, 103
Judging criteria, 317–18
Jumpers. *See* Hunter/jumper horses
Justin Morgan (Figure)
  background, 2–5, 8
  characteristics, 8–9, 12, 19
  Dutch breeding theory, 4–5
  final years, 16–18
  and modern Morgans, 143–44
  owners, 1–2, 3, 8, 10, 14–15, 16, 17
  picture of, 2
  progeny, 15–16, 19–87
  prowess, 10–12
  racing record, 12–14
  and Standardbred and Saddle horses,
    105–107
  statue of, 122
Justin Morgan Class, 216, 218

Kate, 103
Kentucky Prince, 92, 94
Kentucky Queen, 92
King's Genius, 105
Krantz, Earl, 131, 133

Lady de Jarnette, 66, 102–103
Lady Moscow, 66

Lady Suffolk, 66
Lady Sutton, 66
Lead-shanks, 345
Lee Axworthy, 94
Linsley, D.C., 12, 16, 18, 19, 20, 35–36,
    39, 67, 80, 110, 112
Linsley 7233, 124
Longe-lines, 344, 352
Lord Clinton, 91
Lou Berry, 102
Lou Chief, 125
Lute Boyd, 125

Mac, 66
Mace, Don, 62
Magellen, 135
Maggie Marshall, 107
Magna Charta, 66
The Maine Farmer, 80
Mambrino, 61
Mansfield 7255, 125–26, 129
Mares, Morgan ideal, 194, 195, 200–201
  body, 197
  head, 194–95
  judging, 203, 361
  legs and feet, 197–99
  moving in hand, 202–204
  neck, 195–97
  symmetry, overall, 199, 202
  trot, 204
  walk, 202, 204
Marvel King, 103
Mary Boston, 99
Meldert, Leon de, 7
Mentor, 129, 134
Messenger, 54, 61, 78, 79, 81, 87, 88
Miller's Adel, 106
Montgomery Chief, 103
Moon, Owen, 117
Morgan Caesar, 66
Morgan Eagle, 66, 92
The Morgan Horse Club, 113
  impact of, 113–14

local groups, 117–18
and Register, combined, 116–17
Morgan Horse Farm. *See* United States
    Morgan Horse Farm
Morgan Horse Heritage Classes, 332, 334
The Morgan Horse Magazine, 117
The Morgan Horse and Register, 110, 112–
    113, 114, 116
Morgan horses
    See also specific Morgan horses
    breeding. *See* Breeders' guidelines
    characteristics of, 19, 81
    demand for in 1850s, 80–81
    and demands for speed and size, 78,
        80, 94, 138
    Dutch or Frisian influence on, 4–7
    as farming horses, 77–78
    geldings. *See* Geldings, Morgan
    history, 1–5
    influence on other American breeds,
        88–109
    mares. *See* Mares, Morgan ideal
    modern, pictures of, 9, 38
    outcrossing breed, 81, 87, 94
    percentage of Justin Morgan's blood,
        143–44
    rules for admission to the Morgan
        Register, 138–43
    stallions. *See* Stallions, Morgan ideal
    standard of perfection, 147–49
    versatility, 209–14
    as working horses today, 77–78, 136,
        278
    "X" in modern Morgan pedigrees,
        144
Morgan Horses, 12, 110
Morrill family, 81–87
    Jennison Colt, 83–84
    Old Morrill, 84–85
    Randolph Morgan, 83
    and Standardbred horses, 87, 89, 94
    Young Morrill, Winthrop and Fear-
        naught, 85, 87

National Saddle Horse Breeders Associa-
    tion, 97
National Saddle Horse Register, 100
New York State Fair (1847), 70
Nichols horse, 67
Norfolk trotting horse, 8

Old Castor 5833, 128
Old Morrill, 84–85
100-Mile Trail Ride, 128, 129, 325–328

Panfield, 129
Park horses, 209, 211, 212, 216, 233–36
    canter, 245–48
    in harness, 248–57
    harness equipment, 228–29
    manners, 257
    under saddle, 236–48
    saddle equipment, 221–25
    trot, 237–45, 249, 251
    walk, 236–37, 249
    whip, using, 254, 257
Parlin, S.W., 50, 64
Peavine, 105, 106
Pedigree, 146
Perkins' Young Morrill, 85, 87, 89
Peters' Vermont, 143, 148
Pleasure driving, 272–73, 275
    See also Carriage driving
    manners, 274, 276–77
    showing, 273–74
    tack for, 229, 273
Pleasure horses, 209, 212, 216, 257–58
    carriage driving, 328, 332–35
    competitive trail rides, 325–28
    dressage, 328, 329–30
    English, performance of, 260–63
    English, on the trail, 268–72
    English trail classes, 263, 267–68
    fun, 322–25
    in harness, 272–77
    under saddle in the ring, 258–59
    Western, 277–87

Pocahontas, 54
"Porter Colt." *See* Daniel Lambert
Putnam horse, 67

Querido 7370, 128

Racing Hall of Fame, 55
Randolph Morgan, 83
Reata, 279
Red Bird. *See* Billy Root
Red Oak 5249, 124
Red Robin, 51–52
Regent, 6
Reins, 279
Revenge, 20
  owners, 37
  qualities and background, 37–38
Rex Peavine, 105
Richelieu, 103
Road hacks, 293
  appointments, 294–95
  performance, 295–96
Roadsters, 288–89
  in harness, 290–91
  under saddle, 292–93
  training, 289
  trot, 290–91
Road Allen F-38, 107
Royal Morgan, 143

Saddle blankets, 225, 226, 279
Saddlebred horses. *See* American Saddlebred horses
Saddles, 221–22, 225–26, 270, 279
St. Louis Fair (1878), 102
Scharf, Emely Ellen ("Susanne"), 106
Sherman, 20–22
  appearance and early years, 22–23
  compared to Bulrush and Woodbury,
    35–37
  offspring, 20, 25, 40–66
  owners, 22, 23
  picture of, 21

record at stud, 23–25
Show circuit, 303
  ASHA rulebook, 301, 303–304
  carriage driving, 328, 332–35
  championship stakes, 218–21
  competitive trail rides, 325–28
  dressage, 328, 329–30
  English pleasure. *See* English pleasure
  fitting, 303–10
  handling in the ring, 314–18
  hunters/jumpers, 296–302
  introduction to, 214–18
  judging criteria, 317–18
  pleasure driving, 273–74
  road hacks, 293–96
  roadsters, 288–93
  showing in hand, 310–18
  showmanship in practice, 318–21
  tack. *See* Tack and dress requirements
  Western pleasure. *See* Western pleasure
Silvertail, 13
Sir Ethan Allen 6537, 126
Size, 138, 140
Speed, 78, 80, 81, 94, 138
Sprague and Akers Stock Farm, 59
Stables, home, 343
  grooming aids, 347–49
  grooming area, 346–47
  halters and lead-shanks, 345
  stall, 349
  tack area, 347
Stallions, Morgan ideal, 176–78, 188–89
  blemishes, faults and unsoundness, 191
  body, 183, 185
  head, 178–80
  judging them, 193, 361
  legs and feet, 185, 187, 190
  moving in hand, 187–94
  neck, 182–83, 184
  tail-set and croup, 185, 186
  trot, 192, 194
  walk, 187, 192
Standard of perfection, 147–49

Standardbred horses, 61, 88, 98, 108
  and demands for speed and size, 94,
    138
  Ethan Allen 50's contribution, 90–92
  Golddust, 89–90, 91
  and the Morrill family, 87, 89
"Stevenson" mare, 96
Stillman, C. C., 113, 114, 116, 118
Stockholm's American Star, 61
Stone, Charles, 116, 117, 118
Sumpter Denmark, 96
Superb, 91, 95
Sweepstakes, 13

Tack and dress requirements, 336–37,
    343
  English pleasure and park saddle class,
    221–25, 337–40
  English trail class, 270–71
  harness class, 228–29, 342–43
  hunter/jumper class, 299–300, 341
  pleasure driving class, 229, 232, 273
  road hack class, 294–95, 340–41
  roadster class, 291, 292
  on the show circuit, 349–51
  showing in hand, 310–12
  stable, tack for, 343–49
  for tailers, 312
  training equipment, 351–54
  Western pleasure class, 225–28, 279–
    280, 341–43
Tailers, duties of, 312, 314
Tennessee Walking Horse, 96, 98, 107,
    109
Thoroughbreds, 3
300-Mile Endurance Rides, 128, 326
Titan Hanover, 94
Tom Boyd, 98
Tom Hal, 97, 98
Trail rides, competitive, 325–28
Training
  for carriage driving, 333–34
  for dressage, 328

equipment, 351–54
  hunter/jumper horses, 296–98
  roadsters, 289
  and versatility, 211
Traveller. *See* True Briton
Trophy, 129, 135
Trotting horse. *See* American Trotter;
    Standardbred horses
Troubadour, 129
True Briton, 2–3, 4
Tutor, 129

Uhlan, 94
Ulysses, 128
The United States Morgan Horse Farm,
    54, 91, 119, 140
  Bennington, 124–25
  Earl Krantz as superintendent, 131, 133
  export horses from, 135
  as a federal venture, 119, 121
  General Gates and offspring, 121–24
  Mansfield and Ethan Allen 3rd, 125–
    126, 129
  move to Weybridge (Bread Loaf Farm),
    121
  police work horses from, 136
  Querido, Ulysses and Canfield, 128
  results achieved, 128–29
  Vermont takes over, 133–35
University of Vermont, 133–35
Upwey Ben Don, 106
UVM Flash, 134
UVM Promise, 134, 136
UVM Watchman, 134

Vermont Morgan, 89, 143
Vermont State Fair (1854), 75
Versatility of the Morgan horse, 209–14

"Walker horse." See Woodbury
Walker Morrill, 89
Walking horse. *See* Tennessee Walking
    Horse

Wallace's Monthly, 55
Ward, Joseph, 3
Wardner, Henry S., 113
Washington's Denmark, 96
Western pleasure, 277–79, 286–87
  equipment for, 225–28, 279–80, 341–343
  jog, 281–83
  lope, 283–84
  under saddle in the ring, 279–84
  on the trail, 285–86
  walk, 280
Whips, 254, 257, 273
Wildair mare, 4
Willowmoor 6459, 129
Windcrest Dona Lee, 106
Windcrest Madonna, 106
Windcrest Nancy C., 106
Windcrest Rose Marie, 106
Windcrest Sentimental Lady, 106

Winthrop Morrill, 85, 87, 89
Woodbury, 20, 25–26
  compared to Bulrush and Sherman, 35–37
  descendants of, 66–67
  owners, 26, 28, 29, 30
  picture of, 28
  qualities and background, 26–29
  reputation and travels, 29–30
  speed, 66
Woodward's Ethan Allen, 91
Working horses, 77–78, 136, 278

"X" in modern Morgan pedigrees, 144

Young Bulrock, 4
Young Morrill. *See* Perkins' Young Morrill

Zilcaadi, 89